Emergencies in Obstetrics and Gynecology

Editors

PATRICIA S. HUGUELET
HENRY L. GALAN

OBSTETRICS AND GYNECOLOGY CLINICS OF NORTH AMERICA

www.obgyn.theclinics.com

Consulting Editor
WILLIAM F. RAYBURN

September 2022 • Volume 49 • Number 3

ELSEVIER

1600 John F. Kennedy Boulevard • Suite 1800 • Philadelphia, Pennsylvania, 19103-2899

http://www.theclinics.com

OBSTETRICS AND GYNECOLOGY CLINICS OF NORTH AMERICA Volume 49 Number 3
September 2022 ISSN 0889-8545, ISBN-13: 978-0-323-98755-4

Editor: Kerry Holland
Developmental Editor: Hannah Almira Lopez

Obstetrics and Gynecology Clinics (ISSN 0889-8545) is published quarterly by Elsevier Inc., 360 Park Avenue South, New York, NY 10010-1710. Months of issue are March, June, September, and December. Periodicals postage paid at New York, NY, and additional mailing offices. Subscription price per year is $345.00 (US individuals), $963.00 (US institutions), $100.00 (US students), $416.00 (Canadian individuals), $982.00 (Canadian institutions), $100.00 (Canadian students), $473.00 (international individuals), $982.00 (international institutions), and $225.00 (international students). To receive student/resident rate, orders must be accompanied by name of affiliated institution, date of term, and the signature of program/residency coordinator on institution letterhead. Orders will be billed at individual rate until proof of status is received. Foreign air speed delivery is included in all *Clinics* subscription prices. All prices are subject to change without notice. POSTMASTER: Send address changes to *Obstetrics and Gynecology Clinics*, Elsevier Health Sciences Division, Subscription Customer Service, 3251 Riverport Lane, Maryland Heights, MO 63043. **Customer Service: Telephone: 1-800-654-2452 (U.S. and Canada); 314-447-8871 (outside U.S. and Canada). Fax: 314-447-8029. E-mail: journalscustomerservice-usa@elsevier.com (for print support); journalsonlinesupport-usa@elsevier. com (for online support).**

Reprints. For copies of 100 or more of articles in this publication, please contact the Commercial Reprints Department, Elsevier Inc., 360 Park Avenue South, New York, New York 10010-1710. Tel.: 212-633-3874; Fax: 212-633-3820; E-mail: reprints@elsevier.com.

Obstetrics and Gynecology Clinics of North America is also published in Spanish by McGraw-Hill Interamericana Editores S.A., P.O. Box 5-237, 06500, Mexico; in Portuguese by Reichmann and Affonso Editores, Rio de Janeiro, Brazil; and in Greek by Paschalidis Medical Publications, Athens, Greece.

Obstetrics and Gynecology Clinics of North America is covered in MEDLINE/PubMed (Index Medicus), Excerpta Medica, Current Concepts/Clinical Medicine, Science Citation Index, BIOSIS, CINAHL, and ISI/BIOMED.

Contributors

CONSULTING EDITOR

WILLIAM F. RAYBURN, MD, MBA
Affiliate Professor, Department of Obstetrics and Gynecology and College of Graduate Studies Medical University of South Carolina Charleston, South Carolina Emeritus Distinguished Professor, Department of Obstetrics and Gynecology University of New Mexico School of Medicine Albuquerque, New Mexico

EDITORS

PATRICIA S. HUGUELET, MD
Associate Professor, Chief of Pediatric and Adolescent Gynecology, Fellowship Director, Pediatric and Adolescent Gynecology, Department of Obstetrics and Gynecology, University of Colorado Anschutz Medical Campus, Aurora, Colorado

HENRY L. GALAN, MD
Professor, Division of Maternal-Fetal Medicine, Department of Obstetrics and Gynecology, Colorado Fetal Care Center, Children's Hospital of Colorado, University of Colorado Anschutz Medical Campus, Aurora, Colorado

AUTHORS

ALFRED ABUHAMAD, MD
Interim President and Provost Dean of the School of Medicine, Mason C. Andrews Professor of Obstetrics and Gynecology and Radiology, Division of Maternal Fetal Medicine, Department of Obstetrics and Gynecology, Eastern Virginia Medical School, Norfolk, Virginia

ZACHARY ALHOLM, MD
The University of rizona College of Medicine-Phoenix, Department of Obstetrics and Gynecology, Phoenix, Arizona

LINDA A. BARBOUR, MD, MSPH
University of Colorado, School of Medicine, Aurora, Colorado

EMILY BUTTIGIEG, MD
Assistant Professor, University of Wisconsin-Madison School of Medicine and Public Health, Madison, Wisconsin

SUNEET P. CHAUHAN, MD, Hon.D.Sc
Department of Obstetrics and Gynecology, Division of Maternal/Fetal Medicine, The University of Texas Health Sciences Center at Houston McGovern Medical School, Houston, Texas

STEPHANIE M. CIZEK, MD
Clinical Assistant Professor, Pediatric and Adolescent Gynecology, Department of Obstetrics and Gynecology, Stanford University School of Medicine, Center for Academic Medicine, Palo Alto, California

ASHLEY S. COGGINS, MD
Fellow, Division of Maternal-Fetal Medicine, Department of Gynecology and Obstetrics, Johns Hopkins School of Medicine, Baltimore, Maryland

CHRISTINE CONAGESKI, MD, MSc
Associate Professor, Department of Obstetrics and Gynecology, University of Colorado, Aurora, Colorado

SHAD DEERING, MD, CHSE, COL(ret) USA
Associate Dean, Children's Hospital of San Antonio, System Medical Director, CHRISTUS Simulation Institute, Professor, Department of Obstetrics and Gynecology, Baylor College of Medicine

MICHAEL R. FOLEY, MD
Chief Medical Officer, Sera Prognostics, Professor and Former Chairman, Department of Obstetrics and Gynecology, The University of Arizona College Medicine-Phoenix

DANIELLE N. FROCK-WELNAK, MD, MPH, MS
Senior Instructor, Division of Academic Specialists in Obstetrics and Gynecology, University of Colorado School of Medicine, Obstetrics and Gynecology, School of Medicine, CU Anschutz, Aurora, Colorado

ROBERT B. GHERMAN, MD
PA (Department of Obstetrics and Gynecology, Division of Maternal/Fetal Medicine), Wellspan Health System York, Laytonsville, Maryland

DENA GOFFMAN, MD
Chief of Obstetrics, Sloane Hospital for Women, Associate Chief Quality Officer, Obstetrics, NewYork-Presbyterian, Ellen Jacobson Levine and Eugene Jacobson Professor of Women's Health in Obstetrics and Gynecology, Vice Chair for Quality and Patient Safety, Obstetrics and Gynecology, Associate Dean for Professionalism, Columbia University Irving Medical Center

ERIN GOMEZ, MD
Assistant Professor, Diagnostic Imaging Division, Associate Program Director, Diagnostic Radiology Residency, Course Director, JHU SOM Diagnostic Radiology Elective, Department of Radiology, Johns Hopkins Hospital, Baltimore, Maryland

ODESSA P. HAMIDI, MD
University of Colorado, School of Medicine, Aurora, Colorado

MARIA C. HOFFMAN, MD, MSC
Associate Professor of Maternal Fetal Medicine, Departments of Obstetrics and Gynecology, and Psychiatry, University of Colorado School of Medicine, Denver, Colorado

REBECCA HORGAN, MD
Division of Maternal Fetal Medicine, Department of Obstetrics and Gynecology, Eastern Virginia Medical School, Norfolk, Virginia

MEGAN L. HUTCHCRAFT, MD
Gynecologic Oncology Fellow Physician, Division of Gynecologic Oncology, Department of Obstetrics and Gynecology, University of Kentucky Markey Cancer Center, Lexington, Kentucky

BRIDGET KELLY, MD
Assistant Professor, University of Wisconsin-Madison School of Medicine and Public Health, Madison, Wisconsin

RACHEL W. MILLER, MD
Associate Professor, Division of Gynecologic Oncology, Department of Obstetrics and Gynecology, University of Kentucky Markey Cancer Center, Lexington, Kentucky

KELSIE J. OVENELL, DO
The University of Arizona College of Medicine-Phoenix, Department of Obstetrics and Gynecology, Phoenix, Arizona

LUIS D. PACHECO, MD
Department of Obstetrics and Gynecology, Division of Maternal-Fetal Medicine and Anesthesiology, Division of Surgical Critical Care, The University of Texas Medical Branch at Galveston, Galveston, Texas

GEORGE S. SAADE, MD
Department of Obstetrics and Gynecology, Division of Maternal-Fetal Medicine, The University of Texas Medical Branch at Galveston, Galveston, Texas

MARIA SHAKER, MD
University Hospitals Cleveland Medical Center - MacDonald Women's Hospital, Cleveland, Ohio; Assistant Professor, Department of Reproductive Biology, Case Western Reserve University School of Medicine

JEAN-JU SHEEN, MD
Medical Director, Carmen and John Thain Labor and Delivery Unit, NewYork-Presbyterian/Columbia University Irving Medical Center, Director of Obstetric Simulation, Associate Professor of Obstetrics and Gynecology, Columbia University Irving Medical Center

JEANNE S. SHEFFIELD, MD
Professor and Director, Division of Maternal-Fetal Medicine, Department of Gynecology and Obstetrics, Johns Hopkins School of Medicine, Baltimore, Maryland

MEGAN C. SHEPHERD, MD
Department of Obstetrics and Gynecology, Division of Maternal-Fetal Medicine, The University of Texas Medical Branch at Galveston, Galveston, Texas

AYANNA SMITH, MD, MPH
Resident Physician, University Hospitals Cleveland Medical Center - MacDonald Women's Hospital, Cleveland, Ohio

NANCY SOKKARY, MD, FACOG
Associate Professor, Emory University School of Medicine, Children's Healthcare of Atlanta, Atlanta, Georgia

JENNY TAM, MD, FACOG
Assistant Professor, Division of Academic Specialists in Obstetrics and Gynecology, Department of Obstetrics and Gynecology, University of Colorado, School of Medicine, CU Anschutz, Aurora, Colorado

SHAWNA TONICK, MD
Assistant Professor, Department of Obstetrics and Gynecology, University of Colorado, Aurora, Colorado

NICHOLE TYSON, MD
Clinical Associate Professor, Pediatric and Adolescent Gynecology, Department of Obstetrics and Gynecology, Stanford University School of Medicine, Center for Academic Medicine, Palo Alto, California

CYNTHIE K. WAUTLET, MD, MPH
Maternal Fetal Medicine Fellow, Department of Obstetrics and Gynecology, University of Colorado School of Medicine, Denver, Colorado

RUTH E.H. YEMANE, MD, FACOG
Assistant Clinical Professor, University of Wisconsin-Madison, West Clinic, Madison, Wisconsin

KATIE W. ZENG, MD
The University of Arizona College of Medicine-Phoenix, Department of Obstetrics and Gynecology, Phoenix, Arizona

Contents

This article serves to highlight both the common nature and severity of
postpartum hemorrhage (PPH). Identification of etiologies and management of each is reviewed. In addition, the evaluation and administration
of proper blood component therapies and massive transfusion are also explained to help providers become comfortable with early administration
and delivery of blood component therapies.

The incidence of placenta accreta spectrum (PAS) is increasing and is now
about 3 per 1000 deliveries, largely due to the rising cesarean section rate.
Ultrasound is the preferred method for diagnosis of PAS. Ultrasound
markers include multiple vascular lacunae, loss of the hypoechoic retroplacental zone, abnormalities of the uterine serosa–bladder interface, retroplacental myometrial thickness less than 1 mm, increased placental
vascularity, and observation of bridging vessels linking the placenta and
bladder. Patients with PAS should be managed by experienced multidisciplinary teams. Hysterectomy is the accepted management of PAS and
conservative or expectant management of PAS should be considered
investigational.

Venous thromboembolism (VTE) as well as other embolic events including
amniotic fluid embolism (AFE) remain a leading cause of maternal death in
the United States and worldwide. The pregnant patient is at a higher risk of
developing VTE including pulmonary embolism. In contrast, AFE is a rare,
but catastrophic event that remains incompletely understood. Here the authors review the cause of VTE in pregnancy and look at contemporary and
evidence-based practices for the evaluation, diagnosis, and management
in pregnancy. Then the cause and diagnostic difficulty of AFE as well as
what is known regarding the pathogenesis are reviewed.

Diagnosis of gynecologic emergencies in the pediatric and adolescent population requires a high index of suspicion to avoid delayed or incorrect diagnoses. This article aims to dispel common misunderstandings and aid with diagnosis and management of 3 common pediatric and adolescent gynecologic emergencies: adnexal torsion, vulvovaginal lacerations, and nonsexually acquired genital ulcers.

Ectopic pregnancy occurs in 2% of all pregnancies and is a potentially life-threatening emergency. A high level of clinical suspicion is required for any pregnant patient who presents with vaginal bleeding and/or pelvic pain. Workup should begin with immediate triage based on vital signs, a pregnancy test, and transvaginal ultrasound. Ectopic pregnancy can be treated either medically with methotrexate or surgically with either salpingectomy or salpingostomy. Carefully counseled, asymptomatic patients may be candidates for expectant management.

Pelvic inflammatory disease (PID) is an ascending polymicrobial infection of the upper female genital tract. The presentation of PID varies from asymptomatic cases to severe sepsis. The diagnosis of PID is often one of exclusion. Primary treatment for PID includes broad-spectrum antibiotics with coverage against gonorrhea, chlamydia, and common anaerobic and aerobic bacteria. If not clinically improved by antibiotics, percutaneous drain placement can promote efficient source control, as is often the case with large tubo-ovarian abscesses. Ultimately, even with treatment, PID can result in long-term morbidity, including chronic pelvic pain, infertility, and ectopic pregnancy.

Sexual assault and intimate partner violence (IPV) of children, adolescents, and adult women are prevalent in the United States and have long-term physical and mental health, financial, and social effects. Pregnant women and women of color are particularly high-risk populations. Obstetrics and gynecology providers are uniquely situated to assess and treat survivors of IPV and sexual assault. A timely, thorough forensic medical examination, appropriate evaluation, and prophylactic therapy are all vital components in the care of these patients.

Heavy vaginal bleeding is a common, life-altering condition affecting around 30% of women at some point in their reproductive lives. Initial evaluation should focus on hemodynamic stability. A thorough history including the patient's menstrual cycle and personal and family bleeding history should be obtained. Causes are stratified using the structural and nonstructural International Federation of Gynecology and Obstetrics classification system. Further consideration of the patient's age is essential because this can help to narrow the differential diagnosis. Work-up includes laboratory and imaging studies. Treatment approach includes acute stabilization and long-term treatment with medical and surgical modalities.

Initial assessment of vaginal bleeding in gynecologic malignancies includes a thorough history and physical examination, identification of site and extent of disease, and patient goals of care. Patients who are initially hemodynamically unstable may require critical care services. Choice of treatment is disease site specific. Cervical cancer frequently is treated with chemoradiation. Uterine cancer may be treated surgically, with radiation, or pharmacologically. Gestational trophoblastic disease is treated surgically. Alternative treatment modalities include vascular embolization and topical hemostatic agents. Patients with bleeding gynecologic malignancies should be managed as inpatients in facilities with gynecologic oncology, radiation oncology, and critical care services.

First trimester miscarriage, or early pregnancy loss, is a common occurrence in the United States. Miscarriage management includes expectant, medical, or surgical approaches. Decisions about management options should be approached through shared decision making between the patient and provider and with consideration of patient's preferences, hemodynamic stability, cost, gestational age, and effectiveness. Emergencies requiring immediate interventions are rare. Newer developments in management, including a more effective medical regimen with the addition of mifepristone and cost-effective and convenient in-office surgical interventions, have expanded treatment options.

Simulation is a critical part of training for obstetric emergencies. Incorporation of this training modality has been shown to improve outcomes for patients and is now required by national accrediting organizations.

OBSTETRICS AND GYNECOLOGY CLINICS

SERIES OF RELATED INTEREST

Clinics in Perinatology
www.perinatology.theclinics.com
Pediatric Clinics of North America
https://www.pediatrics.theclinics.com

THE CLINICS ARE AVAILABLE ONLINE!
Access your subscription at:
www.theclinics.com

Foreword

Emergencies in Obstetrics and Gynecology: Readiness, Recognition, Response, and Reporting

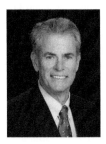

William F. Rayburn, MD, MBA
Consulting Editor

This issue of *Obstetrics and Gynecology Clinics of North America* provides an update in advances and current practice in handling emergencies in obstetrics and gynecology. Capably edited by Patricia Huguelet, MD and Henry Galan, MD from the University of Colorado, the reader is updated with the evaluation and management of emergencies that go beyond descriptions in standard texts. The review is thorough and covers a variety of topics ranging from first-trimester miscarriage and ectopic pregnancy to placenta accreta spectrum disorders and postpartum hemorrhage to acute pelvic inflammatory disease, adolescent gynecology emergencies, and bleeding from gynecologic malignancies.

Managing emergent situations requires teamwork and communication. Many different training methods and evaluation tools have been reported, which makes generalization of results difficult. Crew resource management makes optimum use of all available resources: equipment, procedures, and people. Core concepts of training programs involve communication, leadership, and mutual support while monitoring the situation.

Urgent and emergent problems affect the health care of all women at some time during their lives. This issue provides strategies for individual and team training; simulations and drills; development of protocols, guidelines, and checklists; and use of information technology. These activities and tools apply to outpatient and inpatient settings. Although participants tend to react positively to this continuing education and improve in knowledge, skills, and behavior, more descriptions about patient outcomes are necessary.

Obstet Gynecol Clin N Am 49 (2022) xiii–xiv
https://doi.org/10.1016/j.ogc.2022.04.006
0889-8545/22/© 2022 Published by Elsevier Inc.

Obstetric emergencies have served as excellent examples of simulation training of individuals and multidisciplinary teams to swiftly address conditions that could rapidly deteriorate. Simulation drills reviewed in this issue are nicely summarized in the last article. Examples include hypertension during pregnancy, shoulder dystocia, pulmonary embolism and amniotic fluid embolism, and postpartum hemorrhage. Preparing for and management of women with septic shock, cardiac arrest, endocrine emergencies, and acute pelvic inflammatory disease are also well covered. Annual training is adequate for providers who demonstrate competency after initial training. However, those who are unsuccessful during and after a few weeks of training should undergo remediation and be followed to ensure retention of skills.

A standardized checklist can be a helpful reminder for urgent or emergent conditions in the clinic, operating room, and labor and delivery. Condition-specific checklists provide a set of elements to be checked at sign in, timeout, and sign out. Before an emergent surgery, a surgeon-led preoperative briefing or "timeout" that goes beyond a simple checklist permits more thorough communication among all team members. Debriefings or "huddles" after surgery are useful to understand everyone's role, identify any underappreciated hazards, and acknowledge any mistakes for improvement. Last, formal handoffs through verbal and written communications can be used during the transfer of patient care from one individual or team to another during and after the emergency.

Most emergencies described in this issue occur in or lead to hospitalization. Consistent use of well-developed, evidence-based practice guidelines results in a more consistent application of best practices. Depending on the emergent condition, guidelines can include several components: development of multidisciplinary engagement and pathways, formation of any rapid response teams, and performance of regular simulation drills. Reexamining each case, such as at nonpunitive morbidity and mortality conferences, identifies any deviation from hospital guidelines. These guidelines can then be revised to reduce practice deviation, train staff in management of the emergency condition, and implement more effective practice drills.

Definite progress has occurred since our last issue on this subject. I appreciate the efforts of Dr Huguelet and Dr Galan, along with their team of experienced obstetricians and gynecologists. Their thoughtful and comprehensive recommendations include many scenarios faced by the practitioner at various times in their careers. Providers must be equipped with the medical knowledge, surgical skills, and current scientific evidence to guide their approach to any emergent event. By instituting recommendations provided in this issue, we should be better prepared to be ready, and to recognize, respond, and report our delivery of health care to our compromised patients.

William F. Rayburn, MD, MBA
Department of Obstetrics and Gynecology
Medical University of South Carolina
1721 Atlantic Avenue
Sullivan's Island, SC 29482, USA

E-mail address:
wrayburnmd@gmail.com

Preface

Emergencies in Obstetrics and Gynecology: Advances and Current Practice

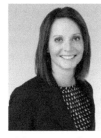 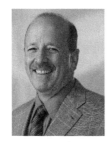

Patricia S. Huguelet, MD   Henry L. Galan, MD
Editors

Welcome to the latest issue of *Obstetrics and Gynecologic Clinics of North America*, focused on emergencies in obstetrics and gynecology. Every medical or surgical specialty encounters the occasional emergency, and the field of obstetrics and gynecology is no exception. Urgent and emergent problems are common events in the reproductive health care of women, and providers must be equipped with the medical knowledge, surgical skills, and most up-to-date scientific evidence to guide their approach to the emergent event. Pregnancy alone presents a unique challenge, where a single emergent event can threaten the life of not just one, but two individuals, the mother and her fetus. Furthermore, an otherwise completely healthy patient without any previous medical history may succumb purely to a pregnancy-related complication.

Providing the most current scientific medical and surgical approaches to care for these patients is the guiding principle in this issue of *Obstetrics and Gynecology Clinics of North America*. We have invited experts to review a variety of topics, with attention to the most recent high-quality evidence, combined with personal experiences, to provide the reader with the knowledge and skills to manage emergencies encountered in routine practice.

This review of obstetric emergencies is thorough and covers a varied array of topics. Foley and colleagues begin by addressing postpartum hemorrhage and blood component therapy, including the challenge of caring for patients who refuse blood products. Abuhamad and Horgan also address postpartum hemorrhage, specifically focusing on placenta accreta spectrum disorders and associated imaging findings. Sheffield and Coggins review thromboembolic disease, including the profound maternal cardiovascular collapse and disseminated intravascular coagulation that can occur in the setting of amniotic fluid embolism. Pacheco reviews septic shock and the approach to

Obstet Gynecol Clin N Am 49 (2022) xv–xvi
https://doi.org/10.1016/j.ogc.2022.04.003
0889-8545/22/© 2022 Published by Elsevier Inc.

cardiopulmonary resuscitation in the pregnant patient. Barbour and Hamidi then guide us through endocrinologic emergencies in pregnancy, specifically diabetic ketoacidosis and thyroid storm. Gehrman and Chauhan review risk factors and management of shoulder dystocia, but primarily focus on challenging common assumptions of shoulder dystocia that need further study. Finally, Hoffman and Wautlet guide the reader through the evaluation and management of hypertensive crises in pregnancy.

Shifting to gynecologic emergencies that occur in routine practice, Tyson and Cizek review emergencies commonly encountered in pediatric and adolescent patients, including the unique but not uncommon occurrence of nonsexually acquired genital ulcers. Tonick and Conageski discuss the ever-present topic of ectopic pregnancy and review the most recent guidelines on ultrasound discriminatory zones, acceptable B-HCG levels in a pregnancy of unknown location, and methotrexate treatment regimens. Frock-Welnak and Tam review the medical and surgical approaches to acute pelvic inflammatory disease and tubo-ovarian abscess. Yemane and Sokkary remind us of the high prevalence of sexual assault and intimate partner violence and how to approach this topic in daily practice. Kelly and Buttigieg discuss management options for one of the most common conditions encountered in practice, heavy menstrual bleeding, including the importance of first assessing hemodynamic stability. This article is appropriately followed by Hutchcraft and Miller, addressing heavy menstrual bleeding in the setting of gynecologic malignancy. Shaker and Smith then guide us through the management of first-trimester miscarriage bleeding. The issue closes with Goffman and Deering reviewing simulation training in obstetrics and gynecology and how it can be used to prepare the provider and medical team for such emergencies.

Remarkable advances have been made since the last issue of emergencies in obstetrics and gynecology, and we hope the reader will find this issue enjoyable and helpful for care provided to their patients. We would like to add a personal note of gratitude to all the gifted individuals contributing to this issue of *Obstetrics and Gynecology Clinics of North America*, to Kerry Holland for her guidance, and to Hannah Almira Lopez of Elsevier for her patience and professionalism. Most of all, we would like to thank our patients and learners from all levels, from whom we learn so much about our beautiful specialty.

Patricia S. Huguelet, MD
Pediatric and Adolescent Gynecology
Department of Obstetrics and Gynecology
University of Colorado Anschutz Medical Campus
13123 East 16th Avenue, Box B467, Room C5125
Aurora, CO 80045
USA

Henry L. Galan, MD
Division of Maternal-Fetal Medicine
Department of Obstetrics and Gynecology
Colorado Fetal Care Center, Children's Hospital of Colorado
University of Colorado Anschutz Medical Campus
13123 East 16th Avenue
Box B467, Room C5125
Aurora, CO 80045, USA

E-mail addresses:
Patricia.Huguelet@cuanschutz.edu (P.S. Huguelet)
Henry.Galan@cuanschutz.edu (H.L. Galan)

Postpartum Hemorrhage Management and Blood Component Therapy

Katie W. Zeng, MD[a], Kelsie J. Ovenell, DO[a],*,
Zachary Alholm, MD[a], Michael R. Foley, MD[b]

KEYWORDS

- Postpartum hemorrhage • Uterotonics • Uterine tamponade • Hemorrhagic shock
- Thromboelastography • Massive transfusion • Blood component therapy

KEY POINTS

- Ongoing maternal risk stratification antepartum and intrapartum is key to team preparedness.
- Simulation and utilization of checklists improve patient care outcomes and communication during postpartum hemorrhage (PPH).
- Active management of the third stage of labor is recommended with prophylactic uterotonics, gentle fundal massage, and early placenta delivery.
- Therapy for atony has high success rates and includes multiple treatment modalities with typically less invasive treatments used initially. There are no clear data regarding the superiority of any treatment over another. Possible management options include uterotonic medications, tamponade techniques, vascular embolization, uterine-sparing surgical management, and hysterectomy.
- When hemorrhage is estimated to be more than 1500 cc, early introduction of directed blood component therapies can reduce the total number of products transfused and minimize the occurrence of transfusion-related reactions.

POSTPARTUM HEMORRHAGE
Introduction/Background/Prevalence

a. Postpartum hemorrhage (PPH) is one of the most common obstetric emergencies and is one of the top causes of maternal mortality in the United States and around the world. The prevalence of PPH is estimated to be around 3.2% and accounts for 11% of all maternal mortality in the United States.[1,2] The incidence of PPH seems to have increased by approximately 25% from 1995 to 2004 and approximately

a Department of OBGYN, University of Arizona College of Medicine-Phoenix, 1111 East McDowell Road, Phoenix, AZ 85006, USA; b Department of OBGYN, University of Arizona College of Medicine-Phoenix
* Corresponding author.
E-mail address: Kelsie.ovenell@bannerhealth.com

Obstet Gynecol Clin N Am 49 (2022) 397–421
https://doi.org/10.1016/j.ogc.2022.02.001
0889-8545/22/© 2022 Elsevier Inc. All rights reserved.

obgyn.theclinics.com

54% of cases may be preventable.[3,4] With early identification and action outcomes could be significantly improved. This reviews the pathology, management, and outcomes associated with PPH and delivery of blood components therapy.

Pregnancy Physiology

a. Women experience the expansion of their plasma volume by 40% to 45% in normal pregnancy.[5] This hypervolemia serves multiple functions, including providing for a growing fetus and placenta and protecting the mother against adverse effects of blood loss at delivery.[6] At term, the average pregnant women have a blood volume of ~5 L.[7]

In near-term gestation, the uterus receives a significant volume of blood of 500 to 750 mL per minute.[8] This is approximately 15% of cardiac output. This blood flows through the spiral arteries, which have no muscular layer due to trophoblastic remodeling to achieve a low-pressure system. After placental separation, spiral vessels at the interface between the placenta and myometrium are avulsed. Hemostasis after delivery first depends on the contraction of the myometrium for mechanical compression of these open vessels[6]

Diagnosis/Definitions

a. According to the American College of Obstetricians and Gynecologists, PPH is defined as excessive blood loss of 1000 mL or greater or bleeding associated with signs of hypovolemia[9]. Primary hemorrhage occurs in the first 24 hours after delivery and secondary hemorrhage occurs between 24 hours and up to 12 weeks after delivery. The use of 1000 mL as a cutoff applies to both vaginal delivery and cesarean delivery. This constitutes a change from historical definitions of PPH, which defined 500 mL or greater blood loss after vaginal delivery and 1000 mL or greater blood loss after cesarean delivery as hemorrhage. Despite new definitions supporting the use of the higher threshold of 1000 mL for both routes of delivery, bleeding beyond 500 mL after vaginal delivery, in our opinion, is still considered abnormal and warrants action.[10]

Risk Assessment

a. There are multiple well-established risk factors for PPH. However, many women who undergo a PPH do not have identifiable risk factors and some women who are considered high risk for hemorrhage do not experience one. Given this unpredictability and the possibility of high subsequent morbidity and mortality, providers should always be prepared to manage PPH.

Risk assessment tools have been shown to identify 60% to 85% of patients who are at risk of hemorrhage[11]. To reduce adverse outcomes associated with hemorrhage, the Joint Commission proposed standards, including the completion of an evidence-based assessment tool for determining the risk of hemorrhage on admission to labor and delivery and the postpartum floor. There are multiple risk scoring systems available; however, only 3 have been shown to have potential. All require further external validation: one for cesarean delivery, one for placenta previa, and one for placenta accreta. Unfortunately, none have been validated for vaginal delivery[12].

An example of a risk assessment tool for PPH is the risk classification scheme developed by the California Maternal Quality Care Collaborative (CMQCC). This tool establishes 3 categories of risk that are outlined in **Fig. 1**.[13] Based on these categorizations, different transfusion preparation options are suggested on admission. In addition to these risks, other risk factors for PPH may develop throughout the labor course including a prolonged second stage, prolonged oxytocin use, active bleeding, chorioamnionitis, the use of magnesium sulfate, operative delivery, urgent or emergent cesarean delivery, and retained placenta.

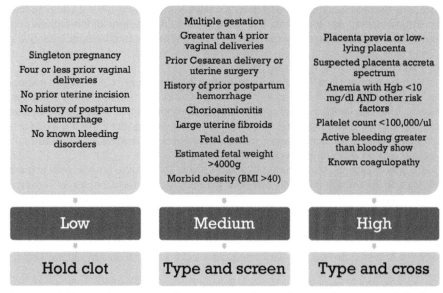

Fig. 1. Predelivery risk assessment for postpartum hemorrhage and recommended admission lab order. (*Data from* Gabel K, AL L, EK M. CMQCC obstetric hemorrhage tool Kit: Risk factor assessment. California Department of health. Available at https://www.cmqcc.org/content/ob-hemorrhage-toolkit-pocket-card.)

Causes

a. Atony occurs when the uterus fails to contract appropriately after delivery. This accounts for 70% to 80% of cases of PPH [11] and should, therefore, be considered and addressed first. Most of the increase in incidence from 1995 to 2004 of PPH is driven by an increase in uterine atony.[3] The diagnosis of atony is typically made when bimanual examination reveals a boggy uterus that does not become firm with the massage. Atony may or may not be associated with retained products that can affect the uterus globally or focally. Many risk factors have been established for uterine atony. Features that lead to a relatively overdistended uterus, such as large for gestational age fetus, multiple gestation, or polyhydramnios, can create a greater risk for atony. Labor course abnormalities such as the use of prostaglandins or prolonged oxytocin are also associated with a higher risk of uterine atony. Other factors associated with atony include primiparity and grand multiparity, chorioamnionitis, the presence of large fibroids, and uterine inversion. Although uterine atony is the most common cause of PPH, it is not the most common etiology underlying the need for massive transfusion at the time of delivery as it responds well to current treatment modalities.[3]

b. Traumatic injury also accounts for a significant portion of cases of hemorrhage. During vaginal delivery, trauma can occur anywhere along the birth canal, including the uterus, cervix, vagina, and perineum. Operative or precipitous delivery can predispose patients to genital tract trauma; however, vulvovaginal and perineal lacerations are common and complicate up to 85% of all vaginal deliveries.[14] Similarly, genital tract hematomas can also be a significant source of blood loss. Diagnosis of both lacerations and hematomas are made via a thorough examination of the upper and lower genital tract after delivery. Uterine rupture is another traumatic etiology of PPH. This can be primary, as in the case of a previously intact or unscarred uterus, or secondary, when associated with previous uterine surgery.

Trauma-related bleeding can complicate cesarean deliveries with the lateral extension of the hysterotomy, as the most common cause. Risks factors for this include prolonged labor before cesarean, incorrect placement of the hysterotomy, or inadequate incision size. Diagnosis is typically made on thorough inspection of the uterus after delivery and is usually managed surgically.

c. Retained products after delivery are another etiology for PPH. A thorough inspection of the placenta and membranes should be routinely performed after all deliveries, although this may not always capture additional products that may be left behind including succenturiate placental lobes or additional membranes. If there is a concern for retained products, then either an intrauterine bimanual examination or bedside ultrasound can be used for diagnosis.

Care should also be taken during this assessment to evaluate for placenta accreta spectrum (PAS), which includes placenta accreta, increta, and percreta. The incidence of PAS is rising with current estimates of 1 in every 272 pregnancies being affected.[15] Risk factors include prior uterine curettage, multiple cesarean sections, and placenta previa.[16] Abnormal imaging findings on sonographic assessment may increase the suspicion for PAS and provide for proactive antenatal preparation for delivery in a tertiary care center, with adequate blood products and available surgical expertise.[17]

d. Coagulopathy complicates approximately 1 in 500 live deliveries in the United States.[1] Coagulopathy can contribute to PPH by worsening bleeding or as a result of severe hemorrhage. Differential diagnosis includes pregnancy-related etiologies such as HELLP syndrome, pre-eclampsia with severe features, placental abruption, and amniotic fluid embolus as well as non–pregnancy-related causes of coagulopathy such as von Willebrand disease.

Pre-eclampsia with severe features and HELLP syndrome can result in thrombocytopenia and platelet dysfunction that can lead to abnormalities in coagulation. Placental abruption can lead to disseminated intravascular coagulation and hypofibrinogenemia as well as uterine atony. While uncommon, this combination of complications makes abruption responsible for 16.7% of cases that use massive transfusion protocols.[18] Amniotic fluid embolus is an extremely rare, poorly understood obstetric complication that classically presents with the triad of hypotension, hypoxia, and coagulopathy.[19] The coagulopathy that results from an amniotic fluid embolus can be severe and confers high risk for PPH when present.

Patients with von Willebrand disease are at higher risk for both antepartum and postpartum bleeding and are more than five times more likely to need a transfusion.[20] Patients with acquired (eg, antiphospholipid syndrome) and inherited thrombophilias (eg, Factor V Leiden, prothrombin gene mutation, Protein C and S deficiency, antithrombin deficiency) are often treated with anticoagulation during pregnancy. Understandably, these patients are also at an increased risk for hemorrhage during delivery.

Measurement of Blood Loss

a. Quantitative methods of estimating blood loss have demonstrated more accuracy than visual or qualitative estimations.[21] Despite this, quantitative methods have not been shown to positively affect clinical outcomes, including the prevention of severe hemorrhage or need for blood transfusion, plasma expanders, or uterotonics.[22] However, obstetric hemorrhage bundles often include quantitative blood loss estimation and have been shown to improve overall morbidity related to hemorrhage.[23] Further studies are needed to show the specific impact of quantitative methods on reducing hemorrhage-related morbidity across diverse health care settings.

Management

Antepartum optimization

i. Predelivery optimization of maternal status includes the treatment of iron deficiency anemia of pregnancy with oral or parenteral iron. Adequate prenatal counseling and discussion in the office relating to PPH, especially for those with risk factors is also beneficial.

Team preparedness

As discussed previously, assessment of risk factors on admission to labor and delivery and ongoing assessment during labor is a vital component to optimizing outcomes from PPH. However, many cases of PPH occur in women without risk factors. Therefore, providers must be prepared for hemorrhage at every delivery.

Institutions with comprehensive hemorrhage protocols have demonstrated improved patient outcomes.[24] This helps standardize the approach for expedited recognition and management of PPH which leads to earlier bleeding resolution and decreased need for transfusions.[24] **Fig. 2** shows an example of a PPH protocol that outlines provider roles and provides step by step care directives as blood loss worsen. Additional protocols are available on the ACOG website. Designated obstetric hemorrhage carts with readily available suture, foley catheters, tamponade balloons, and other supplies can also decrease time to intervention resulting in improved patient outcomes.[25]

Simulation training for managing PPH is also a vital tool to help improve maternal morbidity and mortality. The Joint Commission recommends that all obstetric staff:

a. Undergo team training to teach staff to work together and communicate more effectively when PPH occurs
b. Conduct clinical simulation drills to help staff prepare for PPH, and
c. Conduct debriefings after PPH to evaluate team performance and identify areas for improvement

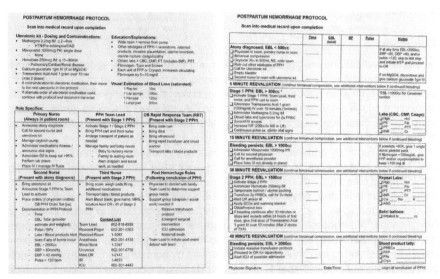

Fig. 2. Example of PPH Hemorrhage checklist from the University of Arizona College of Medicine- Phoenix Department of Obstetrics and Gynecology.

It is also important to consider that these protocols and simulations training drills be adapted to address individual institutions and resources, or lack thereof. Some systems may not have sufficient blood product availability necessary for massive transfusion or interventional radiology resources readily available. Alternative action and/or versus transport to a higher level of care should be considered as part of each institution's protocol.

Patient evaluation overview and management

As stated previously, causes of PPH can be broken down into 4 main categories: Atony, trauma/lacerations, retained products, and coagulopathy. It is important to perform a comprehensive evaluation and address lacerations and retained products as indicated. The remainder of this section will focus primarily on the management of uterine atony as it accounts for 70% to 80% of PPH.

Active management of the third stage of labor has been recommended to reduce PPH related to uterine atony. Compared with expectant management, this seems to reduce the risk of PPH greater than 1000 mL.[26] Active management encompasses a collection of interventions performed in the third stage to prevent hemorrhage from its most common cause, uterine atony. These methods include the administration of prophylactic uterotonics, uterine massage, and active placental delivery.

Routine use of prophylactic uterotonics is recommended by several governing organizations.[10,27] The most used prophylactic uterotonic in the United States is oxytocin. Details regarding oxytocin can be found in **Table 1**. Misoprostol is another option that can be considered in resource-limited settings. While data are limited, oxytocin seems to be the most effective option for the prevention of PPH and has few adverse effects. The use of tranexamic acid (TXA) has not yet been proven for prophylaxis, but current data show potential for future benefit.[28,29]

Data regarding the efficacy of uterine massage and active traction for the delivery of the placenta are from small studies and show mixed results.[30,31] Given low overall risk, especially with uterine massage, these can still be considered as part of the prevention of hemorrhage. Of note, bimanual massage for which the uterus is compressed between the provider's 2 hands can be a useful adjunct for diagnosis as well as the management of atony.

Medications

Uterotonic medications are the first-line treatment of hemorrhage secondary to atony. No specific agent has been shown to be superior so the choice of medication is primarily based on the drug side-effect profile and provider discretion.[32,33] Often, multiple medications are needed to treat atony and can be used in a rapid series. Details regarding the mechanism, dosing, frequency of use, contraindications, and adverse effects are noted in **Table 1**.

Oxytocin is routinely administered as part of active management of the third stage of labor, but the rate of infusion can be increased with the identification of abnormally high volume of bleeding. Adverse effects are rare and the drug is well tolerated. If intravenous access is limited, oxytocin can also be administered intramuscularly.

A second uterotonic medication is required after oxytocin administration in 1.7% to 25% of cases.[34] Carboprost, a synthetic prostaglandin $F_{2\alpha}$ analog, and methylergonovine, an ergot derivative, can also be used to stimulate uterine contractility and treat atony. The decision to use either is primarily driven by contraindications to each medication, which is outlined in **Table 1**. Misoprostol is a synthetic prostaglandin E1 analog that can be used as an adjunctive measure. Optimum dose and route of administration are unclear. Sublingual misoprostol is rapidly absorbed and peaks in 30 minutes and is

Table 1
Medication management of uterine atony

Medication	Mechanism	Dosing	Contraindications	Common Adverse Effects
First Line Agents				
Oxytocin (Pitocin)	Increases intracellular calcium on uterine myofibrils to stimulate contraction	IV: 10–40 units per 500–1000 mL bag continuous infusion IM: 10 units	Hypersensitivity to drug	• Nausea/vomiting • Hyponatremia with prolonged use • Hypotension with IV push
Second Line Agents				
Carboprost (15-methyl PGF2α) (Hemabate)	Stimulates myometrial contractility	IM: 0.25 mg every 15–90 min (max 8 doses) Intramyometrial: same as above	Asthma Relative contraindications: hypertension, active hepatic, pulmonary, or cardiac disease	• Nausea/vomiting • Diarrhea • Transient fever • Headache • Chills • Hypertension • Bronchospasm
Methylergonovine Maleate (Methergine)	Stimulates myometrial smooth muscle contractions	IM: 0.2 mg every 2–4 h	Hypertension, pre-eclampsia, cardiovascular disease, hypersensitivity to drug	• Nausea/vomiting • Severe hypertension (especially IV use)
Misoprostol (PGE1) (Cytotec)		Oral, sublingual, or rectal: 600–1000 mcg once	Hypersensitivity to drug	• Nausea/vomiting • Diarrhea • Shivering • Transient fever • Headache
Tranexamic acid (TXA)	Antifibrinolytic; reversibly binds (inhibits) plasminogen	IV: 1g infused over 10–30 min. Repeated dose can be given if bleeding persists after 30 min.	None	Seizures, ocular changes, thrombotic events (rare)

Data from Bulletins-Obstetrics CoP. Practice Bulletin No. 183: Postpartum Hemorrhage. Obstet Gynecol. 10 2017;130(4):e168-e186. https://doi.org/10.1097/AOG.000000000002351.

sustained for about 3 hours. Oral use is also rapidly absorbed but levels also decline rapidly given hepatic metabolism. Rectal administration reaches peak concentration slower than both sublingual and oral Cytotec but also has a longer duration of action. Vaginal misoprostol is not recommended as heavy bleeding will likely impair absorption. Transient fever is a risk with misoprostol use and should be treated accordingly but may lead to unnecessary work-up for sepsis and antibiotic use.

Tranexamic acid is an anti-fibrinolytic medication that works by reversibly binding to the lysine receptor on plasminogen and inhibiting its conversion to plasmin. The World Maternal Antifibrinolytic Trial (WOMAN) trial was an international randomized, double-blind, placebo-controlled trial that compared the administration of TXA with placebo in the setting of PPH (given within 3h of delivery).[35] This study demonstrated a statistically significant reduction in mortality due to bleeding from 1.7% to 1.2% with the use of TXA, especially in women treated within 3 hours of delivery. Adverse events, such as thromboembolic events did not differ significantly with the administration of TXA.

Tamponade Management

If bleeding persists despite conservative measures and uterotonics, it is reasonable to consider uterine tamponade techniques with intrauterine balloon catheters, intrauterine pack, or vacuum-induced tamponade.

Multiple balloons are available and use is primarily dictated by provider comfort, availability, and cost. Bakri, Ebb, and B-Cath are all FDA approved for use in PPH. These have variable recommended filling capacities usually between 500 and 750 cc. In vitro studies have shown that the risk of device rupture occurs at much higher volumes greater than 2500 cc.[36] Low resource settings may also use Foley catheters for tamponade but these are limited by a maximum recommended fill volume of 10 to 35 cc with in vitro rupture occurring at about 120 cc.[36] After the placement of a balloon for tamponade, vaginal packing may be required as well as urinary Foley catheter placement. Balloons can remain in place for a maximum of 24 hours per manufacturer guidelines before they are recommended to be removed, though the optimal duration of inflation has not been established. Overall success rate for pooled balloon tamponade was 85.9% and was more effective after vaginal delivery than cesarean section. Risks seem to be overall low as well.[37]

Intrauterine packing can be used in a similar fashion to balloon tamponade. Several materials can be used for packing. Plain gauze or laparotomy sponges can be inserted into the uterine cavity. This approach has recently fallen out of favor but can be used in low-resource settings. Hemostatic gauze can also be inserted into the intrauterine cavity with the benefit of hemostasis in addition to physical tamponade. This specialized gauze can be impregnated with various substances, including kaolin, which activates the clotting cascade on contact, and chitosan, which swell and form a gel-like plug to aid hemostasis. Small studies suggest a success rate of approximately 90% with the use of hemostatic gauze.[38]

Several novel methods for tamponade are currently under investigation. One such method is the mini-sponge device, which uses the XStat mini sponge dressing© originally developed for wounds in the trauma setting. An obstetric prototype that encases these mini sponges in a mesh pouch to facilitate removal can be inserted into the uterine cavity whereby they are able to absorb blood rapidly, expand to conform to the uterine cavity, and provide an effective tamponade. In small studies, this seems to be highly effective in cases of hemorrhage.[39,40] Another method is the use of low-level vacuum-induced tamponade with the Jada device. This is thought to rapidly evacuate blood from the uterine cavity and allow for subsequent contraction. The device consists of a 41 cm silicone rod with an intrauterine loop consisting of vacuum pores at the distal end. The device is then connected to wall suction at a level of 80 mm Hg ± 10 mm Hg until about 30 minutes after adequate control of bleeding is obtained. A prospective, multi-center treatment study shows an efficacy of 94% as well as a favorable safety profile. The FDA granted premarket approval for the device in August 2020.[41]

Embolization

When patients have failed less invasive therapies for PPH, uterine (UAE) or hypogastric artery embolization can be considered. Candidates for this method are those who are hemodynamically stable but continue to have slow, ongoing bleeding. The procedure, performed by interventional radiology, involves fluoroscopic evaluation and embolization of uterine arteries with gelatin sponges or coils. Gelfoam, which is an absorbable gelatin sponge, is preferred as it allows for temporary occlusion of about 2 to 6 weeks, which is adequate for control of bleeding but allows for the minimization of long-term side effects of embolization. Small studies have shown a success rate of 58% to 98% and little to no effect on subsequent pregnancies.[33,42]

Surgical Management

When patients with atony have failed less invasive therapies including UAE or are unable to receive embolization due to hemodynamic instability, then surgical management should be considered. Adequate resuscitation, including maintaining adequate oxygen saturation, avoiding hypothermia, treating acidosis, and correcting coagulopathy if present, should be undertaken. Laparotomy is typically performed with a midline vertical incision in the setting of vaginal delivery to optimize exposure. After cesarean deliveries, the surgical incision is typically used for exploration even if a Pfannenstiel incision was used.

On entry, thorough exploration should be performed to identify sources of bleeding. If a laceration in the myometrium or broad ligament is identified, then primary repair may be attempted. Care should be taken in these instances to also evaluate for concomitant bladder injury or retroperitoneal bleeding.

Vascular ligation to reduce blood flow to the uterus is commonly used (**Fig. 3**).[43] Most commonly, uterine artery ligation with O'Leary sutures can be placed at the time of cesarean section for control of bleeding from a lacerated uterine artery or in attempts to control bleeding during ongoing hemorrhage. After the identification of the ureter, a suture is passed 1–2 cm medial to the uterine vessels close to the cervix at the level of the internal os and then through the broad ligament just lateral to the uterine vessels. Similarly, the utero-ovarian ligaments can also be suture ligated. These measures may not completely stop hemorrhage from etiologies such as atony but can reduce bleeding while other techniques are performed. They also do not seem to impact future pregnancy outcomes.[44] Suture ligation of the internal iliac or hypogastric artery can also be used. However, due to surgeon inexperience with retroperitoneal dissection, this is rarely used today.

Uterine compression sutures are another surgical technique used for the management of PPH. Although no compression technique has been proven to be superior, the B-Lynch suture is the most well-known technique. The placement of this suture is detailed in **Fig. 4**.[43] Typically, a large, rapidly absorbable suture such as 0-Chromic is used to minimize the risk of suture breakage and reduce the risk of bowel herniation through remaining suture loops after the involution of the uterus. This seems to be effective for controlling hemorrhage and has minimal long-term risks.[33,45]

Other possible temporizing surgical techniques include uterine tourniquet placement, intrauterine balloon placement as an adjunct to compression sutures, and pelvic

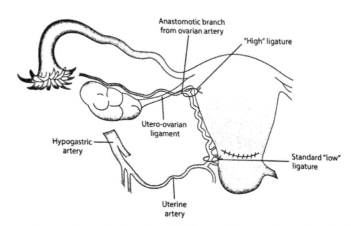

Fig. 3. Areas where uterine artery ligation via O'Leary stitch may be performed. (*From* Foley MR, Strong TH, Garite TJ. Obstetric intensive care manual. Fifth edition ed. New York: McGraw-Hill Education; 2018. with permission.)

packing. In the event of massive hemorrhage with risk of rapid exsanguination, proximal control of bleeding may be considered with manual compression or balloon occlusion of the aorta.

If all other therapies have failed, hysterectomy remains the definitive treatment of uterine bleeding and occurs in about 0.1% of deliveries in the United States.[46] This results in infertility and has increased risk of associated surgical injury. Care should be taken to address and correct coagulopathy as well as ascertain whether other invasive surgical, but fertility-sparing techniques, are feasible before proceeding with hysterectomy. In the case of suspected PAS, early use of hysterectomy may result in the least possible morbidity.

Delayed Sequelae

Sheehan syndrome, also known as postpartum hypopituitarism, is a rare but life-threatening sequela of severe blood loss due to hypoperfusion of the enlarged pituitary gland during pregnancy. Classically, it presents as a failure of lactation after delivery with amenorrhea or oligomenorrhea; however, it can present as a variety of deficiencies in pituitary hormone.

BLOOD COMPONENT THERAPIES

Administration of blood component therapy can be a complicated process and difficult to balance the morbidity of hemorrhage with the risks and morbidity of transfusion. However, early action with transfusion of blood products is a vital component to the reduction in maternal mortality related to significant obstetric hemorrhage. Approximately 3% of women require a blood transfusion postpartum and this number continues to rise.[47] The following portion of this aims to highlight key components for the evaluation and delivery of blood component therapies as well as alternatives to assist providers in clinical decision making.

Clinical Evaluation of Blood Loss

In pregnant women at term, approximately 20% to 25% blood loss, equating to 1000 to 1500 cc may occur before exhibiting vital sign changes. Early vital sign changes are

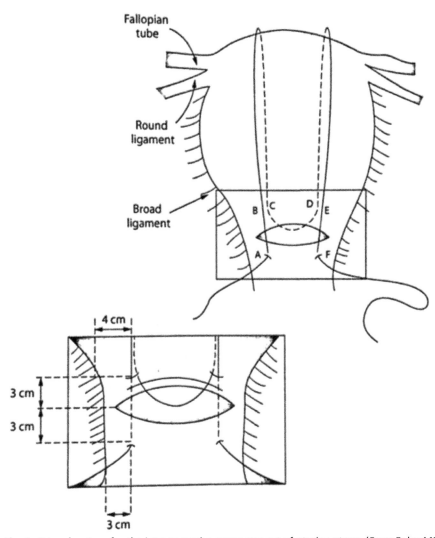

Fig. 4. B-Lynch suture for the intraoperative management of uterine atony. (*From* Foley MR, Strong TH, Garite TJ. Obstetric intensive care manual. Fifth edition ed. New York: McGraw-Hill Education; 2018. with permission.)

subtle, beginning with mild tachycardia and a decrease in blood pressure without overt hypotension. Because of this discrete nature in changes, it is important to have an ongoing assessment of blood loss in addition to the evaluation of clinical signs and symptoms. The WOMAN trial demonstrated that 60% of patients had clinical signs of hemodynamic instability at the time of PPH diagnosis and 4% had signs of end-organ damage.[48] As blood loss continues, moderate to severe shock may present as altered mental status, including restlessness or a decreased level of consciousness, in addition to increasing tachycardia and worsening hypotension. However, in the setting of hypotension related to hemorrhagic shock, trauma literature suggests that outcomes are improved with permissive hypotension to maintain a mean arterial pressure of 40 mm Hg compared with aggressive fluid resuscitation to achieve mean arterial pressure of 80 mm Hg.[49] Allowing for permissive hypotension decreases blood loss and reduces the incidence of the lethal triad of hypothermia, acidosis, and coagulopathy.

Laboratory Evaluation

During PPH when blood loss begins to exceed expectations and is continuing despite ongoing interventions, laboratory evaluation is essential. The following 5 tests should always be included to guide the delivery of appropriate blood component therapies and repeated at regular intervals throughout and after the care process. In addition, if routine Type and Screen is not a part of your institutional policy for labor admissions then it should also be sent at this time to not further delay cross-matching, as needed.

Hemoglobin/Hematocrit

Commonly, anemia of pregnancy results in reduced starting hemoglobin/hematocrit on admission to labor and delivery units. The recommendation level for transfusion is for hemoglobin less than 7 g/dL or hemoglobin levels between 8 and 10 (Hematocrit 21%–24%) when ongoing bleeding or symptomatic anemia is occurring.[50] However, it is important to note that hemoglobin change can be delayed 4 to 6 hours due to diffusion and that in an unstable hemorrhaging patient, normal hemoglobin levels should not delay transfusion.

Platelets

In pregnant women at term, the platelet count usually is between 150,000 and 450000/μL. Thrombocytopenia is considered at levels less than 150,000/μL; however, this does not significantly impact care plans until much lower levels occur. In actively bleeding patients or patients undergoing surgical intervention; transfusion of platelets should be considered at levels less than 50,000/μL. Before vaginal deliveries, platelets should be transfused to achieve levels above 30,000/μL. Otherwise, platelet transfusion should not be considered unless levels are less than 10,000/μL OR spontaneous bleeding is occurring.

Prothombin Time/International Normalized Ratio (PT/INR)

Prothrombin Time/International Normalized Ratio (PT/INR) measures the time for plasma to clot when it is exposed to tissue factor. This assesses both the extrinsic and common pathways of coagulation. It is clinically used to assess unexplained bleeding, disseminated intravascular coagulation, and factor deficiencies including fibrinogen, factor II, V, VII, and or X. The PT/INR is always abnormal before the activated partial thromboplastin time (aPTT) in patients with DIC. Goal INR levels during active and ongoing hemorrhage should be 1.5 to 2.0.

Activated Partial Thromboplastin Time

Activated partial thromboplastin time measures the time to clot using the intrinsic and common pathways of coagulation. Similar to the PT/INR can be used to identify worsening DIC and factor deficiencies when prolonged. Transfusion of fresh frozen plasma (FFP) should be considered during active hemorrhage requiring massive transfusion with aPTT greater than 1.5 times the upper limit of normal.

Fibrinogen

While typically increased during pregnant women at term compared with nonpregnant populations ranging between 4 and 6 g/L, fibrinogen remains a crucial independently associated component during obstetric hemorrhage. A recent study identified that for every 1 g/L decrease in fibrinogen the risk of severe PPH increased 2.6-fold. A baseline fibrinogen level less than 200 mg/dL had a positive predictive value of 100% for PPH.[51] Multiple other studies have also identified that fibrinogen <2 g/L predicted the need for further intervention including UAE, packing, vessel ligation, or hysterectomy.

While preemptive transfusion of fibrinogen has not been shown to be effective, early intervention with cryoprecipitate or fibrinogen concentrates during PPH may reduce the need for the transfusion of other products.[52] During ongoing bleeding goal levels greater than 150 to 200 mg/dL should be maintained.

THROMBOELASTOGRAPHY AND OTATIONAL HROMBOELASTOMETRY

Thromboelastography (TEG) and rotational thromboelastometry (ROTEM) have also grown in use across care centers given that they can quickly and simultaneously assess five parameters of hemostasis on 0.35 mL fresh whole blood samples. TEG has been validated and used in obstetric hemorrhage to guide providers to which blood factors may be most indicated for transfusion.[53] Though a TEG graph can be difficult to interpret, **Fig. 5** can serve as a quick resource for directed replacement.

BLOOD COMPONENT THERAPY

Once comprehensive laboratory evaluation or TEG/ROTEM results have been obtained, this information can be used to guide the directed replacement of various blood components. Using direct replacement may reduce over-treating hemorrhage and decrease the incidence of posttransfusion complications. The following represent different blood components and alternative therapies that may be considered during PPH and a further summarized in **Table 2**.

Whole Blood

Despite containing all necessary components in a physiologic appropriate ratio, whole blood is not universally available for transfusion and has not been well studied in the setting of PPH.

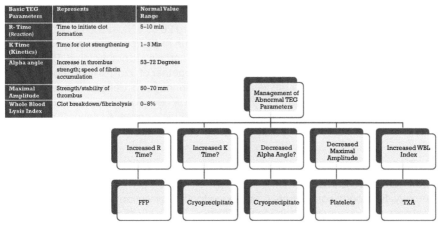

Fig. 5. Thromboelastography for blood component replacement during hemorrhage. (*Data from* Jackson DL, DeLoughery TG. Postpartum Hemorrhage: Management of Massive Transfusion. Obstet Gynecol Surv. Jul 2018;73(7):418-422. https://doi.org/10.1097/OGX. 0000000000000582.)

Packed Red Blood Cells

Packed red blood cells (PRBCs) are most often the key product for transfusion during postpartum hemorrhage to correct anemia, preserve blood volume and oncotic pressure, and maintain oxygen-carrying capacity of blood.[50] To avoid hemolytic reactions and RH alloimmunization, patients should be given type matched blood. In the setting of massive transfusion when blood type is not known, all women of child-bearing potential should be given O-RH negative blood. If there is a shortage, RH positive blood may be used and then RhoGAM administered if the patient subsequently is RH negative.[50]

Platelets

Platelets are key to clot formation. During active bleeding or ongoing surgery, it is important to maintain a goal level greater than 50,000/μL. One unit of single donor apheresis platelets or 4 to 6 pooled units will increase the platelet count by 30,000 to 50,000/μL platelets within 1-hour posttransfusion.[50]

Fresh Frozen Plasma

Fresh Frozen Plasma, or FFP, contains all the clotting factors and other proteins and is derived from the processing of a whole blood sample. It is generally stored frozen at −18C for approximately 1 year. Once thawed the product is useable for up to 5 days. Fresh frozen plasma is best used during massive transfusion for the replacement of multiple coagulation factor deficits which may occur during severe hemorrhage and hemodilution by PRBCs and crystalloids. It is important to note that for INR less than 1.5 it takes significantly more FFP to improve laboratory numbers without significant clinical change for coagulopathy.

However, plasma contains antibodies which may lead to the risk of alloimmunization if incompatible blood is administered as well as febrile and allergic reactions. In addition, patients who receive plasma are at increased risk of lung injury and volume overload to be described later.

Cryoprecipitate

A single unit of cryoprecipitate consists of only 10 to 20 cc of fluid and increases fibrinogen by 10 to 15 mg/dL compared with the volume of 250 cc required by FFP. Cryoprecipitate does not contain antibodies so cross-matching is not required. Because of its small volume, cryoprecipitate is often pooled together of 5 to 10 units depending on the institution and can more efficiently replace fibrinogen[50] deficits with less risk of fluid overload compared with FFP.[50] It also can be used for bleeding related to von Willebrand's disease and hemophilia A given the high concentrations of von Willebrand's factor and factor VIII, respectively.

Specific Factors

Fibrinogen concentrates

Currently, fibrinogen concentrate is approved for the correction of hypofibrinogenemia in patients with congenital fibrinogen deficiency. The is insufficient support for use of early fibrinogen concentrate to improve PPH outcomes. Data comparing the use of fibrinogen concentrates to cryoprecipitate in the correction of hypofibrinogenemia, subsequent transfusion requirements, and mortality are limited.[52] Further investigation is required for optimal timing, dosage, and benefit for use in the obstetric setting.

Table 2
Blood component indications, dosing, and expected response

Table Product	Indication	Key Components	Shelf Life	Volume	Dosing	Expected Response (for a 75 kg Patient)	Risk
Whole Blood	Acute Blood Loss Massive Transfusion	Red cells, platelets, clotting factors	35–42 d	500 cc	1 Unit	Hb 1–1.5 g/dL Hct 3%–5%	TACO, TRALI, alloimmunization, infection, anaphylaxis, hemolytic and nonhemolytic reaction
Packed Red Blood Cells (PRBCs)	Correct Anemia, Hb < 7 g/DL, Hct <	Red cells, some plasma, few WBCs	42 d at ~ 4C	300 cc	1 Unit of Matched ABO and Rh	Hb 1–1.5 g/dL Hct 3%–5%	TACO, TRALI, alloimmunization, infection, anaphylaxis, hemolytic and nonhemolytic reaction
Fresh Frozen Plasma	Evidence of coagulopathy (abnormal PT/ INR > 2, PTT 1.5 x normal, Massive transfusion	Factors II, VII, IX, X, Fibrinogen	1 y @ −18 C 5 d thawed	200–250 cc	1 Unit of Matched ABO and RH (10–20 mL/kg)	May Decrease PT/ INR, aPTT Increase Fibrinogen by 10–15 mg/dL/U Increases clotting factors by 20*	TACO, TRALI, anaphylaxis, alloimmunization, transfusion-transmitted infection
Platelets	Thrombocytopenia, <50k during ongoing bleeding/ procedure	Platelets	5 d at room temperature	50 cc	1 unit of platelets (6 pooled pack or single apheresis)	Single unit: 7000–10,000 platelets/UL Pooled/Apheresis: 30,000–50,000	Bacterial Contamination and transfusion-related sepsis

(continued on next page)

Table 2
(continued)

Table Product	Indication	Key Components	Shelf Life	Volume	Dosing	Expected Response (for a 75 kg Patient)	Risk
Cryoprecipitate	Fibrinogen < 200 Hemophilia A, Von Willebrand Disease	5–10 mg/dL of fibrinogen, Factor V, VIII, XIII, vWF	1 y at −18 4–6 h thawed	15 cc (Pooled up to 150 cc)	5–10 pooled Units	Each unit in pool Increase total fibrinogen 10–15 mg/dL/U	Rare TRALI, allergic reactions, infection

Data from Storch EK, Custer BS, Jacobs MR, Menitove JE, Mintz PD. Review of current transfusion therapy and blood banking practices. Blood Rev. 11 2019;38:100593. https://doi.org/10.1016/j.blre.2019.100593; Kogutt BK, Will S, Ferrell J, Sheffield JS. 1180: Development of an obstetric hemorrhage response intervention: The postpartum hemorrhage cart. American journal of obstetrics and gynecology. 2020;222(1):S725-S726. https://doi.org/10.1016/j.ajog.2019.11.1192; and Foley MR, Strong TH, Garite TJ. Obstetric intensive care manual. Fifth edition ed. New York: McGraw-Hill Education; 2018.

Recombinant factor VIIA

Recombinant Factor VIIA is approved in the US for the treatment of patients with hemophilia. There are limited data to support use with a significant risk of thromboembolism and maternal myocardial infarction.[54] It is not a recommended therapy but may be used when other methods to control bleeding and multiple transfusions have failed and there is a delay in ability to perform a hysterectomy. rFVIIA is dosed as 60 to 90 mg/kg and can be repeated after 30 minutes.

Prothrombin complex concentrates

Prothrombin complex concentrates (PCCs) replace 3 to 4 Vitamin K-dependent clotting factors, usually II, VII, IX, and X. It is predominantly used to reverse bleeding related to anticoagulation with warfarin. There are little to no data in obstetric, trauma, or cardiovascular surgery literature to support off-label use to improve outcomes in hemorrhage not related to anticoagulation.

Special Considerations

For patients with the documented refusal of blood products, limited resource settings, or blood antibodies making it difficult for appropriate cross-matching there are alternative therapy options. While the following methods yield fewer febrile reactions, reduced opportunity for sensitization to foreign antigens, and can mimic the closed-circuit requirement for Jehovah's witnesses, they do not completely eliminate the potential need for allogeneic blood products.

i. Cell salvage can be safely used for PPHs related to both vaginal and cesarean deliveries with minimal risk. The use had been previously contraindicated due to theoretic risk of amniotic fluid embolism and bacteremia; however, a review of more than 400 documented uses of cell salvage noted no amniotic fluid embolisms had occurred.[55,56] Cell savage can be offered to patients who either due to blood antibodies or limited resources a cross-matched product is unavailable. It is also a possible option for those who refuse allogeneic blood products.

ii. In pregnant women in which extensive blood is anticipated or have blood antibodies that may complicate cross-matching, predelivery collection of products for autologous blood transfusion may be beneficial and has been shown to be safe in pregnancy.[57] The patient must have starting hemoglobin of 11 g/dL and no active seizure disorders or cardiopulmonary disease. Collection cannot begin before 6 weeks before and may occur weekly until 2 weeks before planned use. This also may lead to anemia and does not eliminate the possibility of allogeneic transfusion.

iii. Preoperative planning for acute euvolemic hemodilution can be used for procedures in which significant blood loss is anticipated, such as PAS. Blood is taken at the time of procedure from the patient and stored with an anticoagulant while the equivalent volume is replaced with crystalloid. This provides a more hemodiluted blood loss during the procedure. Once hemostasis is achieved, the previously stored blood is then transfused back to the patient. This technique preserves clotting factors and may limit the need and risks associated with allogeneic transfusions.[58]

iv. In accordance with current trauma and critical care guidelines it is recommended to restrict crystalloid resuscitation to match the volume of blood lost that is, for blood loss of 1000 mL, give 1000 to 2000 mL of crystalloid.[49,59,60] Over correction with crystalloids does not improve oxygen-carrying capacity of blood, further dilutes clotting factors, and may contribute to hypothermia and acidosis which exacerbates coagulopathy and can also result in fluid overload.[49,60]

v. Colloid solutions such as albumin increase oncotic pressure with less extracellular extravasation, this benefit, however, is transient.[43] Compared with crystalloids, colloid solutions are expensive, less common, and have an increased risk of anaphylaxis. There are limited data in obstetric literature to support the use of colloids.

Massive Transfusion

The most widely accepted definition of massive transfusion is the need to administer 10 units of PRBCs in a 24-h period or greater than 4 units within 1 hour. This relates to a hemorrhage event whereby loss is greater than 50% of the patient's blood volume and is associated with a high mortality rate. Initiation of Massive Transfusion Protocol in obstetrics often occurs after a patient has experienced a loss of 20% or more of her blood volume with continued active or uncontrolled bleeding.[61] Pregnancy-related increase in fibrinolysis as well as hemorrhages related to abruption, abnormal placentation or amniotic fluid embolism propagate more significant coagulopathy as blood loss continues. It is important to understand and be proactive with this process to decrease the morbidity and mortality that accompany prolonged delays in care while awaiting laboratory results and blood product matching.

Implementation of institutional massive transfusion protocols has demonstrated a decrease in mortality during hemorrhage and decreasing time to transfusion.[62] This is in part due to streamlining communication between the interdisciplinary teams which expedites delivery of products. While the optimal ratio of red blood cells: plasma: platelets: varies among subspecialty literature—many institutions have adopted a 1:1:1 ratio after the PROPPR study identified faster achievement of hemostasis and stability at 24 hours.[63] Other ratios had previously been proposed to mimic true physiology blood ratios, such as 6:4:1, and 2:1:1; however, more recent data state that the rate of hemodilution of clotting factors is higher than expected and there is no difference in 30-day mortality rates.[63] The typical delivered pack of products contains: 4 to 6 U PRBCs, 4 to 6 units FFP and 1 units of platelet apheresis or a pooled 6-pack of platelets. If cross-matching had not previously occurred, the products given to obstetric patients must be RH negative to reduce the risk of alloimmunization. If RH negative blood is not available and the maternal blood type is RH negative, then Rhogam can be administered. It is also important to note that standard massive transfusion protocols do not include cryoprecipitate which may be an important consideration given the significant role fibrinogen levels play in PPH. As stated previously, crystalloid resuscitation should match the volume of product transfused and a temporary allowance for hypotension is permitted to achieve hemodynamic stabilization and minimize complications. Once stabilization is achieved, a continued restrictive clinical and laboratory-directed approach should be utilized.

COMPLICATIONS/SEQUELAE OF TRANSFUSIONS

a. The Lethal Triad is when coagulopathy is further exacerbated by acidosis and hypothermia during ongoing hemorrhage and massive transfusion which leads to an increased morality. Ongoing hemorrhage leads to organ hypoperfusion and rising lactic acid. This can reduce clotting factor activity by greater than 50% depending on the level of acidemia.[64] In conjunction, the rapid transfusion of blood products and IV fluids can decrease body temperature resulting in further coagulopathy. The impact of defects on clot formation occurs at 34° Celsius and at 33°, hemostasis is at 50% activity.[64] This is mitigated through transfusion through blood warmers and minimizing surgical intervention until the patient is fully warmed and resuscitated. Behr Huggers or warmed blankets should also be used to ensure the patient does not experience further heat loss.

Metabolic Derangements

i. Hypocalcemia, hyperkalemia, hypomagnesaemia may occur and correction of this should be based on measured levels. Most prevalent, hypocalcemia, results from hemodilution and the binding of calcium to the anticoagulant citrate within PRBCs and FFP. Calcium is a necessary component of both the clotting cascade and cardiac function. While not driven by clinical trial or guidelines, it is common practice to monitor ionized calcium levels throughout large volume transfusion and consider administering 2 g of calcium gluconate for every 2 to 4 units of PRBCs transfusions.[64]

c. Transfusion of blood component therapy, even in the setting of ongoing hemorrhage, is not without risk. While most consultation with patients before transfusion regards the low risk of viral transmission of blood-borne illness such as HIV and Hepatitis B. 40% to 50% of transfusion-related deaths in the united states is actually caused by either bacterial contamination leading to sepsis, anaphylaxis, acute hemolytic transfusion reactions, transfusion-related acute lung injury (TRALI) or transfusion-associated circulatory overload (TACO).[65] All of the aforementioned potential consequences of transfusion require interprofessional health care teams to adequately assess and care for these patients.

In the United States, each donated blood component is universally screened for a composite number of viral infections including but not limited to HIV, Hepatitis B, Hepatitis C, Human T-lymphotropic Virus. The composite risk of transmission of all 4 viruses is estimated to be less than 1:30,000.[43] The risks of each individual virus is listed in **Table 3**.[43,66] In addition to viral transmission, bacterial contamination of blood products can also occur. Most often this contamination occurs in platelets and accounts for 17% to 22% of infectious deaths related to transfusion.[66–68]

While adequate cross-matching and pretreatment with antipyretics and antihistamines can minimize fevers, allergic reaction, and significant hemolytic reactions related to transfusion, they do not exclude severe consequences of acute transfusion-related lung injury or TACO.

TRALI occurs in about 0.04% to 0.1% of transfused patients within 6 to 12 hours of transfusion. It also accounts for a 6% risk of mortality which has the highest mortality of all transfusion-related complications.[69] While the mechanism of action is unclear, it occurs with rapid onset of respiratory distress, pulmonary edema, fever, and hypotension often requiring ventilatory support and cessation of current transfusion. However, those who need an additional transfusion of products can receive products from a different donor product.

Table 3	
Frequency of infectious transmissions related to transfusion	
Hepatitis B	1: 100,0000–1: 400,000
Hepatitis C	1: 1,600,000–1: 3,100,000
HIV	1: 1,400,000–1:4, 700,000
HTLV	1: 500,000–1:3,000,000
Bacterial Contamination PRBCS	1: 28,000–1:143,000
Bacterial Contamination Platelets	1:2000–1:8000

From Foley MR, Strong TH, Garite TJ. Obstetric intensive care manual. Fifth edition ed. New York: McGraw-Hill Education; 2018. with permission.

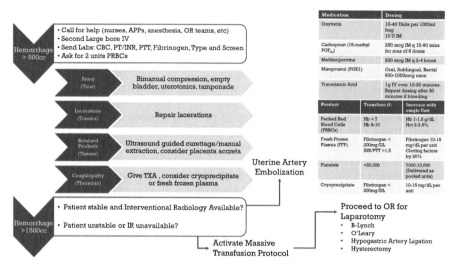

Fig. 6. Postpartum hemorrhage and transfusion of blood component therapy.

Transfusion-associated circulatory overload can occur within 12 hours of transfusion and as associated respiratory distress, pulmonary edema, elevated brain natriuretic protein, and other unexplained cardiovascular changes. The risk of TACO increases as the volume of products transfused increases and is less likely to occur with cryoprecipitate than with FFP. It is managed through supportive care through oxygen or ventilatory support and diuresis. Once volume status is corrected and the patient still requires transfusion of products then transfusion can be resumed.

SUMMARY/DISCUSSION/FUTURE DIRECTIONS

PPH continues to be a leading cause of maternal morbidity and mortality worldwide. It results from a variety of causes, can be difficult to predict, and can have devastating consequences if not proactively managed. Broad differentials, effective interprofessional communication, and fast action are key to success in reducing risks associated with PPH. An ongoing evaluation and invention of innovative devices and new medications is needed to reduce the need for allogeneic transfusions and hysterectomy.

CLINICS CARE POINTS

> **Fig. 6** provides a summary of the following keys to reducing morbidity and mortality related to PPH include:
>
> - Awareness of risk factors and optimization of maternal status before and during delivery is important for management.
>
> - Multidisciplinary team preparedness through simulation and utilization of checklists improves patient care outcomes and communication.
>
> - Active management of the third stage of labor is recommended with prophylactic uterotonics, gentle fundal massage, and early placenta delivery.

- Therapy for atony has high success rates and includes multiple methods of treatment. There are no clear data regarding the superiority of any treatment over another. Typically, less invasive treatments are used first. Possible treatments include uterotonic medications, tamponade techniques, vascular embolization, uterine-sparing surgical management, and hysterectomy.

- Early introduction of directed blood component therapies, when hemorrhage is anticipated to extend beyond 1500 cc, can reduce the total number of products transfused and minimize the occurrence of transfusion-related reactions.

DISCLOSURE

The authors have nothing to disclose.

REFERENCES

1. Reale SC, Easter SR, Xu X, et al. Trends in Postpartum Hemorrhage in the United States From 2010 to 2014. Anesth Analg 2020;130(5):e119–22.
2. Creanga AA, Syverson C, Seed K, et al. Pregnancy-Related Mortality in the United States, 2011-2013. Obstet Gynecol 2017;130(2):366–73.
3. Bateman BT, Berman MF, Riley LE, et al. The epidemiology of postpartum hemorrhage in a large, nationwide sample of deliveries. Anesth Analg 2010;110(5): 1368–73.
4. Della Torre M, Kilpatrick SJ, JU Hibbard, et al. Assessing preventability for obstetric hemorrhage. Am J Perinatol 2011;28(10):753–60.
5. Zeeman GG, Cunningham FG, Pritchard JA. The magnitude of hemoconcentration with eclampsia. Hypertens Pregnancy 2009;28(2):127–37.
6. Cunningham FG, Leveno KJ, Bloom SL, et al. Williams obstetrics. 25th edition. New York, N.Y: McGraw Hill Medical; 2018.
7. Lund CJ, Donovan JC. Blood volume during pregnancy. Significance of plasma and red cell volumes. Am J Obstet Gynecol 1967;98(3):394–403.
8. Pates JA, Hatab MR, McIntire DD, et al. Determining uterine blood flow in pregnancy with magnetic resonance imaging. Magn Reson Imaging 2010;28(4): 507–10.
9. Menard MK, Main EK, Currigan SM. Executive summary of the reVITALize initiative: standardizing obstetric data definitions. Obstet Gynecol 2014;124(1): 150–3.
10. Bulletins-Obstetrics CoP. Practice Bulletin No. 183: Postpartum Hemorrhage. Obstet Gynecol 2017;130(4):e168–86.
11. Kramer MS, Berg C, Abenhaim H, et al. Incidence, risk factors, and temporal trends in severe postpartum hemorrhage. Am J Obstet Gynecol 2013;209(5): 449.e1-7.
12. Neary C, Naheed S, McLernon DJ, et al. Predicting risk of postpartum haemorrhage: a systematic review. BJOG 2021;128(1):46–53.
13. Lyndon A., Lagrew D., Shields L., Main E., Cape V., Improving Health Care Response to Obstetric Hemorrhage. (California Maternal Quality Care Collaborative Toolkit to Transform Maternity Care) Developed under contract #11-10006 with the California Department of Public Health; Maternal, Child and Adolescent Health Division; Published by the California Maternal Quality Care Collaborative, 3/17/15.
14. Frohlich J, Kettle C. Perineal care. BMJ Clin Evid 2015;10:2015.

15. Mogos MF, Salemi JL, Ashley M, et al. Recent trends in placenta accreta in the United States and its impact on maternal-fetal morbidity and healthcare-associated costs, 1998-2011. J Matern Fetal Neonatal Med 2016;29(7): 1077–82.

16. Bowman ZS, Eller AG, Bardsley TR, et al. Risk factors for placenta accreta: a large prospective cohort. Am J Perinatol 2014;31(9):799–804.

17. Shainker SA, Coleman B, Timor-Tritsch IE, et al. Special Report of the Society for Maternal-Fetal Medicine Placenta Accreta Spectrum Ultrasound Marker Task Force: Consensus on definition of markers and approach to the ultrasound examination in pregnancies at risk for placenta accreta spectrum. Am J Obstet Gynecol 2021;224(1):B2–14.

18. Mhyre JM, Shilkrut A, Kuklina EV, et al. Massive blood transfusion during hospitalization for delivery in New York State, 1998-2007. Obstet Gynecol 2013; 122(6):1288–94.

19. Clark SL, Romero R, Dildy GA, et al. Proposed diagnostic criteria for the case definition of amniotic fluid embolism in research studies. Am J Obstet Gynecol 2016;215(4):408–12.

20. James AH, Jamison MG. Bleeding events and other complications during pregnancy and childbirth in women with von Willebrand disease. J Thromb Haemost 2007;5(6):1165–9.

21. Al Kadri HM, Al Anazi BK, Tamim HM. Visual estimation versus gravimetric measurement of postpartum blood loss: a prospective cohort study. Arch Gynecol Obstet 2011;283(6):1207–13.

22. Diaz V, Abalos E, Carroli G. Methods for blood loss estimation after vaginal birth. Cochrane Database Syst Rev 2018;9:CD010980.

23. Main EK, Cape V, Abreo A, et al. Reduction of severe maternal morbidity from hemorrhage using a state perinatal quality collaborative. Am J Obstet Gynecol 2017;216(3):298.e1–11.

24. Shields LE, Wiesner S, Fulton J, et al. Comprehensive maternal hemorrhage protocols reduce the use of blood products and improve patient safety. Am J Obstet Gynecol 2015;212(3):272–80.

25. Kogutt BK, Will S, Ferrell J, et al. 1180: Development of an obstetric hemorrhage response intervention: The postpartum hemorrhage cart. Am J Obstet Gynecol 2020;222(1):S725–6.

26. Begley CM, Gyte GM, Devane D, et al. Active versus expectant management for women in the third stage of labour. Cochrane Database Syst Rev 2019;2: CD007412.

27. WHO recommendations. Uterotonics for the prevention of postpartum haemorrhage. Geneva: World Health Organization; 2018.

28. Sentilhes L, Deneux-Tharaux C, Roberts I, et al. Tranexamic acid for the prevention of postpartum hemorrhage in women undergoing cesarean delivery. Am J Obstet Gynecol 2021. https://doi.org/10.1016/j.ajog.2021.12.039.

29. Saccone G, Della Corte L, D'Alessandro P, et al. Prophylactic use of tranexamic acid after vaginal delivery reduces the risk of primary postpartum hemorrhage. J Matern Fetal Neonatal Med 2020;33(19):3368–76.

30. Hofmeyr GJ, Abdel-Aleem H, Abdel-Aleem MA. Uterine massage for preventing postpartum haemorrhage. Cochrane Database Syst Rev 2013;(7): CD006431.

31. Hofmeyr GJ, Mshweshwe NT, Gülmezoglu AM. Controlled cord traction for the third stage of labour. Cochrane Database Syst Rev 2015;1:CD008020. https://doi.org/10.1002/14651858.CD008020.pub2.

32. Parry Smith WR, Papadopoulou A, Thomas E, et al. Uterotonic agents for first-line treatment of postpartum haemorrhage: a network meta-analysis. Cochrane Database Syst Rev 2020;11:CD012754. https://doi.org/10.1002/14651858.CD012754.pub2.
33. Likis FE, Sathe NA, Morgans AK, et al. Management of Postpartum Hemorrhage. Rockville, MD: Agency for Healthcare Research and Quality US; 2015.
34. Bateman BT, Tsen LC, Liu J, et al. Patterns of second-line uterotonic use in a large sample of hospitalizations for childbirth in the United States: 2007-2011. Anesth Analg 2014;119(6):1344–9.
35. Collaborators WT. Effect of early tranexamic acid administration on mortality, hysterectomy, and other morbidities in women with post-partum haemorrhage (WOMAN): an international, randomised, double-blind, placebo-controlled trial. Lancet 2017;389(10084):2105–16.
36. Antony KM, Racusin DA, Belfort MA, et al. Under Pressure: Intraluminal Filling Pressures of Postpartum Hemorrhage Tamponade Balloons. AJP Rep 2017; 7(2):e86–92.
37. Suarez S, Conde-Agudelo A, Borovac-Pinheiro A, et al. Uterine balloon tamponade for the treatment of postpartum hemorrhage: a systematic review and meta-analysis. Am J Obstet Gynecol 2020;222(4):293.e1–52.
38. Rezk M, Saleh S, Shaheen A, et al. Uterine packing versus Foley's catheter for the treatment of postpartum hemorrhage secondary to bleeding tendency in low-resource setting: A four-year observational study. J Matern Fetal Neonatal Med 2017;30(22):2747–51.
39. Rodriguez MI, Jensen JT, Gregory K, et al. A novel tamponade agent for management of post partum hemorrhage: adaptation of the Xstat mini-sponge applicator for obstetric use. BMC Pregnancy Childbirth 2017;17(1):187.
40. Rodriguez MI, Bullard M, Jensen JT, et al. Management of Postpartum Hemorrhage With a Mini-Sponge Tamponade Device. Obstet Gynecol 2020;136(5): 876–81.
41. D'Alton ME, Rood KM, Smid MC, et al. Intrauterine Vacuum-Induced Hemorrhage-Control Device for Rapid Treatment of Postpartum Hemorrhage. Obstet Gynecol 2020;136(5):882–91.
42. Sentilhes L, Gromez A, Clavier E, et al. Fertility and pregnancy following pelvic arterial embolisation for postpartum haemorrhage. BJOG 2010;117(1):84–93.
43. Foley MR, Strong TH, Garite TJ. Obstetric intensive care manual. Fifth edition. New York: McGraw-Hill Education; 2018.
44. Doumouchtsis SK, Nikolopoulos K, Talaulikar V, et al. Menstrual and fertility outcomes following the surgical management of postpartum haemorrhage: a systematic review. BJOG 2014;121(4):382–8.
45. Sentilhes L, Gromez A, Razzouk K, et al. B-Lynch suture for massive persistent postpartum hemorrhage following stepwise uterine devascularization. Acta Obstet Gynecol Scand 2008;87(10):1020–6.
46. Govindappagari S, Wright JD, Ananth CV, et al. Risk of Peripartum Hysterectomy and Center Hysterectomy and Delivery Volume. Obstet Gynecol 2016;128(6): 1215–24.
47. Ekeroma AJ, Ansari A, Stirrat GM. Blood transfusion in obstetrics and gynaecology. Br J Obstet Gynaecol 1997;104(3):278–84.
48. Shakur H, Elbourne D, Gülmezoglu M, et al. The WOMAN Trial (World Maternal Antifibrinolytic Trial): tranexamic acid for the treatment of postpartum haemorrhage: an international randomised, double blind placebo controlled trial. Trials 2010;11:40. https://doi.org/10.1186/1745-6215-11-40.

49. Morrison CA, Carrick MM, Norman MA, et al. Hypotensive Resuscitation Strategy Reduces Transfusion Requirements and Severe Postoperative Coagulopathy in Trauma Patients With Hemorrhagic Shock: Preliminary Results of a Randomized Controlled Trial. J Trauma 2011;70(3):652–63.

50. Storch EK, Custer BS, Jacobs MR, et al. Review of current transfusion therapy and blood banking practices. Blood Rev 2019;38:100593.

51. Charbit B, Mandelbrot L, Samain E, et al. The decrease of fibrinogen is an early predictor of the severity of postpartum hemorrhage. J Thromb Haemost 2007; 5(2):266–73.

52. Zaidi A, Kohli R, Daru J, et al. Early Use of Fibrinogen Replacement Therapy in Postpartum Hemorrhage-A Systematic Review. Transfus Med Rev 2020;34(2): 101–7.

53. Toffaletti JG, Buckner KA. Use of Earlier-Reported Rotational Thromboelastometry Parameters to Evaluate Clotting Status, Fibrinogen, and Platelet Activities in Postpartum Hemorrhage Compared to Surgery and Intensive Care Patients. Anesth Analg 2019;128(3):414–23.

54. Alfirevic Z, Elbourne D, Pavord S, et al. Use of recombinant activated factor VII in primary postpartum hemorrhage: the Northern European registry 2000-2004. Obstet Gynecol 2007;110(6):1270–8.

55. Esper SA, Waters JH. Intra-operative cell salvage: a fresh look at the indications and contraindications. Blood Transfus 2011;9(2):139–47.

56. Allam J, Cox M, Yentis SM. Cell salvage in obstetrics. Int J Obstet Anesth 2008; 17(1):37–45.

57. Droste S, Sorensen T, Price T, et al. Maternal and fetal hemodynamic effects of autologous blood donation during pregnancy. Am J Obstet Gynecol 1992; 167(1):89–93.

58. Rebarber A, Lonser R, Jackson S, et al. The safety of intraoperative autologous blood collection and autotransfusion during cesarean section. Am J Obstet Gynecol 1998;179(3 Pt 1):715–20.

59. Lange NMd, Schol P, Lance M, et al. Restrictive Versus Massive Fluid Resuscitation Strategy (REFILL study), influence on blood loss and hemostatic parameters in obstetric hemorrhage: study protocol for a randomized controlled trial. Trials 2018;19(1):166.

60. Fodor GH, Habre W, Balogh AL, et al. Optimal crystalloid volume ratio for blood replacement for maintaining hemodynamic stability and lung function: An experimental randomized controlled study. BMC anesthesiology 2019;19(1):21.

61. Jackson DL, DeLoughery TG. Postpartum Hemorrhage: Management of Massive Transfusion. Obstet Gynecol Surv 2018;73(7):418–22.

62. Riskin DJ, Tsai TC, Riskin L, et al. Massive transfusion protocols: the role of aggressive resuscitation versus product ratio in mortality reduction. J Am Coll Surg 2009;209(2):198–205.

63. Holcomb JB, Tilley BC, Baraniuk S, et al. Transfusion of plasma, platelets, and red blood cells in a 1:1:1 vs a 1:1:2 ratio and mortality in patients with severe trauma: the PROPPR clinical trial. JAMA 2015;313(5):471–82.

64. Elmer J, Wilcox SR, Raja AS. Massive transfusion in traumatic shock. J Emerg Med 2013;44(4):829–38.

65. Shander A. Emerging risks and outcomes of blood transfusion in surgery. Semin Hematol 2004;41(1 Suppl 1):117–24.

66. Busch MP, Kleinman SH, Nemo GJ. Current and emerging infectious risks of blood transfusions. JAMA 2003;289(8):959–62.

67. Dodd RY. Current risk for transfusion transmitted infections. Curr Opin Hematol 2007;14(6):671–6.
68. Wagner SJ. Transfusion-transmitted bacterial infection: risks, sources and interventions. Vox Sang 2005;88(1):60.
69. Sayah DM, Looney MR, Toy P. Transfusion reactions: newer concepts on the pathophysiology, incidence, treatment, and prevention of transfusion-related acute lung injury. Crit Care Clin 2012;28(3):363–72, v.

Placenta Accreta Spectrum
Prenatal Diagnosis and Management

Rebecca Horgan, MD*, Alfred Abuhamad, MD

KEYWORDS

- Placenta accreta spectrum • Abnormal placentation • Ultrasound • Diagnosis
- Management

KEY POINTS

- Cesarean section and placenta previa confer the greatest risk for placenta accreta spectrum (PAS).
- Ultrasound is the preferred imaging modality for diagnosing PAS and maintaining a high level of clinical suspicion is essential, particularly in patients with significant risk factors.
- Ultrasound markers of PAS include multiple vascular lacunae, loss of the hypoechoic retroplacental zone, abnormalities of the uterine serosa–bladder interface, retroplacental myometrial thickness less than 1 mm, increased placental vascularity, and observation of bridging vessels linking the placenta and bladder.
- Patients with PAS should be managed by a multidisciplinary team with experience in PAS and delivered at 34 to 35 + 6 weeks gestational age in a level III or level IV center with adequate subspecialists and critical care facilities.
- Hysterectomy is the accepted management of PAS and conservative or expectant management of PAS should be considered investigational.

INTRODUCTION

Placenta accreta spectrum (PAS) is a term used to describe placenta accreta, increta, and percreta. Placenta accreta occurs when the placental villi adhere directly to the myometrium, placenta increta occurs when placental villi invade into the myometrium, and placenta percreta occurs when the placental villi invade through the myometrium into the serosa. A 2019 meta-analysis demonstrated that among patients with PAS, 63% are placenta accreta, 15% are placenta increta, and 22% are placenta percreta.[1] Placenta accreta can be further categorized as total placenta accreta, partial placenta accreta, or focal placenta accreta according to the amount of placental tissue adhered to the myometrium. The pathogenesis of PAS remains unclear. The most prominent theory is that following uterine surgery, abnormal vascularization during the scarring

Division of Maternal Fetal Medicine, Department of Obstetrics & Gynecology, Eastern Virginia Medical School, 825 Fairfax Avenue, Suite 528, Norfolk, VA 23507, USA
* Corresponding author.
E-mail address: horganr@evms.edu

Obstet Gynecol Clin N Am 49 (2022) 423–438
https://doi.org/10.1016/j.ogc.2022.02.004
obgyn.theclinics.com

process leads to secondary localized hypoxia and resultant defective decidualization, thus allowing excessive trophoblastic invasion to occur during placentogenesis.[2–4]

PAS is a major complication of pregnancy with substantial maternal morbidity and mortality, in particular due to life threatening hemorrhage. Seventy percent of patients diagnosed with PAS undergo cesarean hysterectomy.[5] Complications of PAS include damage to local organs, postoperative bleeding, amniotic fluid embolism, consumptive coagulopathy, transfusion-related complications, acute respiratory distress syndrome, postoperative thromboembolism, infectious morbidities, multisystem organ failure, and maternal death.[6] Of women who undergo cesarean hysterectomy, 84% will require a blood transfusion and 25% will lose greater than 5 L of blood.[5,7] The overall mortality rate from cesarean hysterectomy is 1.6% but may be as high as 10% for patients with placenta percreta.[5]

The incidence of PAS has increased significantly during the past several decades, and the incidence is now around 3 per 1000 deliveries.[6,8] The increasing incidence of PAS is largely attributed to the rising cesarean section rate in recent decades.[9] PAS is now the most common reason for cesarean hysterectomy in developed countries.[5] There are several risk factors for the development of PAS. Prior cesarean delivery and placenta previa confer the greatest risk of PAS. Furthermore, the number of previous cesarean deliveries is directly proportional to the risk of PAS, with the risk reaching 67% for those patients with 4 previous cesarean deliveries and a placenta previa.[10] It is important to note that even among patients with no prior cesarean delivery, the presence of placenta previa is associated with a 3% risk of PAS. In the absence of placenta previa, a systematic review demonstrated that the rate of PAS increased from 0.3% in women with 1 previous cesarean delivery to 6.74% for women with 5 or more cesarean deliveries.[11] Additional risk factors for PAS include advanced maternal age, multiparity, prior uterine surgery, prior uterine radiation, endometrial ablation, Asherman syndrome, leiomyomas, uterine anomalies, hypertensive disorders, and smoking. Cesarean scar pregnancy is generally considered a risk factor for PAS. However, given the similar histology between the 2 conditions, they may represent a continuum of the same condition.[12–14] Overall, 80% of patients with PAS have a history of a prior cesarean delivery, uterine curettage, or myomectomy.[3]

PATIENT EVALUATION OVERVIEW

Accurate prenatal diagnosis of PAS is essential in order to allow surgical planning, to coordinate multidisciplinary care, and to enable patient transfer of care to a tertiary center, when appropriate. Delivery before onset of labor and avoidance of placental disruption are essential to optimize maternal outcome. A 2018 meta-analysis demonstrated that a PAS diagnosis before delivery was associated with a significantly lower blood loss (mean difference 0.9 L) and fewer units of red blood cells transfused (mean difference 1.5 units) in comparison with women who have an intraoperative diagnosis of PAS.[15] Prenatal diagnosis of PAS is generally by ultrasound because most patients with placenta accreta are asymptomatic. Patients may report vaginal bleeding and cramping because most PAS cases occur in the presence of a placenta previa. However, intraoperative diagnosis also occurs frequently, most commonly in patients with significant risk factors. Thus, maintaining a high level of clinical suspicion is essential, particularly in patients with significant risk factors.

Ultrasound is the most commonly used imaging modality for the diagnosis of PAS. Ultrasound has been demonstrated to have a sensitivity of 90.72% (95% CI, 87.2–93.6) and specificity of 96.94% (95% CI, 96.3%–97.5%) for the PAS diagnosis.[16] It is important to note that no ultrasound features of PAS or combination of features reliably predict the depth of invasion of PAS,[17] with the exception of demonstration of penetrating placental tissue into adjoining pelvic organs. Patients at risk of PAS should be referred to centers with expertise in the condition because significant interobserver variability and lower sensitivities for diagnosis have been demonstrated in some studies.[18] A transvaginal sonographic approach for the evaluation of the placenta allows for a higher resolution, which enhances visualization. This allows an associated placenta previa to be confirmed, assessment of the posterior bladder wall, and assessment of the extent of placental invasion into cervical tissue. Greater than 80% of cases of PAS occur in association with placenta previa.[19–21] Placental and lower segment vascularization can be further assessed by the application of color Doppler in low velocity.

First Trimester Ultrasound

First trimester sonographic findings of PAS include a gestational sac that is implanted in the lower uterine segment, and/or in a cesarean section scar, and the presence of multiple lacunae within the placenta.[22] Lower uterine segment implantation is defined as a gestational sac implanted in the lower third of the uterus between 8 and 10 weeks or primarily occupying the lower uterine segment from 10 weeks onward.[23] It is important to note that not all gestational sacs that implant in the lower uterine segment result in PAS. In a normal pregnancy, thick anterior myometrium superior to the gestational sac and the bladder–uterine wall interface will be seen on ultrasound.[24] In cases of PAS, the anterior myometrium seems thin and the placental–myometrial and bladder–uterine wall interfaces often seem irregular.[25] In first trimester sonography, it is important to differentiate suspected PAS from a cesarean scar pregnancy. In a true cesarean scar pregnancy, implantation is within the myometrium and the fibrous tissue of the cesarean scar, and the gestational sac is typically ellipsoid or triangular in shape (**Figs. 1–3**).

Second and Third Trimester Ultrasound

The presence of *multiple vascular lacunae* within the placenta in the second and third trimester of pregnancy has a high sensitivity and a low false-positive rate for the presence of PAS.[26] Placental lacunae are believed to develop due to placental tissue alterations because of a long-term exposure to high-velocity, pulsatile blood flow.

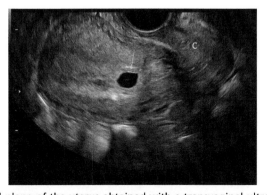

Fig. 1. Midsagittal plane of the uterus obtained with a transvaginal ultrasound showing a low implantation of a gestational sac at 6 weeks gestation in a patient without a prior cesarean section. Note that the gestational sac is circular in shape (*arrow*) and is located in the central portion of the lower uterine segment. C, cervix.

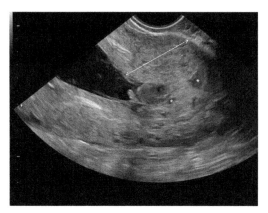

Fig. 2. Midsagittal plane of the uterus obtained with a transvaginal ultrasound showing thickening of placenta (*double arrow*) over the cervix and lacunae (*asterisks*) at 9 weeks in a patient with 3 prior cesarean sections. These findings are suggestive of abnormal implantation in the first trimester with a risk for placenta accreta spectrum.

However, it is important to note that placental lacunae may be present in normal placentas, particularly in the absence of placenta previa, and not all cases of PAS will demonstrate placental lacunae. Placental lacunae have a sensitivity of 73% to 100% and a negative predictive value of 88% to 100% for the diagnosis of PAS.[26] A greater number of placental lacunae, particularly more than 4, confer a higher risk of placenta accreta[27] in pregnancies with placenta previa. The presence of multiple vascular lacunae within the placenta, often referred to as a swiss-cheese appearance, is one of the most important sonographic findings of placenta accreta in the second and third trimester. Color flow Doppler will demonstrate turbulent lacunar blood flow. It is important to note that placental lacunae have the most significance in association with a placenta previa and especially when lacunae are closest to the cervical region.

Loss of the hypoechoic retroplacental zone is another sonographic marker for PAS with a sensitivity of 52% and a specificity of 57%.[28,29] With a false-positive rate of 21%, the true value of this sonographic finding is in its negative predictive value of

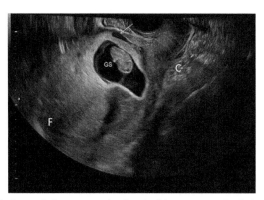

Fig. 3. Midsagittal plane of the uterus obtained with a transvaginal ultrasound showing a cesarean scar pregnancy at 9 weeks gestation. Note the ellipsoid shape of the gestational sac (GS) and thinning of the anterior myometrium (*arrow*). C, cervix; F, fundus.

96% to 100%. Thus, PAS is unlikely in the presence of a hypoechoic retroplacental clear space that extends the length of the placenta.[27,30] It is important to note, however, that this marker is difficult to evaluate and requires scanning along the longitudinal aspect of the placenta with minimal abdominal pressure by the transducer. It is an important marker for the evaluation of focal accretas, however, because these pregnancies typically lack many of the classic markers of PAS (**Fig. 4**).

Abnormalities of the uterine–serosa–bladder interface is another sonographic marker for PAS. These include interruption of the interface, thickening of the interface, irregularity of the interface, or increased vascularity on color Doppler.[26,31] With the use of a transvaginal sonographic approach and color Doppler, the specificity for abnormalities of the serosa–bladder interface reaches 99%, and the positive and negative predictive values are 96% and 92%, respectively.[30]

A *retroplacental myometrial thickness less than 1 mm* is a sonographic marker for PAS with a reported sensitivity of 22% to 100% and a specificity of 72% to 100%.[32,33] It is important to note that the myometrium in the lower uterine segment will thin with advancing gestational age and that patients with a prior cesarean delivery will have a thinner lower uterine segment with a median myometrial thickness of 2.4 mm in the third trimester[34] (**Fig. 5**).

Increased placental vascularity demonstrated on color Doppler has been described in the literature as a marker for PAS because it differentiates normal subplacental venous complexes from markedly dilated peripheral subplacental vascular channels with pulsatile venous-type flow, suggestive of PAS. It is important to note that with advancement in the ultrasound technology and the current ability to display low-velocity flow, most normal placentas will show extensive vascularity, thus rendering the ability to differentiate a normal from a PAS placenta somewhat difficult.

Finally, the *observation of bridging vessels linking the placenta and bladder* with high diastolic arterial blood flow is also suggestive of PAS.[35,36] This is an important finding because it suggests the presence of percreta with vascular flow accompanying placental tissue outside of the uterine cavity.

In the sonographic evaluation of pregnancies at risk for PAS, we recommend an initial ultrasound in the first trimester, followed by an ultrasound at 18 to 20 weeks and then monthly thereafter given the possibility of progression of placental invasion

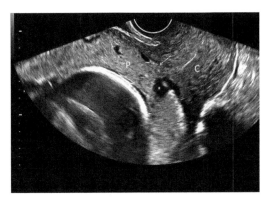

Fig. 4. Midsagittal plane of the uterus obtained with a transvaginal ultrasound at 28 weeks of gestation showing the presence of a placenta previa, a large lacuna (*asterisk*) and a focal loss of the hypoechoic retroplacental zone (*arrow*). These findings are concerning for placenta accreta spectrum. C, cervix; P, placenta.

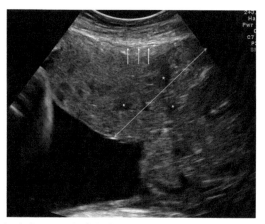

Fig. 5. Transabdominal ultrasound of the lower uterine segment in the late second trimester showing several sonographic markers of placenta accreta spectrum including placental thickening (*double arrow*), multiple lacunae (*asterisks*), and loss of the retroplacental hypo-echoic zone (*small arrows*).

with advancing gestation. We strongly recommend having a protocol and ensuring a thorough evaluation of the placenta in multiple planes.[37] A transvaginal ultrasound is critically important in the evaluation of the cervical region and lower-uterine segment in PAS-at risk pregnancies (**Figs. 6–8**).

Magnetic Resonance Imaging

Magnetic resonance imaging (MRI) features associated with PAS include dark intra-placental bands on T2-weighted imaging, abnormal bulging of the placenta or uterus, disruption of the zone between the uterus and the placenta, and abnormal or disorga-nized placental blood vessels.[16,38] Research to date shows that MRI does not seem superior to ultrasound in the diagnostic accuracy of PAS.[39] MRI may possibly be use-ful as an adjunct to ultrasound in cases of suspected PAS where the placenta is pos-terior or lateral.[40] In addition, MRI may be useful to assess the depth of invasion of the placenta, discerning placenta accreta from increta.[41] However, this would only be of

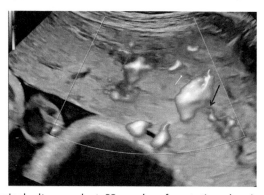

Fig. 6. Transabdominal ultrasound at 33 weeks of gestation showing the presence of crossing vessels in an anterior placenta (*red and blue large arrows*). Moreover, note the loss of the retroplacental hypoechoic zone in a focal area of the placenta (*small arrow*). These findings are concerning for placenta accreta spectrum.

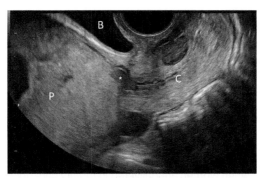

Fig. 7. Midsagittal plane of the uterus obtained with a transvaginal ultrasound at 26 weeks of gestation showing the presence of a placenta previa, a large vascular lacuna (*asterisk*) is seen crossing from the placenta to the cervical tissue and placental thickening. These findings are concerning for placenta accreta spectrum. B, bladder; C, cervix; P, placenta.

clinical utility if the patient's management was dependent on the degree of placental invasion. Furthermore, there is some concern that MRI may even result in ultrasound-based diagnosis of PAS being revised incorrectly.[40] Therefore, further research on the potential use of MRI in the diagnosis of PAS is required because most studies to date have been underpowered. MRI is more expensive than ultrasound, less widely available, and few clinicians have expertise in placental assessment on MRI. Therefore, we do not recommend the routine use of MRI for the evaluation of possible PAS.

An unexplained elevated Maternal serum alpha-fetoprotein (MSAFP) (>2.5 multiple of the median (MOM)) has been associated with PAS.[42,43] However, it is not a consistent finding and should not be used by itself for diagnosis because a normal MSAFP does not exclude a diagnosis of PAS. Preliminary data may suggest a role for biochemical markers in the diagnosis of PAS.[37]

MANAGEMENT OF PLACENTA ACCRETA SPECTRUM
Preoperative Management of Placenta Accreta Spectrum

It is recommended that patients with PAS be delivered at a level III or level IV center due to the availability of appropriate medical staff with training in managing complex

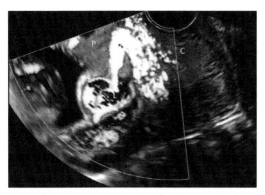

Fig. 8. Midsagittal plane of the cervix obtained with a transvaginal ultrasound at 22 weeks of gestation showing the presence of a placenta previa, a large vascular lacuna (*L*) with vascular invasion into the cervical tissue. These findings are concerning for placenta accreta spectrum. C, cervix; P, placenta.

obstetric conditions, including PAS, in addition to access to subspecialists and critical care facilities.[44] Management of patients with PAS should involve a standardized approach with multidisciplinary team care with experience in the management of PAS. Team members may include maternal fetal medicine, experienced pelvic surgeons, neonatology, skilled nursing team, blood bank team, anesthesia team, intensivist, urology, and interventional radiology. Any patient at high risk of PAS should also be transferred to centers of excellence for their delivery. This may include patients with suspected PAS on sonogram, placenta previa with an abnormal ultrasound appearance, placenta previa with a history of 3 or more prior cesarean sections, history of a classic cesarean section and anterior placentation, pregnancy with a history of endometrial ablation, or pelvic irradiation.[45] Improvement in maternal morbidity has been demonstrated when women are delivered in tertiary care hospitals with multidisciplinary teams experienced in the management of PAS.[19,46]

PAS is a potentially life-threatening condition due to the risk of massive hemorrhage. Massive hemorrhage may lead to disseminated intravascular coagulation, adult respiratory distress syndrome, transfusion-related acute lung injury, renal failure, and even death. Therefore, when PAS is diagnosed or suspected in the previable period, women should be counseled regarding the option of pregnancy termination. However, no data exists regarding the magnitude of risk reduction with pregnancy termination in cases of PAS because termination itself carries substantial risk for women with PAS. Blood transfusion is the most common morbidity associated with PAS followed by bladder injury.[47] Injury to ureters, genitourinary fistulas, bowel injury, thrombosis, postoperative infections, hemorrhagic shock, and renal failure occur in less than 2% of patients.[47] The level of maternal morbidity associated with PAS is related to the depth of placental invasion. There is an 86% risk of composite maternal morbidity in patients with placenta percreta versus 27% risk in patients with placenta accreta.[48] This is likely due to placental invasion of extrauterine anatomic structures such as pelvic vasculature. Placenta percreta can also predispose to uterine rupture due to invasion through a previous uterine scar, an event that may be catastrophic to the patient.

Timing of delivery in patients with PAS needs to consider both maternal and fetal risks versus benefits. Cesarean hysterectomy before the onset of labor has been shown to improve maternal outcomes.[49] The Society for Maternal Fetal Medicine recommends delivery between 34 and 35 + 6 weeks gestational age because more than half of patients with PAS will experience vaginal bleeding beyond 36 weeks of gestation.[44] Earlier delivery is indicated in patients with persistent vaginal bleeding, severe preeclampsia, onset of labor, preterm premature rupture of membranes, or evidence of fetal compromise. Patients with PAS should receive antenatal corticosteroids for fetal lung maturation before delivery, consistent with current gestational age-based recommendations.[50] Avoidance of pelvic examinations is recommended as well as avoiding vigorous physical activity. Consider hospitalization if vaginal bleeding or contractions occur or if the patient is in the third trimester and lives remote from a center of excellence for management of PAS. Small for gestational age infants and preterm birth are more common in pregnancies complicated by PAS.[28] However, neonatal outcome seems to be related to the gestational age at delivery as opposed to the depth of placental invasion.[51]

It is essential that patients with PAS deliver at hospitals with blood banks capable of using massive transfusion protocols. The mean blood loss at the time of cesarean hysterectomy for PAS is 3000 to 5000 cc. Therefore, notification and collaboration with your blood bank is recommended due to the frequent need for massive transfusion in cases of PAS. We recommend crossmatching 4 to 6 units of packed red blood cells upon the patient's admission for delivery and ensuring adequate availability of fresh frozen plasma (FFP), cryoprecipitate, and platelets before the procedure. Optimization of the patient's hemoglobin before delivery is essential. In patients with iron deficiency anemia, every effort should be made to adequately treat it before delivery. This may include oral iron replacement, intravenous infusions and, occasionally the use of erythropoietin stimulating agents.[44]

Intraoperative Management of Placenta Accreta Spectrum

Before proceeding with surgical management of PAS, it is important to have adequate IV access with a minimum of 2 large bore IV cannulas. An arterial line may be also useful for invasive blood pressure monitoring intraoperatively. Pneumatic compression devices should be used intraoperatively because hemorrhage, blood transfusion, and prolonged surgery are all risk factors for deep venous thrombosis. General anesthesia is most commonly used but regional anesthesia is also reasonable.[52] Placement of a 3-way foley is useful if the urinary tract needs to be assessed intraoperatively. We do not recommend the routine use of cystoscopy for all PAS patients. However, cystoscopy is useful to discern anatomy if bladder involvement is suspected. In these cases, we recommend collaboration with urology or gynecology oncology. The placement of preoperative ureteral stents is often performed in cases of PAS with bladder involvement, but their value remains unclear.[53]

The use of prophylactic endovascular interventions in PAS such as placement of bilateral balloon catheters in the iliac arteries, uterine artery embolization or a combination of the 2 in an attempt to reduce blood loss remains controversial.[54,55] It is not currently possible to predict which patients may benefit from endovascular interventions.[56] Some case series have demonstrated decreased blood loss with iliac artery occlusion whereas others have not.[54,57-59] A meta-analysis examining the use of endovascular interventional radiology interventions in more than 950 patients with PAS demonstrated reduced blood loss (mean difference -1.02 L, 95% CI, -1.6 to -0.43 L), but this did not translate into a statistically significant decrease in transfusion of blood products and 5% of patients were noted to have a procedure-related complication.[60] Groin and retroperitoneal hematomas are the most common associated complications but rare events such as thrombotic or embolic complications have been reported.[59] In the event an endovascular intervention is planned, delivery should occur on a fluoroscopy table so that the procedure can occur immediately after delivery of the fetus.

There is a lack of comparative data regarding the optimal skin incision for patients with PAS. Many providers will use a vertical incision for access and visualization, but transverse incisions such as a Maylard or Cherney incision is also a reasonable option. Ultrasound mapping of the placental site pre/intraoperatively may be useful to aid uterine incision planning in order to avoid disruption of the placenta and hemorrhage at the time of delivery of the fetus. Efforts to avoid the placenta may require a nontraditional uterine incision.[44] Following clamping and cutting of the umbilical cord, we recommend tying off the umbilical cord and closing the uterine incision in a timely manner to aid hemostasis before proceeding to complete the cesarean hysterectomy with the placenta in situ. Avoidance of forced placental removal is essential because profuse hemorrhage often occurs.[53, 21] If there is uncertainty regarding the diagnosis of PAS, a period of observation for spontaneous placental separation is appropriate in the presence of hemodynamic stability. Prophylactic oxytocin should not be used after delivery of the neonate as partial placental separation and profuse bleeding may occur.[56] Tranexamic acid is an antifibrinolytic drug that has been shown to reduce maternal mortality in cases of postpartum hemorrhage and to decrease bleeding when used prophylactically at the time of cesarean delivery.[61,62] No randomized control trials to data have examined the use of tranexamic acid in the management of PAS. However, we believe it is reasonable to use 1g of tranexamic after cord clamping based on current data and the major risk for hemorrhage in PAS. In general, a total hysterectomy is recommended because lower uterine segment or cervical bleeding frequently precludes a supracervical hysterectomy.[63] Intraoperatively, the use of autologous cell-saver technology is an option. Current filtering technologies have reduced theoretic concerns regarding the risk of contamination with fetal blood and other debris.[64–66]

During cesarean hysterectomy for PAS, close monitoring of volume status, maternal electrolytes, especially potassium, urine output, ongoing blood loss, and overall hemodynamics is essential. Patients should be kept warm because many clotting factors function poorly if the body temperature is less than 36° Celsius. In the event of hemorrhage with a blood loss of 1,500 cc or more, redosing of prophylactic antibiotics is recommended.[67] Initial intraoperative laboratories in the setting of hemorrhage should include hemoglobin, platelet count, prothrombin time, partial thromboplastin time, and fibrinogen levels. Although laboratory results can aid in transfusion management, it is vital to remember to treat the clinical scenario and not the laboratory results. Should massive transfusion be required, transfusion of packed red blood cells at a rate of 1:1 with FFP is recommended.

In the event there is unexpectedly a concern for PAS during a cesarean delivery based on the intraoperative appearance of the uterus, notification of the relevant multidisciplinary team members should occur before proceeding with delivery, if the patient is in a stable condition. This should include notifying anesthesiology about the possibility of requiring general anesthesia, notifying blood bank and crossmatching of 4 to 6 units of packed red blood cells, obtaining additional intravenous access, notifying critical care, and obtaining assistance from an expert pelvic surgeon when required. If concern for PAS arises during a case in a hospital without appropriate resources to optimize patient outcome, patient stabilization and transfer to an appropriate tertiary care facility is recommended. Similarly, if concern for PAS arises following delivery of a fetus at a cesarean section due to failure of separation of the placenta, rapid uterine closure and progression to hysterectomy should occur while the relevant multidisciplinary team is mobilized concurrently.

Postoperative Management of Placenta Accreta Spectrum

Following cesarean hysterectomy for PAS, intensive hemodynamic monitoring is required in the early postoperative period. A period of postoperative monitoring in the intensive care unit is often required because PAS patients are at significant risk of ongoing abdominopelvic bleeding, fluid overload from resuscitation, and multiorgan damage depending on the degree of blood loss. A low threshold for reoperation is recommended, postoperatively, if there is concern for ongoing bleeding. In the presence of intractable bleeding and suspected disseminated intravascular coagulation (DIC), blue-towel closure is recommended with packing of the abdomen and pressure closure of the skin with dressing with drains, followed by permanent fascial and skin closure in 24 to 48 hours. In the setting of massive hemorrhage, evaluation for Sheehan syndrome is also advised.

Alternative Management

Uterine preservation is usually defined as removal of placenta without removal of the uterus and expectant management is defined as leaving the placenta either partially or totally in situ.[6] The Society for Maternal Fetal Medicine recommends that the uterine preservation or expectant management only be considered in rare circumstances and should be on a case-by-case basis due to the life threatening nature of PAS because of hemorrhage.[6] In the presence of focal PAS, the removal of the placenta by manual extraction or by surgical excision of the adherent placenta and uterine tissue followed by repair of the resulting defect has been previously attempted as a method of conservative management.[68,69] Attempts at conservative management are with the goal of reducing the loss of future fertility, hemorrhage, and injury to other pelvic organs that may occur during cesarean hysterectomy.[68,70] Other authors have reported avoidance of hysterectomy in 84% of patients with PAS by the manual placental removal and Bakri balloon placement.[71] When considering conservative management, it is important to note that no randomized control trials exist for conservative management options in patients with PAS and that the conservative management does not allow confirmation of the diagnosis of PAS. Therefore, we cannot be certain of the diagnosis of PAS and thus the efficacy of conservative management options. Furthermore, a definitive decision preoperatively to proceed with cesarean hysterectomy has been associated with decreased blood loss and associated complications.[21,53]

Expectant management of PAS should be considered investigational because data are limited to small case series. In general, the umbilical cord is ligated near its insertion before closure of the uterus. Previous case series have demonstrated successful uterine preservation rates between 6% and 78%.[72–74] Most primary and delayed failures in the conservative management are due to increased bleeding necessitating hysterectomy. The largest case series demonstrated severe maternal morbidity and mortality rate of 6% with most cases because of sepsis in the delayed hysterectomy group.[72] It is also important to be aware that the risk of recurrent placenta accreta in women who undergo successful conservative management is high at 13.3% to 28.6%.[75–77] We believe that the conservative management of placenta accreta should only be undertaken in carefully selected patients with a small focal accreta after thorough counseling on the associated risks. Delayed interval hysterectomy for patients with placenta percreta with the goal of reducing blood loss and maternal morbidity has also been attempted with some promising results from small single center case series.[78] The largest case series included 13 patients and demonstrated a transfusion rate of 46% and average blood loss of 1600 cc (900 cc at time of cesarean delivery and 700 cc at time of hysterectomy).[79] Another potential advantage of delayed interval hysterectomy is that several patients in the series were able to undergo a minimally invasive hysterectomy. However, given the limited data, delayed interval hysterectomy remains investigational at this time and is not routinely recommended.

SUMMARY

PAS is a life-threatening condition due to hemorrhage. The incidence of PAS is rising due to the increased rates of cesarean deliveries. Identification of patients with PAS preoperatively is crucial to allow preoperative planning and coordination of multidisciplinary team care. Hysterectomy is the accepted management of PAS, and conservative or expectant management of PAS should be considered investigational. The optimal combination of medical, surgical, and imaging strategies for patients with PAS requires further investigation.

CLINICS CARE POINTS

Risk factors for PAS
- Placenta previa and prior cesarean section

- Advanced maternal age
- Multiparity
- Prior uterine surgery
- Prior uterine radiation
- Endometrial ablation
- Asherman syndrome
- Leiomyomas
- Uterine anomalies
- Hypertensive disorders
- Smoking

Sonographic markers of PAS
- Multiple vascular lacunae
- Loss of the hypoechoic retroplacental zone
- Abnormalities of the uterine serosa-bladder interface
- Retroplacental myometrial thickness less than 1 mm
- Increased placental vascularity
- Observation of bridging vessels linking the placenta and bladder

Complications of PAS
- Damage to local organs
- Postoperative bleeding
- Amniotic fluid embolism
- Consumptive coagulopathy
- Transfusion-related complications
- Acute respiratory distress syndrome
- Postoperative thromboembolism
- Infectious morbidities
- Multisystem organ failure
- Maternal death

DISCLOSURE

The authors report no conflicts of interest to disclose.

REFERENCES

1. Jauniaux E, Bunce C, Gronbeck L, et al. Prevalence and main outcomes of placenta accreta spectrum: a systematic review and meta-analysis. Am J Obstet Gynecol 2019;221(3):208–18.
2. Gafvels ME, Coukos G, Sayegh R, et al. Regulated expression of the trophoblast alpha 2-macroglobulin receptor/low density lipoprotein receptor-related protein. Differentiation and cAMP modulate protein and mRNA levels. J Biol Chem 1992;267(29):21230–4.
3. Tantbirojn P, Crum CP, Parast MM. Pathophysiology of placenta creta: the role of decidua and extravillous trophoblast. Placenta 2008;29(7):639–45.
4. Wehrum MJ, Buhimschi IA, Salafia C, et al. Accreta complicating complete placenta previa is characterized by reduced systemic levels of vascular endothelial growth factor and by epithelial-to-mesenchymal transition of the invasive trophoblast. Am J Obstet Gynecol 2011;204(5):411 e411.
5. Shellhaas CS, Gilbert S, Landon MB, et al. The frequency and complication rates of hysterectomy accompanying cesarean delivery. Obstet Gynecol 2009;114(2 Pt 1):224–9.
6. Publications Committee SfM-FM, Belfort MA. Placenta accreta. Am J Obstet Gynecol 2010;203(5):430–9.

7. Miller DA, Chollet JA, Goodwin TM. Clinical risk factors for placenta previa-placenta accreta. Am J Obstet Gynecol 1997;177(1):210–4.

8. Hull AD, Resnik R. Placenta accreta and postpartum hemorrhage. Clin Obstet Gynecol 2010;53(1):228–36.

9. Jauniaux E, Chantraine F, Silver RM, et al. Diagnosis FPA, Management Expert Consensus P. FIGO consensus guidelines on placenta accreta spectrum disorders: Epidemiology. Int J Gynaecol Obstet 2018;140(3):265–73.

10. Silver RM, Landon MB, Rouse DJ, et al. Maternal morbidity associated with multiple repeat cesarean deliveries. Obstet Gynecol 2006;107(6):1226–32.

11. Marshall NE, Fu R, Guise JM. Impact of multiple cesarean deliveries on maternal morbidity: a systematic review. Am J Obstet Gynecol 2011;205(3):262 e261–268.

12. Pekar-Zlotin M, Melcer Y, Levinsohn-Tavor O, et al. Cesarean Scar Pregnancy and Morbidly Adherent Placenta: Different or Similar? Isr Med Assoc J 2017;19(3):168–71.

13. Timor-Tritsch IE, Monteagudo A, Cali G, et al. Cesarean scar pregnancy and early placenta accreta share common histology. Ultrasound Obstet Gynecol 2014;43(4):383–95.

14. Timor-Tritsch IE, Monteagudo A, Cali G, et al. Cesarean scar pregnancy is a precursor of morbidly adherent placenta. Ultrasound Obstet Gynecol 2014;44(3):346–53.

15. Buca D, Liberati M, Cali G, et al. Influence of prenatal diagnosis of abnormally invasive placenta on maternal outcome: systematic review and meta-analysis. Ultrasound Obstet Gynecol 2018;52(3):304–9.

16. D'Antonio F, Iacovella C, Bhide A. Prenatal identification of invasive placentation using ultrasound: systematic review and meta-analysis. Ultrasound Obstet Gynecol 2013;42(5):509–17.

17. Jauniaux E, Collins S, Burton GJ. Placenta accreta spectrum: pathophysiology and evidence-based anatomy for prenatal ultrasound imaging. Am J Obstet Gynecol 2018;218(1):75–87.

18. Bowman ZS, Eller AG, Kennedy AM, et al. Interobserver variability of sonography for prediction of placenta accreta. J Ultrasound Med 2014;33(12):2153–8.

19. Eller AG, Bennett MA, Sharshiner M, et al. Maternal morbidity in cases of placenta accreta managed by a multidisciplinary care team compared with standard obstetric care. Obstet Gynecol 2011;117(2 Pt 1):331–7.

20. Shamshirsaz AA, Fox KA, Salmanian B, et al. Maternal morbidity in patients with morbidly adherent placenta treated with and without a standardized multidisciplinary approach. Am J Obstet Gynecol 2015;212(2):218 e211–219.

21. Warshak CR, Ramos GA, Eskander R, et al. Effect of predelivery diagnosis in 99 consecutive cases of placenta accreta. Obstet Gynecol 2010;115(1):65–9.

22. Abinader RR, Macdisi N, El Moudden I, Abuhamad A. First-trimester ultrasound diagnostic features of placenta accreta spectrum in low-implantation pregnancies. Ultrasound Obstet Gynecol 2021. https://doi.org/10.1002/uog.24828. Epub ahead of print.

23. Ballas J, Pretorius D, Hull AD, et al. Identifying sonographic markers for placenta accreta in the first trimester. J Ultrasound Med 2012;31(11):1835–41.

24. Comstock CH, Lee W, Vettraino IM, et al. The early sonographic appearance of placenta accreta. J Ultrasound Med 2003;22(1):19–23.

25. Comstock CH, Bronsteen RA. The antenatal diagnosis of placenta accreta. BJOG 2014;121(2):171–81.

26. Comstock CH, Love JJ Jr, Bronsteen RA, et al. Sonographic detection of placenta accreta in the second and third trimesters of pregnancy. Am J Obstet Gynecol 2004;190(4):1135–40.

27. Wong HS, Cheung YK, Zuccollo J, et al. Evaluation of sonographic diagnostic criteria for placenta accreta. J Clin Ultrasound 2008;36(9):551–9.

28. Gielchinsky Y, Mankuta D, Rojansky N, et al. Perinatal outcome of pregnancies complicated by placenta accreta. Obstet Gynecol 2004;104(3):527–30.

29. Hudon L, Belfort MA, Broome DR. Diagnosis and management of placenta percreta: a review. Obstet Gynecol Surv 1998;53(8):509–17.

30. Cali G, Giambanco L, Puccio G, et al. Morbidly adherent placenta: evaluation of ultrasound diagnostic criteria and differentiation of placenta accreta from percreta. Ultrasound Obstet Gynecol 2013;41(4):406–12.

31. Warshak CR, Eskander R, Hull AD, et al. Accuracy of ultrasonography and magnetic resonance imaging in the diagnosis of placenta accreta. Obstet Gynecol 2006;108(3 Pt 1):573–81.

32. Twickler DM, Lucas MJ, Balis AB, et al. Color flow mapping for myometrial invasion in women with a prior cesarean delivery. J Matern Fetal Med 2000;9(6):330–5.

33. Wong HS, Cheung YK, Strand L, et al. Specific sonographic features of placenta accreta: tissue interface disruption on gray-scale imaging and evidence of vessels crossing interface- disruption sites on Doppler imaging. Ultrasound Obstet Gynecol 2007;29(2):239–40.

34. Rac MW, Dashe JS, Wells CE, et al. Ultrasound predictors of placental invasion: the Placenta Accreta Index. Am J Obstet Gynecol 2015;212(3):343 e341–347.

35. Comstock CH. Antenatal diagnosis of placenta accreta: a review. Ultrasound Obstet Gynecol 2005;26(1):89–96.

36. Chou MM, Ho ES, Lee YH. Prenatal diagnosis of placenta previa accreta by transabdominal color Doppler ultrasound. Ultrasound Obstet Gynecol 2000;15(1):28–35.

37. Shainker SA, Coleman B, Timor-Tritsch IE, et al. Special Report of the Society for Maternal-Fetal Medicine Placenta Accreta Spectrum Ultrasound Marker Task Force: Consensus on definition of markers and approach to the ultrasound examination in pregnancies at risk for placenta accreta spectrum. Am J Obstet Gynecol 2021;224(1):B2–14.

38. Baughman WC, Corteville JE, Shah RR. Placenta accreta: spectrum of US and MR imaging findings. Radiographics 2008;28(7):1905–16.

39. Dwyer BK, Belogolovkin V, Tran L, et al. Prenatal diagnosis of placenta accreta: sonography or magnetic resonance imaging? J Ultrasound Med 2008;27(9):1275–81.

40. Einerson BD, Rodriguez CE, Kennedy AM, et al. Magnetic resonance imaging is often misleading when used as an adjunct to ultrasound in the management of placenta accreta spectrum disorders. Am J Obstet Gynecol 2018;218(6):618 e611–7.

41. Maldjian C, Adam R, Pelosi M, et al. MRI appearance of placenta percreta and placenta accreta. Magn Reson Imaging 1999;17(7):965–71.

42. Zelop C, Nadel A, Frigoletto FD Jr, et al. Placenta accreta/percreta/increta: a cause of elevated maternal serum alpha-fetoprotein. Obstet Gynecol 1992;80(4):693–4.

43. Kupferminc MJ, Tamura RK, Wigton TR, et al. Placenta accreta is associated with elevated maternal serum alpha-fetoprotein. Obstet Gynecol 1993;82(2):266–9.

44. Society of Gynecologic Oncology, American College of Obstetricians and Gynecologists and the Society for Maternal–Fetal Medicine, Cahill AG, et al. Placenta Accreta Spectrum. Am J Obstet Gynecol 2018;219(6):B2–16.
45. Silver RM, Fox KA, Barton JR, et al. Center of excellence for placenta accreta. Am J Obstet Gynecol 2015;212(5):561–8.
46. Esakoff TF, Sparks TN, Kaimal AJ, et al. Diagnosis and morbidity of placenta accreta. Ultrasound Obstet Gynecol 2011;37(3):324–7.
47. Morlando M, Schwickert A, Stefanovic V, et al. Maternal and neonatal outcomes in planned versus emergency cesarean delivery for placenta accreta spectrum: A multinational database study. Acta Obstet Gynecol Scand 2021;100(Suppl 1):41–9.
48. Marcellin L, Delorme P, Bonnet MP, et al. Placenta percreta is associated with more frequent severe maternal morbidity than placenta accreta. Am J Obstet Gynecol 2018;219(2):193 e191.
49. Silver RM, Barbour KD. Placenta accreta spectrum: accreta, increta, and percreta. Obstet Gynecol Clin North Am 2015;42(2):381–402.
50. Committee on Obstetric P. Committee Opinion No. 713: Antenatal Corticosteroid Therapy for Fetal Maturation. Obstet Gynecol 2017;130(2):e102–9.
51. Seet EL, Kay HH, Wu S, et al. Placenta accreta: depth of invasion and neonatal outcomes. J Matern Fetal Neonatal Med 2012;25(10):2042–5.
52. Lilker SJ, Meyer RA, Downey KN, et al. Anesthetic considerations for placenta accreta. Int J Obstet Anesth 2011;20(4):288–92.
53. Eller AG, Porter TF, Soisson P, et al. Optimal management strategies for placenta accreta. BJOG 2009;116(5):648–54.
54. Bodner LJ, Nosher JL, Gribbin C, et al. Balloon-assisted occlusion of the internal iliac arteries in patients with placenta accreta/percreta. Cardiovasc Intervent Radiol 2006;29(3):354–61.
55. Greenberg JI, Suliman A, Iranpour P, et al. Prophylactic balloon occlusion of the internal iliac arteries to treat abnormal placentation: a cautionary case. Am J Obstet Gynecol 2007;197(5):470 e471–474.
56. Collins SL, Alemdar B, van Beekhuizen HJ, et al. Evidence-based guidelines for the management of abnormally invasive placenta: recommendations from the International Society for Abnormally Invasive Placenta. Am J Obstet Gynecol 2019; 220(6):511–26.
57. Ballas J, Hull AD, Saenz C, et al. Preoperative intravascular balloon catheters and surgical outcomes in pregnancies complicated by placenta accreta: a management paradox. Am J Obstet Gynecol 2012;207(3):216 e211–215.
58. Cali G, Forlani F, Giambanco L, et al. Prophylactic use of intravascular balloon catheters in women with placenta accreta, increta and percreta. Eur J Obstet Gynecol Reprod Biol 2014;179:36–41.
59. Shrivastava V, Nageotte M, Major C, et al. Case-control comparison of cesarean hysterectomy with and without prophylactic placement of intravascular balloon catheters for placenta accreta. Am J Obstet Gynecol 2007;197(4):402 e401–405.
60. D'Antonio F, Iacovelli A, Liberati M, et al. Role of interventional radiology in pregnancy complicated by placenta accreta spectrum disorder: systematic review and meta-analysis. Ultrasound Obstet Gynecol 2019;53(6):743–51.
61. Collaborators WT. Effect of early tranexamic acid administration on mortality, hysterectomy, and other morbidities in women with post-partum haemorrhage (WOMAN): an international, randomised, double-blind, placebo-controlled trial. Lancet 2017;389(10084):2105–16.

62. Simonazzi G, Saccone G, Berghella V. Evidence on the use of tranexamic acid at cesarean delivery. Acta Obstet Gynecol Scand 2016;95(7):837.
63. Clark SL, Phelan JP, Yeh SY, et al. Hypogastric artery ligation for obstetric hemorrhage. Obstet Gynecol 1985;66(3):353–6.
64. Committee on Practice B-O. Practice Bulletin No. 183: Postpartum Hemorrhage. Obstet Gynecol 2017;130(4):e168–86.
65. Bernstein HH, Rosenblatt MA, Gettes M, et al. The ability of the Haemonetics 4 Cell Saver System to remove tissue factor from blood contaminated with amniotic fluid. Anesth Analg 1997;85(4):831–3.
66. Waters JH, Biscotti C, Potter PS, et al. Amniotic fluid removal during cell salvage in the cesarean section patient. Anesthesiology 2000;92(6):1531–6.
67. ACOG Practice Bulletin No. 120. Use of prophylactic antibiotics in labor and delivery. Obstet Gynecol 2011;117(6):1472–83.
68. Fox KA, Shamshirsaz AA, Carusi D, et al. Conservative management of morbidly adherent placenta: expert review. Am J Obstet Gynecol 2015;213(6):755–60.
69. Palacios Jaraquemada JM, Pesaresi M, Nassif JC, et al. Anterior placenta percreta: surgical approach, hemostasis and uterine repair. Acta Obstet Gynecol Scand 2004;83(8):738–44.
70. Perez-Delboy A, Wright JD. Surgical management of placenta accreta: to leave or remove the placenta? BJOG 2014;121(2):163–9.
71. Pala S, Atilgan R, Baspinar M, et al. Comparison of results of Bakri balloon tamponade and caesarean hysterectomy in management of placenta accreta and increta: a retrospective study. J Obstet Gynaecol 2018;38(2):194–9.
72. Sentilhes L, Ambroselli C, Kayem G, et al. Maternal outcome after conservative treatment of placenta accreta. Obstet Gynecol 2010;115(3):526–34.
73. Agostini A, Vejux N, Bretelle F, et al. Value of laparoscopic assistance for vaginal hysterectomy with prophylactic bilateral oophorectomy. Am J Obstet Gynecol 2006;194(2):351–4.
74. Kayem G, Davy C, Goffinet F, et al. Conservative versus extirpative management in cases of placenta accreta. Obstet Gynecol 2004;104(3):531–6.
75. Eshkoli T, Weintraub AY, Sergienko R, et al. Placenta accreta: risk factors, perinatal outcomes, and consequences for subsequent births. Am J Obstet Gynecol 2013;208(3):219 e211–217.
76. Sentilhes L, Kayem G, Ambroselli C, et al. Fertility and pregnancy outcomes following conservative treatment for placenta accreta. Hum Reprod 2010; 25(11):2803–10.
77. Kabiri D, Hants Y, Shanwetter N, et al. Outcomes of subsequent pregnancies after conservative treatment for placenta accreta. Int J Gynaecol Obstet 2014; 127(2):206–10.
78. Lee PS, Kempner S, Miller M, et al. Multidisciplinary approach to manage antenatally suspected placenta percreta: updated algorithm and patient outcomes. Gynecol Oncol Res Pract 2017;4:11.
79. Clausen C, Lonn L, Langhoff-Roos J. Management of placenta percreta: a review of published cases. Acta Obstet Gynecol Scand 2014;93(2):138–43.

Pulmonary Embolism and Amniotic Fluid Embolism

Ashley S. Coggins, MD[a],*, Erin Gomez, MD[b], Jeanne S. Sheffield, MD[a]

KEYWORDS

- Pulmonary embolism • Amniotic fluid embolism • Deep vein thrombosis
- Venous thromboembolism • Disseminated intravascular coagulopathy • Pregnancy
- Anticoagulation • Diagnostic imaging

KEY POINTS

- VTE incidence approximately 1 to 2 per 1000 births; 20% are PE.
- Pregnancy predisposes VTE formation.
- No best diagnostic algorithm for PE.
- Anticoagulation is mainstay of treatment of PE.
- Prompt management of AFE improves outcomes.

INTRODUCTION

Venous thromboembolism (VTE) as well as other embolic events including amniotic fluid embolism (AFE) remain a leading cause of maternal death in the United States and worldwide.[1] The pregnant patient is at a higher risk of developing VTE including pulmonary embolism (PE). In contrast, AFE is a rare, but catastrophic event that remains incompletely understood. Here the authors review the cause of VTE in pregnancy and look at contemporary and evidence-based practices for the evaluation, diagnosis, and management in pregnancy. Then the cause and diagnostic difficulty of AFE as well as what is known regarding the pathogenesis are reviewed.

PULMONARY EMBOLISM
Background and Prevalence

VTE is a term referring to both PE and deep vein thrombosis (DVT). Normal physiologic changes in the pregnant patient predispose these individuals to blood clot formation and the development of VTE. Pregnant patients are at 4-fold increased risk of

ᵃ Division of Maternal-Fetal Medicine, Department of Gynecology and Obstetrics, Johns Hopkins University School of Medicine, 600 North Wolfe Street, Phipps 228, Baltimore, MD 21287-4922, USA; ᵇ Diagnostic Imaging Division, Diagnostic Radiology Residency, JHU SOM Diagnostic Radiology Elective, Department of Radiology, Johns Hopkins Hospital, Baltimore, 600 N. Wolfe St. Nelson MRI Building #143 Baltimore, MD 21287, USA
* Corresponding author.
E-mail address: acoggin1@jhmi.edu

Obstet Gynecol Clin N Am 49 (2022) 439–460
https://doi.org/10.1016/j.ogc.2022.02.015
0889-8545/22/Published by Elsevier Inc.

developing VTE than their nonpregnant counterparts with the highest risk time frame occurring in the first few weeks postpartum.[2] The overall incidence of VTE in pregnancy is estimated to be between 0.5 and 1.9 per 1000 births.[2–4] DVT accounts for 80% of VTEs in pregnancy, and the remainder are caused by PE (20%).[5] Overall mortality from VTE is low at 1.1 per 100,000 deliveries; however, when stratified, mortality from PE is estimated to be as high as 2.4%.[3]

Pathophysiology

The central premise of VTE formation is the Virchow triad, which includes venous stasis, vascular injury, and hypercoagulable state. Vascular injury can occur during the course of normal labor and delivery as well as at the time of cesarean delivery. In addition, there are multiple physical, hormonal, and chemical changes that occur in pregnancy that increase the risk of VTE. Venous stasis in the lower extremities progressively increases until term and continues for 6 weeks postpartum. This effect is due to mechanical compression of the inferior vena cava by the gravid uterus as well as due to hormonal influences. Estrogen affects the nitric oxide pathway resulting in dilation and increased capacity in the deep venous system of the lower extremities. Altogether, venous flow in the lower extremities is decreased by approximately 50%. Owing to the anatomic orientation and crossover of the iliac veins, most DVTs in pregnancy will be left sided.[6]

The pregnant state is associated with multiple changes in coagulation factors that result in increased clotting potential, and decreased anticoagulation potential. The pregnant state is also associated with decreased fibrinolysis and increased rates of VTE.[6]

Changes associated with pregnancy:
- Doubling of fibrinogen levels
- Progressively increasing levels of factors VII, VIII, IX, X, and XII
- Increased von Willebrand factor level
- Decreased levels of factors XIII and XI and protein S
- Increased resistance to activated protein C
- Prothrombin and factor V Leiden levels remain unchanged

Risk Factors

A personal history of prior VTE confers the highest risk of recurrent VTE in pregnancy. In fact, 15% to 25% of all VTE that occur in pregnancy are recurrent events.[5] However, the absolute risk of recurrence depends greatly on the nature of the first event and if it was provoked or nonprovoked. Up to 40% of cases of VTE in pregnancy will be found to have an inherited thrombophilia.[7] The most common thrombophilia diagnoses in the obstetric population include factor V Leiden (FVL) mutation, prothrombin gene mutation, antithrombin deficiency, protein C deficiency, and protein S deficiency.[7]

The most common inherited thrombophilia is FVL, and mutations in this gene account for a large proportion of VTE seen in pregnancy (approximately 40%).[6,8] The risk of patients developing VTE in pregnancy with known mutations in the FVL gene depends on zygosity and personal or family history of VTE. For example, heterozygous patients with no personal or family history of VTE have approximately 1% risk of VTE in pregnancy compared with 10% if such a history is present.[6,9] Homozygous FVL mutation without history of VTE confers a 1% to 2% risk of VTE in pregnancy versus those with history of VTE being greater than 10%.

Mutations in the prothrombin gene enhance transcription and cause increased levels of prothrombin accounting for 17% of VTE in pregnancy. Similar to FVL, mutations in the prothrombin gene also depend on zygosity and personal history for their clinical impact. In a heterozygous patient with no personal or family history of VTE, the pregnancy risk for VTE is less than 1% versus 10% if such a history is present. Homozygous patients with no history of VTE have approximately 3% risk of VTE in pregnancy versus greater than 15% likelihood of VTE in pregnancy if history is present.[6]

Antithrombin mutations are the most thrombogenic form of inherited thrombophilia but are much less common, only accounting for approximately 1% of VTE in pregnancy. Without personal or family history of VTE, individuals with antithrombin deficiency are at 3% to 7% risk of developing VTE in pregnancy. When history is present, VTE risk increases as much as 10-fold.[6,8]

Protein C and protein S activities steadily decrease over the course of pregnancy until term. Thus, a diagnosis of protein C or S deficiency should ideally be made outside of pregnancy. Women with no personal or family history of VTE and protein C or S deficiency are at low risk of VTE in pregnancy (<1%). If protein activity levels are markedly low and there is a personal or family history of VTE, risk of VTE in pregnancy may be between 1% and 3%.[9]

Other medical risk factors include advanced maternal age, smoking, varicose veins, obesity, immobility, and any other medical conditions that increase the risk for VTE (diabetes, heart disease, sickle cell disease, systemic lupus erythematosus, inflammatory bowel disease, and so on.) Antiphospholipid antibody syndrome (APLS) is an autoimmune phenomenon predisposing individuals to thromboembolism and obstetric complications. Both DVT and PE can manifest in the setting of APLS with a 5% to 12% risk of VTE during pregnancy.[10] Anticoagulation is recommended in these patients for the duration of pregnancy and the postpartum period.[6]

Maternal age has been associated with increased risk of VTE with a 38% increase for women older than 35 years compared with those younger than 35 years; this may be due to the presence of other comorbidities more likely to be present in older patients such as cardiac disease, diabetes, and hypertension.[3] Smoking is notably a modifiable risk factor with patients who have ever smoked showing a 2.6-fold increase in postpartum VTE rates over their have-never-smoked counterparts.[11] There have been conflicting data regarding a history of superficial vein thrombosis as an independent risk factor with some studies showing no significance and some showing definite significance.[11]

Obstetric risk factors include multiple gestations,[7] in vitro fertilization and ovarian hyperstimulation syndrome, nephrotic syndrome, antepartum or postpartum hemorrhage, postpartum infection, preeclampsia, and placental previa.[3] Cesarean delivery is an independent risk factor showing not only increased percentage of VTEs than vaginal deliveries by approximately 2-fold but also possibly increased mortality from PE when they occur postpartum.[3,12]

Presentation and Initial Evaluation

Pregnant patients with PE have a clinically similar presentation as their nonpregnant counterparts overall. However, symptoms of PE in pregnant patients may be more nonspecific and a high index of suspicion is required. In one study looking at maternal deaths due to PE, 34.7% of women presented with shortness of breath, tachycardia was present in 30.4%, leg pain or weakness was present in 19.6%, and chest pain in only 13%. At least 2 symptoms were reported by 21.7% of patients in the days leading up to their death.[13] Other presenting signs can include hemoptysis and decreased oxygen saturation.

Diagnosis of PE in the nonpregnant population relies on evaluations of pretest probability to guide imaging and intervention. Unfortunately, many of these pretest probability calculations remain unvalidated in the pregnant population. More recently, work has been done to improve the ability to clinically assess the likelihood of PE in the pregnant population. One such calculator is the pregnancy-adapted Geneva score (PAG score). A multicenter prospective study including 395 women with suspected PE was performed using the modified Geneva score, which excluded cancer and age greater than 65 years. In their analysis, the PAG score showed a high discriminative power to stratify patients between low, intermediate, and high risk for PE.[14] Scoring criteria and predictive values are detailed in **Tables 1** and **2**.

D-dimer evaluation is frequently used for VTE evaluation in nonpregnant individuals. In pregnancy, utility has been historically limited because pregnancy is known to have increased values for D-dimer even in the absence of VTE. Owing to its low specificity and sensitivity, D-dimer is not recommended by American College of Obstetricians and Gynecologists (ACOG) for use in evaluation of pregnant patients suspected to have VTE. More recent work has been done to evaluate the possible use of D-dimer in pregnant patients in efforts to avoid unnecessary imaging and radiation exposure to the mother and fetus. One study from the Netherlands developed the "YEARS" clinical decision tool using differential D-dimer cutoffs to reduce unnecessary computed tomographic (CT) pulmonary angiography (CTPA) studies. This study was performed in the nonpregnant population and showed a 14% decrease in CTPA examinations.[15] In a prospective study of pregnant women with suspected PE, a pregnancy-adapted YEARS algorithm was developed to guide management in 510 pregnant patients. The investigators found a 39% decrease in CTPA usage with no missed diagnoses of PE.[16] Overall, the pregnancy-adapted YEARS algorithm showed a greater reduction in chest

Table 1
The Geneva score and the pregnancy-adapted Geneva score for assessment of pretest clinical probability of pulmonary embolism in pregnant women

Geneva Score		Pregnancy-Adapted Geneva Score	
Item	Points	Item	Points
Age>65 y	+1	Age 40 y and older	+1
Active malignant condition	+2		
Surgery (under GA) or lower limb fracture in past month	+2	Surgery (under GA) or lower limb fracture in past month	+2
Previous DVT or PE	+3	Previous DVT or PE	+3
Unilateral lower limb pain	+3	Unilateral lower limb pain	+3
Hemoptysis	+2	Hemoptysis	+2
Pain on lower limb palpation and unilateral edema	+4	Pain on lower limb palpation and unilateral edema	+4
Heart rate 75–94	+3	Heart rate>110 bpm	+5
≥95	+5		
Maximal point number	22	Maximal point number	20
ROC curve AUC	0.684	ROC curve AUC	0.795
95% CI	0.563–0.805	95% CI	0.690–0.899

Abbreviations: AUC, area under the curve; CI, confidence interval; DVT, deep vein thrombosis; GA, general anesthesia; ROC, receiver operating characteristic.

From Robert-Ebadi H, Elias A, Sanchez O, et al. Assessing the clinical probability of pulmonary embolism during pregnancy: The Pregnancy-Adapted Geneva (PAG) score. J Thromb Haemost. 2021;19(12):3044-3050. https://doi.org/10.1111/jth.15521; with permission.

Table 2
Patients' distribution and corresponding prevalence of pulmonary embolism according to the pregnancy-adapted Geneva score

Points	Category	Distribution	Distribution %	Confirmed PE, n	Prevalence of PE, %	95% CI
0–1	Low	265/390	67.9%	6/265	2.3%	10%–4.9%
2–6	Intermediate	112/390	28.7%	13/112	11.6%	6.9%–18.9%
≥7	High	13/390	3.3%	8/13	61.5%	35.5%–82.2%

Abbreviation: CI, confidence interval.
From Robert-Ebadi H, Elias A, Sanchez O, et al. Assessing the clinical probability of pulmonary embolism during pregnancy: the pregnancy-adapted Geneva (PAG) score. J Thromb Haemost. 2021;19(12):3044-3050. https://doi.org/10.1111/jth.15521; with permission.

imaging than the PAG score with less utilization of lower extremity ultrasonography. The pregnancy-adapted YEARS algorithm, however, has been met with some controversy. When applied by an external facility, 5 of 12 women ultimately diagnosed with PE would have been missed using this algorithm.[17] Ultimately, research continues in the search for a universal pregnancy PE diagnostic calculator. This search is driven by a desire to avoid unnecessary radiation exposure in the pregnant population, which is usually encountered with traditional imaging options for PE including ventilation-perfusion $(\dot{V} - \dot{Q})$ and CT scans.

When a patient presents with symptoms of PE, a physical examination and a lower extremity compression ultrasonography should be performed. If evidence of DVT is present, empirical treatment of PE may be initiated. If the result of compression ultrasonography is negative or if there are no signs of DVT on examination, then the ACOG recommends initial evaluation for PE with a chest radiograph based on guidelines from the American Thoracic Society and the Society of Thoracic Radiology. If the results of radiography are normal, $\dot{V} - \dot{Q}$ scan or CTPA is indicated (**Fig. 1**).[5] $\dot{V} - \dot{Q}$ scan is preferred by some providers due to decreased radiology dosage to maternal breast tissue, but it is not known if a true association to increased breast cancer risk exists.[4,18] In addition, the fetal radiation dose for $\dot{V} - \dot{Q}$ scan is actually higher (0.019 rad) than that for CT (0.013 rad). CT angiography has also been shown to

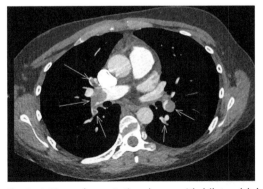

Fig. 1. Pregnant patient at 40 weeks gestational age with bilateral lobar, segmental and subsegmental PEs (arrows). Crescentic and circumferential contrast surrounding the clot as well as expansion of the vessels confirm acuity. (*Courtesy of* Erin Gomez, MD, Baltimore, MD.)

have increased sensitivity for inconclusive intermediate-probability $\dot{V} - \dot{Q}$ scan results.[19] Ultimately both $\dot{V} - \dot{Q}$ scan and CT angiography are considered safe in pregnancy[20] and could be used for PE evaluation based on individual facility capabilities. MRI has been suggested as an alternative imaging modality for PE in the setting of pregnancy, but is not in widespread use due to a relative contraindication to gadolinium-based contrast. Alternative, iron-based contrast agents are under investigation, but do not have long-term feasibility or safety data.[17]

Initial work should also include complete blood cell count, arterial or venous blood gas, and electrocardiography. Echocardiography, pro-bone natriuretic peptide (BNP), and cardiac enzymes should be obtained if initial imaging is concerning for massive PE or right heart strain.

Medical Management

The mainstay of medical management of PE in pregnancy is anticoagulation. In general, heparin compounds are preferred in pregnancy, including unfractionated heparin (UFH) and low-molecular-weight heparin (LMWH). As of yet, there is insufficient evidence to recommend direct oral anticoagulants due to lack of safety and efficacy studies in pregnant women.

In patients without a history of VTE, but who are at risk for VTE in pregnancy, the decision for prophylactic anticoagulation is not always straightforward. In many cases, when taking into account patient preference, thromboprophylaxis may be foregone in favor of vigilant monitoring.[5,9] The ACOG has published guidance for patient selection as well as medication dosing for thromboprophylaxis in pregnancy (**Tables 3** and **4**).

Most cases of new-onset PE in pregnancy can be managed as an outpatient with initiation of anticoagulation, most commonly with therapeutic enoxaparin at 1 mg/kg every 12 hours. Factors that should prompt inpatient management include large clot burden, medical instability, or concern for imminent delivery or need for thrombectomy or thrombolysis. UFH as a continuous infusion is more appropriate in these settings because it can quickly reach therapeutic levels, has a shorter half-life, and is reversible if needed.[7] Facility protocols for heparin infusion should be used until a therapeutic target activated partial thromboplastin time is reached (1.5–2.5 times control).[5]

In the outpatient setting, many providers transition patients who are on therapeutic or prophylactic LMWH to UFH in the third trimester to allow for epidural placement should they present in labor and to decrease the risk of bleeding. Alternatively, as recommended by the American Society of Hematology (ASH), women receiving therapeutic dosing of LMWH may be continued on their regimen through the third trimester with a scheduled delivery and time-appropriate discontinuation of LMWH before admission and epidural placement.[20] For prophylactic LMWH dosing, the ACOG recommends waiting 12 hours after the last dose before neuraxial blockade placement. For therapeutic dosing, the recommended wait time is 24 hours from the last dose (**Table 5**).[5] The decision for switching from LMWH to UFH or continuing on LMWH should be guided by patient preference and provider experience with appropriate counseling of risks. When therapeutic LMWH is used, the ASH recommends against surveillance with anti-factor Xa levels due to no difference in VTE events between monitored and unmonitored groups.[20]

Interventional Management

There are some situations in which anticoagulation alone will be insufficient management for a patient critically ill from VTE. According to the ASH guideline panel, thrombolytic therapy is suggested (in addition to UFH) in pregnant women with acute PE and life-

Table 3
Recommended pharmacologic thromboprophylaxis in pregnancy and the postpartum period

Clinical Scenario	Antepartum Management	Postpartum Management
No history of VTE, no thrombophilia	Surveillance[a] without anticoagulation therapy	Surveillance without anticoagulation therapy or postpartum prophylactic anticoagulation therapy if the patient has multiple risk factors[b]
VTE diagnosed during pregnancy	Adjusted-dose LMWH/UFH	Adjusted-dose LMWH/UFH for a minimum of 6 wk postpartum. Longer duration of therapy may be indicated depending on the timing of VTE during pregnancy, prior VTE history, or presence of a thrombophilia. Oral anticoagulants may be considered postpartum based on planned duration of therapy, lactation, and patient preference
Single provoked VTE (precipitated by a specific event such as surgery, trauma, or immobility) unrelated to estrogen or pregnancy due to a transient (resolved) risk factor, no thrombophilia	Surveillance[a] without anticoagulation therapy	Surveillance without anticoagulation therapy or postpartum prophylactic anticoagulation therapy if the patient has additional risk factors[b]
History of single unprovoked VTE (no identified precipitating factor present: includes prior VTE in pregnancy or associated with hormonal contraception), not on long-term anticoagulation	Prophylactic, intermediate dose, or adjusted-dose LMWH/UFH	Prophylactic, intermediate-dose, or adjusted-dose LMWH/UFH regimen for 6 wk postpartum
Low-risk thrombophilia[c] without previous VTE	Surveillance[a] without anticoagulation therapy	Surveillance without anticoagulation therapy or postpartum prophylactic anticoagulation therapy if the patient has additional risk factors[b]
Low-risk thrombophilia[c] with a family history (first-degree relative) of VTE	Surveillance[a] without anticoagulation therapy or prophylactic LMWH/UFH	Postpartum prophylactic anticoagulation therapy or intermediate-dose LMWH/UFH

(continued on next page)

Table 3
(continued)

Clinical Scenario	Antepartum Management	Postpartum Management
Low-risk thrombophilia[c] with a single previous episode of VTE: not receiving long-term anticoagulation therapy	Prophylactic or intermediate-dose LMWH/UFH	Postpartum prophylactic anticoagulation therapy or intermediate-dose LMWH/UFH
High-risk thrombophilia[d] without previous VTE	Prophylactic or intermediate-dose LMWH/UFH	Postpartum prophylactic anticoagulation therapy or intermediate-dose LMWH/UFH
High-risk thrombophilia[d] with a single previous episode of VTE or an affected first-degree relative: not receiving long-term anticoagulation therapy	Prophylactic, intermediate dose, or adjusted-dose LMWH/UFH	Postpartum prophylactic anticoagulation therapy or intermediate or adjusted-dose LMWH/UFH for 6 wk (therapy level should be equal to the selected antepartum treatment)
Two or more episodes of VTE: not receiving long-term anticoagulation therapy (regardless of thrombophilia)	Intermediate-dose or adjusted-dose LMWH/UFH	Postpartum anticoagulation therapy with intermediate-dose LMWH/UFH for 6 wk (therapy level should be equal to the selected antepartum treatment)
Two or more episodes of VTE: receiving long-term anticoagulation therapy (regardless of thrombophilia)	Adjusted-dose LMWH or UFH	Resumption of long-term anticoagulation therapy. Oral anticoagulants may be considered postpartum based on planned duration of therapy, lactation, and patient preference

[a] VTE risk assessment should be performed prepregnancy or early in pregnancy and repeated if complication develops, particularly those necessitating hospitalization or prolonged immobility.
[b] First-degree relative with a history of a thrombotic episode, or other major thrombotic risk factors (eg, obesity, prolonged, immobility, cesarean delivery).
[c] Low-risk thrombophilia: factor V Leiden heterozygote, prothrombin G20210 A mutation heterozygote, protein C or protein S deficiency, antiphospholipid antibody.
[d] High-risk thrombophilias include factor V Leiden homozygosity, prothrombin gene G20210 A mutation homozygosity, heterozygosity for factor V Leiden and prothrombin G20210 A mutation, or antithrombin deficiency.
Reprinted with permission from Thromboembolism in pregnancy. ACOG Practice Bulletin No. 196. American College of Obstetricians and Gynecologists. Obstet Gynecol 2018;132:e1–17.

threatening hemodynamic instability (systolic blood pressure <90 mm Hg) if bleeding risk is low. Evidence for thrombolysis use in pregnancy is limited to case reports at this time. In a review of the literature by Heavner and colleagues,[21] no maternal deaths were reported following thrombolytic used. Two cases of fetal death were noted and ultimately not attributed to thrombolytic usage. Catheter-directed thrombolysis may have advantages over systemic thrombolysis given the lower dosage used, but systemic thrombolysis is still preferred in patients without a high risk of bleeding.[21] Therapy

Table 4
Anticoagulation regimen definitions

Anticoagulation Regimen	Anticoagulation Dosage
Prophylactic LMWH[a]	Enoxaparin, 40 mg SC once daily Dalteparin, 5000 units SC once daily Tinzaparin, 4500 units SC once daily Nadroparin, 2850 units SC once daily
Intermediate-dose LMWH	Enoxaparin, 40 mg SC once daily Dalteparin, 5000 units SC once daily
Adjusted-dose (therapeutic) LMWH[b]	Enoxaparin, 1 mg/kg every 12 h Dalteparin, 200 units/kg once daily Tinzaparin, 175 units/kg once daily Dalteparin, 100 units/kg every 12 h Target an anti-Xa level in the therapeutic range of 0.6–1.0 U/mL 4 h after last injection for twice-daily regimen; slightly higher doses may be needed for a once-daily regimen
Prophylactic UFH	UFH, 5000–7,500 units SC every 12 h in first trimester UFH, 7500–10,000 units SC every 12 h in the second trimester UFH 10,000 units SC every 12 h in the third trimester, unless the aPTT is elevated
Adjusted-dose (therapeutic) UFH[b]	UFH 10,000 units or more SC every 12 h in doses adjusted to target aPTT in the therapeutic range (1.5–2.5 × control) 6 h after injection
Postpartum anticoagulation	Prophylactic, intermediate, or adjusted dose LMWH for 6–8 wk as indicated. Oral anticoagulants may be considered postpartum based on planned duration of therapy, lactation, and patient preference
Surveillance	Clinical vigilance and appropriate objective investigation of women with symptoms suspicious of deep vein thrombosis or pulmonary embolism. VTE risk assessment should be performed prepregnancy or early in pregnancy and repeated if complications develop, particularly those necessitating hospitalization or prolonged immobility

Abbreviations: aPTT, activated partial thromboplastin time; INR, international normalized ratio; SC, subcutaneously.
[a] Although at extremes of body weight, modification of dose may be required.
[b] Also referred to as weight adjusted, full treatment dose.
Reprinted with permission from Thromboembolism in pregnancy. ACOG Practice Bulletin No. 196. American College of Obstetricians and Gynecologists. Obstet Gynecol 2018;132:e1–17.

should not be delayed when indicated because prolonged maternal hypoxia can worsen pregnancy outcomes.

Surgical thrombectomy is an indicated therapy for massive PE in the nonpregnant population; however, it is associated with risk for maternal bleeding and fetal compromise in the pregnant patient. No randomized studies exist for its use in the setting of pregnancy. In their review of the literature, Martillotti and colleagues[22] reviewed 36 cases of patients with PE who underwent surgical thrombectomy. Diagnosis was before delivery in 21 cases. Seven of those cases underwent emergency cesarean

Table 5
Timing of neuraxial anesthesia in relation to pharmacologic anticoagulation

Dosage	Intrapartum, Elective Procedure	Intrapartum, Urgent/ Emergent Procedure	Postpartum
UFH prophylaxis (7500 units SC twice daily or 10,000 units SC twice daily)	Hold dose for 12 h and assess coagulation status before administering neuraxial anesthesia	Hold dose for 12 h and assess coagulation status before administering neuraxial anesthesia. However, in urgent cases with greater competing risks from general anesthesia placement of neuraxial anesthesia may be appropriate	Wait at least 1 h after neuraxial blockade and catheter removal before restarting heparin
UFH adjusted dose (>10,000 units per dose or > 20,000 units per day)	Hold dose for 24 h and access coagulation status before administering neuraxial anesthesia	If at least 24 h since last dose and aPTT within normal limits or undetectable anti-Xa, likely low risk for neuraxial blockade	Wait at least 1 h after neuraxial blockade or catheter removal before restarting heparin
Low-dose LMWH prophylaxis	Wait 12 h after last dose before neuraxial blockade	Insufficient data to make a recommendation for placement of neuraxial blockade <12 h from last dose of LMWH. In high-risk situations in which intervention is needed, risks of general anesthesia may outweigh risks of spinal epidural hematoma	Wait at least 12 h after neuraxial blockade and at least 4 h after catheter removal LMWH prophylaxis
LMWH intermediate-dose or adjusted-dose	Wait 12 h after last dose before neuraxial blockade	If <24 h, insufficient evidence to recommend proceeding with neuraxial blockade	Consider waiting at least 24 h after neuraxial blockade *and* at least 4 h after catheter removal to restart LMWH anticoagulation

Abbreviation: SC, subcutaneously.
Reprinted with permission from Thromboembolism in pregnancy. ACOG Practice Bulletin No. 196. American College of Obstetricians and Gynecologists. Obstet Gynecol 2018;132:e1–17.

delivery followed by thrombectomy. The remainder of the patients underwent thrombectomy as a primary intervention. Maternal survival for massive PE was 84%. Major bleeding was seen in 20% of cases. Fetal demise was attributable to the intervention in 20% of cases of women who underwent intervention while pregnant.[22]

Recently extracorporeal membrane oxygenation (ECMO) has also been suggested as a possible intervention for "lung rest" in massive PE. ECMO has limited data for use in pregnancy or for use in PE. The most common indications for ECMO during pregnancy are acute respiratory distress syndrome (49%), cardiac failure (18%), and cardiac arrest (15.9%). Maternal survival at 1 year after requiring ECMO is 74.3%, and the associated fetal survival is 64%.[23,24] The decision to proceed with ECMO should be multidisciplinary.

Complications

The mortality rate of acute PE that is promptly managed with anticoagulation is less than 10%. If patients present with hemodynamic instability, mortality rates increase to 50% or more.[6] A retrospective cohort study looked at rates of long-term complications including postthrombotic syndrome and chronic PE in the obstetric population. Postthrombotic syndrome is a condition affecting the lower extremities after a DVT that is composed of leg pain, edema, and superficial ulcers. Most patients presented with DVT (61.8%), followed by PE (25.8%). The remainder of patients presented with both DVT and PE. It was found that when compared with the general population, the risk of postthrombotic syndrome was lower (1.1% at 12 months), and the rates of chronic PE were similar (3.3% at 12 months) to the general population.[25]

Summary

Pregnancy and the associated physiologic changes predispose individuals to VTE while concurrently making it difficult to accurately diagnose when a VTE, particularly PE, is present. There is ongoing research to determine the best pregnancy-appropriate scoring system and treatment algorithms to optimize diagnostic sensitivity and patient outcomes while also minimizing unnecessary imaging and radiation to the maternal-fetal dyad. Heparin compounds are preferred for both prophylactic and therapeutic anticoagulation save for in the setting of mechanical heart valves when warfarin may be used with caution. Chemical thrombolysis or invasive thrombectomy are not well studied in pregnancy and are reserved for life-threatening clinical scenarios.

Care Points

- Pregnancy predisposes to PE formation
- Imaging including chest radiograph, V/Q perfusion scans, and CTPA may all be used in pregnancy
- No best diagnostic algorithm exits
- Anticoagulation is the mainstay of management and improves outcomes
- Interventional management and thrombolysis should be reserved for critically ill and unstable patients

AMNIOTIC FLUID EMBOLISM
Background and Prevalence

AFE is a rare but catastrophic event occurring during labor or immediately postpartum. Diagnostic criteria vary, but presentation typically includes shortness of breath, fetal distress, cardiorespiratory collapse, dissemination intravascular coagulation, altered mental status, and maternal death. Pathophysiology has historically been described to include fetal skin cells and other components in the maternal circulation leading to an anaphanaphylactoid reaction and maternal collapse. Studies are ongoing to attempt to further clarify the cause, pathogenesis, and risk factors of this, as of yet, incompletely understood syndrome.

AFE is one of the most catastrophic obstetric emergencies that providers encounter and has been described in the obstetric literature since it was first reported in a Brazilian journal in 1926.[26] Despite scientific and medical advances, this condition remains incompletely characterized with multiple different criteria being used for diagnosis and lack of a "gold-standard" laboratory or imaging modality for a definitive diagnosis.

AFE is a rare condition with incidence estimated to be approximately 1 in 40,000; however, this estimate is made difficult given variations in diagnostic criteria and reporting methods and likely underreporting of nonfatal cases.[27] One Canadian database study reviewing 120 confirmed AFE cases showed an incidence of 2.5 per 100,000.[28]

Maternal mortality is estimated to be high, although there is variation in reported rates of maternal death attributed to AFE. Original data reported from the US national registry examined 46 cases of AFE over 5 years with a mortality rate of 61% and a neurologically intact maternal survival rate of 15%.[29] As diagnostic criteria were redefined, these statistics were challenged after formation of the US international registry. Charts were submitted to this registry between August 2013 and September 2017 with 129 final charts being available for review. Of these, 27 cases were found to be misclassified as AFE when an alternative diagnosis was available. An additional 28 cases were deemed to be misclassified but with an unclear alternative diagnosis. Accounting for these cases, a much lower maternal mortality rate of 10% with a much higher neurologically intact survival of 46% was found.[30]

In the review of the older US national registry 30 years ago, fetal death rates were close to 60% with one-half of the survivors developing neurologic sequelae. On more recent evaluation of the new US international registry, only 3 neonatal deaths (5%) were seen in women with AFE suggesting that prompt diagnosis and delivery is a driving determinant of outcome.[30]

Pathophysiology

The pathophysiology of AFE is incompletely understood and remains an area of interest for researchers across many specialties. Early studies describe the histologic presence of amniotic fluid components in lung tissue of obstetric patients with unexplained death.[31] The presence of fetal components in maternal circulation alone does not adequately explain the full scope of AFE because elements of amniotic fluid have also been isolated in the blood and sputum of pregnant women without clinical evidence of AFE.[32–34] The endocervix, lower uterine segment, endocervical veins, and placental attachment sites have all been implicated as entry sites for amniotic fluid components.[34–36] It is most likely an individual's response to the breach between the maternal-fetal barriers and the subsequent inflammatory response cascade that dictate severity of the AFE syndrome.[35]

In 1995 Clark[27] proposed to rename AFE as "anaphylactoid syndrome of pregnancy." A history of atopy or allergic reactions is present more commonly in patients with AFE than those without. In evaluation of the US registry, 66% of patients with AFE reported a history of atopy or latex, medication, or food allergy compared with 34% of the general obstetric population during the study period.[30] Allergic reaction and complement activation both point to an immune-mediated response in the pathophysiology of AFE. Anaphylaxis as a general term refers to both IgE-mediated immediate hypersensitivity reactions and non-IgE-mediated anaphylactoid reactions.[37] A typical anaphylactic reaction may ensue in response to mast cell and basophil release of mediators such as histamine, tryptase, and leukotrienes; this leads to bronchial smooth muscle contraction, systemic vasodilation, capillary leak, and edema.[37] However, mast cell mediation as the pathogenesis of AFE has conflicting data in the literature. In early studies, immunohistochemical staining in postmortem cases of AFE showed elevated numbers of mast cells in the pulmonary vasculature.[38] Subsequent studies further examined tryptase as a factor involved in anaphylaxis because it is specific to mast cells and has a longer half-life than histamine. In one study by Benson and colleagues,[39] several patients had negative tryptase results and no evidence of mast cell degranulation; however, C3 and C4 were decreased implicating the complement pathway in AFE pathogenesis. Foreign inflammatory molecules can be recognized by maternal antigen-presenting cells and subsequently activate the complement pathway leading to the decreased C3 and C4 seen in AFE and secondary inflammation.[37,38,40] The subsequent immune storm in sensitized individuals involves the cross-activation between immune cells, complement, and cytokines in an overlapping and interconnected fashion to lead to large-scale release of damaging mediators such as reactive oxygen species, leukotrienes, histamine, and so forth. This release results in the observed clinical symptoms including systemic hypotension, edema, cardiovascular collapse, and disseminated intravascular coagulation (DIC).[37]

In the past, DIC related to AFE was hypothesized to be due to procoagulants present in amniotic fluid. Amniotic fluid contains thromboplastin, urokinaselike plasminogen activator, thrombin-antithrombin complexes, and plasminogen activator inhibitor-1.[41] The presence of vasoactive substances such as platelet-activating factor in the placenta and amniotic fluid have been shown to cause increased vascular permeability, bronchoconstriction, platelet aggregation, recruitment of leukotrienes, cytokines, thromboxanes, and the cascade of prostaglandin production.[42] Both consumptive coagulopathy and hyperfibrinolysis have been demonstrated in AFE with new data suggesting that hyperfibrinolysis may be present very early on in the process followed by profound coagulopathy.[43–45] Tissue factor and activation of the extrinsic pathway mediated by factor VII has also been implicated as a mechanism of consumptive coagulopathy.[46]

Although both increased fibrinolysis and consumptive coagulopathy may be present during AFE, this does not explain bleeding associated with AFE. Tamura and colleagues[36] published a case report in which they performed Alcian blue (marker for AFE derived mucin) and zinc coproporphyrin (meconium marker) immunostaining. The investigators found significantly more emboli material burden in the uterus than the pulmonary vasculature; they also found diffuse tryptase immunostaining around activated mast cells in the uterus and cervix. The presence of mast cells was associated with stromal edema and myometrial swelling when compared with nonpregnant controls. However, they did not compare these to pregnant controls without AFE. Tryptase-positive cells were also found in the pulmonary vasculature, but in much lower proportion than those found in the uterus, which suggests focal tissue anaphylaxis. Staining for C5aR (marker for leukocytes and other inflammatory cells) was present in uterine stroma and associated with edematous myometrium, implicating complement activation and inflammation leading to uterine atony.[36] When studied in primates, AFE syndrome was unable to be reproduced with direct injection of amniotic fluid into the circulation, and no appropriate animal model currently exists.[47]

Overall, the pathophysiology of the various aspects of AFE remains incompletely characterized and continues to be an area of research interest.

Risk Factors

Early reports did not find any strong maternal demographic risk factors for AFE; however, more recently several associations have been found. Older maternal age, grand multiparity, multiple birth, polyhydramnios, hypertensive disorders (eclampsia, pre-eclampsia), placenta previa, and abruption were all significantly associated with AFE. In addition, obstetric complications including premature rupture of membranes, medical induction, fetal distress, cesarean delivery, operative vaginal delivery, uterine rupture, and cervical laceration have all been noted to increase the risk for AFE.[28] One international study has reported findings of increased postnatal AFE following cesarean delivery or operative vaginal delivery (adjusted odds ratio of 9.82 and 14.02, respectively). In this same study, increased risk of AFE was also seen in patients with multifetal gestation, polyhydramnios, placenta previa, abruption, and induction of labor.[48] In analysis of the more recent US international registry, 10% of women with AFE had placenta previa as a pregnancy complication as opposed to the population background of less than 1% at term. In vitro fertilization was found in 8% of cases.[30]

Presentation and Initial Evaluation

AFE should be suspected in any laboring or recently postpartum patient who presents with sudden-onset hypoxia and hypotension, particularly if rapidly followed by coagulopathy. Although AFEs typically occur peripartum, there are case reports of AFE following first- or second-trimester termination and amniocentesis.[49–51]

Historically, respiratory distress is described as the presenting symptom of AFE occurring before delivery. Of patients reviewed in the US national registry, the initial symptom was seizure or seizurelike activity in 30% of patients followed by dyspnea (27%), fetal bradycardia (17%), and hypotension (13%). It is important to point out that in AFE cases occurring postpartum, more than 50% of patients presented with postpartum hemorrhage secondary to coagulopathy.[29]

The diagnosis of AFE is difficult to make given historical variation in diagnostic criteria. Using the uniform diagnostic criteria for research reporting of AFE published in 2016 by Clark and colleagues,[52] AFE is now commonly characterized by:

1. Sudden cardiorespiratory collapse
   Or
   Both hypotension and respiratory compromise followed by
2. Documentation of overt DIC not caused by hemorrhage
3. Onset during labor or within 30 minutes of placental delivery
4. No fever during labor

Owing to the vast overlap of symptoms between AFE and other conditions, a large differential must be kept in mind during evaluation of a possible AFE (**Fig. 2**).

A clinical hallmark of AFE is profound cardiovascular change. Hypotension is present in 100% of patients with AFE according to the US national registry. Three phases of AFE syndrome have been described in the literature. In the early phase, transient pulmonary and systemic vasoconstriction can be seen within the first 30 minutes; this results in a $\dot{V} - \dot{Q}$ mismatch, hypoxemia, and right-sided heart failure. This is a time period of high mortality because myocardial injury may occur concurrently.[35] The second phase demonstrates marked impairment of left ventricular function, and it is during this time that pulmonary arterial pressures may return to normal with subsequent development of pulmonary edema. Further myocardial injury may involve coronary artery spasm and direct ischemia as well as intrapulmonary shunting and a respiratory distress syndrome-type lung injury. The final phase is hallmarked by fulminant heart failure, acute respiratory distress, and coagulopathy.[35,41] Echocardiographic findings at the time of AFE evaluation support the idea of myocardial injury and dysfunction with evidence of right-sided heart failure including

Pulmonary thromboembolism	Placental abruption
Transfusion reaction	Peripartum cardiomyopathy
Hemorrhage	Eclampsia
Air embolism	Myocardial infarction
Anaphylaxis	Septic shock
High spinal anesthesia	Uterine rupture

Fig. 2. Differential diagnosis for patients presenting with possible AFE.

a "D-shaped septum" and acute pulmonary hypertension and right systolic dysfunction.[53]

Respiratory findings including hypoxia, tachypnea, and respiratory distress can be caused by acute pulmonary vasoconstriction as well as ultimate left-sided heart failure, but this is likely to be multifactorial due to the underlying pathophysiology of AFE including mast cell activation and capillary leak. CTPA can be useful in ruling out non-AFE causes of dyspnea (**Fig. 3**).[41]

Profound hematologic dysfunction and coagulopathy is a hallmark of AFE. According to the US international registry, 83% to 100% of patients demonstrate clinical and laboratory findings consistent with DIC.[30] This finding of DIC is likely due to the maternal inflammatory reaction to amniotic fluid components and mediators, but the exact mechanism is still incompletely understood.

Neurologic symptoms including agitation, altered mental state, seizures, and encephalopathy are suspected to be secondary to hypoxia due to the underlying respiratory and cardiovascular collapse. Subsequent permanent neurologic injury is a risk factor with studies showing neurologic sequelae in approximately 60% to 80% of cases, which can be exacerbated with seizure activity.[30,54]

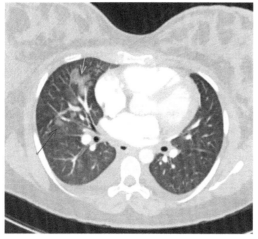

Fig. 3. Thirty-four-year-old patient developed shortness of breath following cesarean delivery. Confluent (*blue arrow*) and nodular (*red arrow*) ground-glass opacities suggest diagnosis of AFE. (*Courtesy of* Erin Gomez, MD, Baltimore, MD.)

Medical Management

As patients who develop AFE often rapidly progress to fulminant cardiopulmonary collapse, the mainstay of initial management is to provide prompt and high-quality cardiopulmonary resuscitation (CPR) in accordance with local advanced cardiac life support protocols. Eighty-seven percent of patients in the original national registry suffered from cardiac arrest, 40% of which occurred within 5 minutes of symptom onset.[29] In a patient with a palpable uterine fundus at the umbilicus, left lateral uterine displacement should also be used.[55] Intraosseous access may be required. If so, access should be placed in the humeral head as placement in the tibia may result in resuscitative products not reaching the central circulation in patients with pelvic bleeding.[56] If the patient is undelivered, delivery should be facilitated either by instrumented vaginal delivery if situationally amenable, or by perimortem cesarean delivery after 4 to 5 minutes of CPR efforts without return of spontaneous circulation.

In the acute phase of AFE, right-sided heart failure develops secondary to acute pulmonary hypertension. When the expertise is available, point-of-care transthoracic echocardiography can readily identify evolving right-sided heart dysfunction and allow for intervention.[53] Hypoxemia and hypercarbia should be actively avoided with proactive ventilator management to avoid further pulmonary constriction.[56] Vasopressors are preferred over aggressive fluid resuscitation for the management of systemic hypotension. Overaggressive fluid resuscitation causes increased right ventricular dilation, coronary compression, and compression of the left ventricle leading to decreased cardiac output. Inotropic agents such as milrinone or dobutamine can be used to improve right ventricular contractility as well as decrease pulmonary vascular resistance. Pharmacologic agents and their dosages used to treat right ventricular failure include[56]:

- Norepinephrine 0.05 to 3.3 µg/kg/min
- Dobutamine 2.5 to 5 µg/kg/min
- Milrinone 0.25 to 0.75 µg/kg/min
- Sildenafil 20 mg orally every 8 hours
- Inhaled nitric oxide 5 to 40 parts per million
- Inhaled prostacyclin 10 to 50 ng/kg/min
- Intravenous prostacyclin 1 to 2 ng/kg/min

Initial laboratory data should include complete blood cell count, arterial blood gas, electrolytes, coagulation profile, and a thromboelastogram if available. If cardiac ischemia or dysfunction is suspected, cardiac enzymes and an electrocardiography should be performed if the patient is not yet on telemetry monitoring. Management of the often-present profound coagulopathy is the next critical step in maternal management. Clotting status should be evaluated early and managed aggressively with standard massive transfusion protocols (MTP), using a 1:1:1 ratio of packed red blood cells, fresh frozen plasma (FFP), and platelets. Cryoprecipitate is favored over FFP if available to avoid worsening fluid overload.[46,56] There is an expanding role for viscoelastic tests such as thromboelastography (TEG) in guiding blood product resuscitation in AFE; this is based on studies of TEG in trauma settings, which demonstrated improved survival when used to guide MTP resuscitation.[57] Hyperfibrinolysis is common in DIC and not normally corrected with normal product resuscitation. However, by using TEG in AFE management, hyperfibrinolysis may be identified and lead to the administration of tranexamic acid thereby avoiding unnecessary volume overload.[56] Uterine atony leading to ongoing hemorrhage and worsening coagulopathy

This checklist is a sample only. Each facility should modify it to fit the facility-specific circumstances

Manage circulatory collapse
- ☐ ABCs: manage airway, breathing, and circulation
- ☐ Designate a timekeeper to call out times at 1-min intervals
- ☐ If no pulse, start CPR
  - ○ Manually displace uterus or lateral tilt
  - ○ Use backboard
- ☐ Consider move to operating room only if this can be accomplished in 2 min or less
- ☐ If no pulse at 4 min, START perimortem cesarean delivery (resuscitative hysterotomy)
  - ○ Splash prep only, do not wait for antibiotics
  - ○ Goal is to improve chances of resuscitation

Anticipate uterine atony, DIC, hemorrhage
- ☐ Oxytocin prophylaxis plus other uterotonics as needed
- ☐ Consider intraosseous line if needed for large-bore IV access
- ☐ Initiate massive transfusion protocol
  - ○ Cryoprecipitate preferred over FFP to reduce volume overload
- ☐ Consider thromboelastometry if available
- ☐ Tranexamic acid (1 g IV over 10 min) if DIC or hemorrhage occurs

Manage pulmonary hypertension and right ventricular failure
(Anesthesiology, Critical Care, or Cardiology)
- ☐ Consider echocardiography (thoracic or esophageal)
- ☐ Avoid fluid overload (eg, 500 mL boluses and reassess)
- ☐ Vasopressor if needed: norepinephrine 0.05–3.3 μg/kg/min
- ☐ Inotropes if needed:
  - ○ Dobutamine 2.5–5.0 μg/kg/min or
  - ○ Milrinone 0.25–0.75 μg/kg/min
- ☐ Pulmonary vasodilator if needed to unload right ventricle
  - ○ Inhaled nitric oxide 5–40 ppm or
  - ○ Inhaled epoprostanol 10–50 ng/kg/min) or
  - ○ IV epoprostanol 1–2 ng/kg/min (via central line) or
  - ○ Sildenafil 20 mg orally (if awake/alert)
- ☐ Consider ECMO if prolonged CPR or refractory right heart failure
- ☐ Wean FiO_2 to maintain O_2 saturation 94% to 98%

Postevent debrief (entire team)
- ☐ Identify opportunities for improvement including any need for revisions to checklist
- ☐ Discuss family and staff support needs
- ☐ Report case to Amniotic Fluid Embolism Registry

Fig. 4. Checklist for the initial management of AFE. FiO2, inhaled fraction of O2; IV, intravenous. (*From* Patient Safety and Quality Committee, Society for Maternal-Fetal Medicine. Electronic address: smfm@smfm.org, Combs CA, Montgomery DM, Toner LE, Dildy GA. Society for Maternal-Fetal Medicine Special Statement: checklist for initial management of amniotic fluid embolism. Am J Obstet Gynecol. 2021;224(4):B29-B32. https://doi.org/10.1016/j.ajog.2021.01.001; with permission.)

should be actively managed with standard obstetric interventions including uterotonics, balloon tamponade, and in refractory cases, uterine artery ligation and hysterectomy.

The Society for Maternal-Fetal Medicine published a checklist for the initial management of AFE that can be adapted to facility-specific circumstances[58] (**Fig. 4**). The use of a checklist for rare clinical emergencies has been shown to standardize practice and improve patient morbidity and mortality.

Interventional Treatment

ECMO is an invasive modality that has been used with success in cases of AFE with refractory low cardiac output and hypotension despite adequate volume resuscitation and inotropic agents. The use of ECMO and the concurrent requirement for aggressive anticoagulation during use complicates the applicability in the setting of AFE due to often-present coagulopathy. In addition, ECMO may not be available in all clinical settings where AFEs take place. Nevertheless, ECMO may be considered in facilities that have this capability.[59]

Continuous hemofiltration has also been suggested as a management strategy in an effort to remove chemical mediators and cytokines responsible for the widespread immunologic response. Case reports showed rapid recovery from shock shortly after initiating hemofiltration.[60–62] Hemofiltration as a mainstay of management for AFE, however, is still under investigation. High-dose corticosteroids have been suggested as a possible moderator of immune response, but effectiveness is controversial.[62]

Future Directions

No laboratory test or biomarker exists for the definitive diagnosis of AFE, and it remains a clinical diagnosis of exclusion. A recent case report from Japan noted successful use of C1 inhibitor concentrate (C1INH) when low levels of C3 and C4 were identified during an AFE.[63] The use of this intervention was based on previous work that showed a low activity of C1INH in AFE cases. As a known inhibitor of C1 esterase, factor XIIa and kallikrein C1INH was hypothesized to mitigate complement activation and to modulate fibrinolysis and the kallikrein-kinin systems.[64] The use of C1INH remains experimental.

Recurrence Risk

There are no good data for the risk of recurrence of AFE because the case is rare and associated with a high mortality rate. There are case reports of patients having uneventful subsequent pregnancies, but small sample size prevents the drawing of any reliable conclusions.[46]

SUMMARY

As stated best by the Society for Maternal-Fetal Medicine, AFE is best managed by a multidisciplinary team including anesthesia, respiratory therapy, critical care, and maternal-fetal medicine specialists.[46] High index of suspicion and prompt intervention with high-quality CPR, blood product resuscitation, and point of care echocardiography can guide management and improve outcomes. There is no gold-standard diagnostic test for AFE. Ongoing research and new developments hope to further clarify cause and pathogenesis because it yet remains unclear.

CLINICS CARE POINTS

- Immediate high-quality CPR and recruitment of multidisciplinary team
- Immediate delivery if patient is undelivered
- Prompt laboratory workup and management of DIC
- Aggressive blood product resuscitation (guided by TEG when available, following local MTP when TEG is not available)
- Avoiding fluid overload

- Management of uterine atony
- Point-of-care echocardiography to evaluate cardiac function and further guide pharmacotherapies
- Consideration for ECMO where available for refractory cases

DISCLOSURE

The authors have nothing to disclose.

REFERENCES

1. Collier AY, Molina RL. Maternal mortality in the United States: updates on trends, causes, and solutions. Neoreviews 2019;20(10):e561–74.
2. Heit JA, Kobbervig CE, James AH, et al. Trends in the incidence of venous thromboembolism during pregnancy or postpartum: a 30-year population-based study. Ann Intern Med 2005;143(10):697–706.
3. James AH, Jamison MG, Brancazio LR, et al. Venous thromboembolism during pregnancy and the postpartum period: incidence, risk factors, and mortality. Am J Obstet Gynecol 2006;194(5):1311–5.
4. Malhamé I, Tagalakis V, Dayan N. Diagnosing pulmonary embolism in pregnancy: synthesis of current guidelines and new evidence. J Obstet Gynaecol Can 2020; 42(12):1546–9.
5. ACOG Practice Bulletin No. 196: Thromboembolism in Pregnancy. Obstet Gynecol 2018;132(1):e1–17.
6. Silver R, Lockwood C. Thrombosis, thrombophilia, and thromboembolism. Am Coll Obstricians Gynecologists Clin Updates Women's Care 2016;15(3):5–17.
7. James AH. Venous thromboembolism in pregnancy. Arterioscler Thromb Vasc Biol 2009;29(3):326–31.
8. Franco RF, Reitsma PH. Genetic risk factors of venous thrombosis. Hum Genet 2001;109(4):369–84.
9. Skeith L. Preventing venous thromboembolism during pregnancy and postpartum: crossing the threshold. Hematology Am Soc Hematol Educ Program 2017;2017(1):160–7.
10. ACOG Practice Bulletin No. 118: antiphospholipid syndrome. Obstet Gynecol 2011;117(1):192–9.
11. Danilenko-Dixon DR, Heit JA, Silverstein MD, et al. Risk factors for deep vein thrombosis and pulmonary embolism during pregnancy or post partum: a population-based, case-control study. Am J Obstet Gynecol 2001;184(2):104–10.
12. Park JE, Park Y, Yuk JS. Incidence of and risk factors for thromboembolism during pregnancy and postpartum: a 10-year nationwide population-based study. Taiwan J Obstet Gynecol 2021;60(1):103–10.
13. Heyl PS, Sappenfield WM, Burch D, et al. Pregnancy-related deaths due to pulmonary embolism: findings from two state-based mortality reviews. Matern Child Health J 2013;17(7):1230–5.
14. Robert-Ebadi H, Elias A, Sanchez O, et al. Assessing the clinical probability of pulmonary embolism during pregnancy: the pregnancy-adapted geneva (PAG) score. J Thromb Haemost 2021;19(12):3044–50.
15. van der Hulle T, Cheung WY, Kooij S, et al. Simplified diagnostic management of suspected pulmonary embolism (the YEARS study): a prospective, multicentre, cohort study. Lancet 2017;390(10091):289–97.

16. van der Pol LM, Tromeur C, Bistervels IM, et al. Pregnancy-adapted YEARS algorithm for diagnosis of suspected pulmonary embolism. N Engl J Med 2019; 380(12):1139–49.

17. Goodacre S, Hunt BJ, Nelson-Piercy C. Diagnosis of suspected pulmonary embolism in pregnancy. N Engl J Med 2019;380(25):e49.

18. Cohen SL, Wang JJ, Chan N, et al. CT pulmonary angiography in pregnancy: Specific conversion factors to estimate effective radiation dose from dose length product: A retrospective cross-sectional study across a multi-hospital integrated healthcare network. Eur J Radiol 2021;143:109908.

19. Cueto SM, Cavanaugh SH, Benenson RS, et al. Computed tomography scan versus ventilation-perfusion lung scan in the detection of pulmonary embolism. J Emerg Med 2001;21(2):155–64.

20. Bates SM, Rajasekhar A, Middeldorp S, et al. American Society of Hematology 2018 guidelines for management of venous thromboembolism: venous thromboembolism in the context of pregnancy. Blood Adv 2018;2(22):3317–59.

21. Heavner MS, Zhang M, Bast CE, et al. Thrombolysis for Massive Pulmonary Embolism in Pregnancy. Pharmacotherapy 2017;37(11):1449–57.

22. Martillotti G, Boehlen F, Robert-Ebadi H, et al. Treatment options for severe pulmonary embolism during pregnancy and the postpartum period: a systematic review. J Thromb Haemost 2017;15(10):1942–50.

23. Naoum EE, Chalupka A, Haft J, et al. Extracorporeal life support in pregnancy: a systematic review. J Am Heart Assoc 2020;9(13):e016072.

24. Pacheco LD, Saade GR, Hankins GDV. Extracorporeal membrane oxygenation (ECMO) during pregnancy and postpartum. Semin Perinatol 2018;42(1):21–5.

25. O'Shaugnessy F, Govindappagari S, Huang Y, et al. Post-Thrombotic syndrome and chronic pulmonary embolism after obstetric venous thromboembolism. Am J Perinatol 2021;22. https://doi.org/10.1055/s-0041-1739471.

26. Meyer JR. Embolia pulmonar amniocaseosa. Brazil Med 1926;2:301–3.

27. Clark SL. Amniotic fluid embolism. Obstet Gynecol 2014;123(2 Pt 1):337–48.

28. Kramer MS, Rouleau J, Liu S, et al. Amniotic fluid embolism: incidence, risk factors, and impact on perinatal outcome. BJOG 2012;119(7):874–9.

29. Clark SL, Hankins GD, Dudley DA, et al. Amniotic fluid embolism: analysis of the national registry. Am J Obstet Gynecol 1995;172(4 Pt 1):1158–67 [discussion: 1167-9].

30. Stafford IA, Moaddab A, Dildy GA, et al. Amniotic fluid embolism syndrome: analysis of the Unites States International Registry. Am J Obstet Gynecol MFM 2020; 2(2):100083.

31. Steiner PE, Lushbaugh CC. Landmark article, Oct. 1941: Maternal pulmonary embolism by amniotic fluid as a cause of obstetric shock and unexpected deaths in obstetrics. In: By Paul E, Steiner and C, Lushbaugh C, editors. JAMA 1986; 255(16):2187–203.

32. Clark SL, Pavlova Z, Greenspoon J, et al. Squamous cells in the maternal pulmonary circulation. Am J Obstet Gynecol 1986;154(1):104–6.

33. Lee W, Ginsburg KA, Cotton DB, et al. Squamous and trophoblastic cells in the maternal pulmonary circulation identified by invasive hemodynamic monitoring during the peripartum period. Am J Obstet Gynecol 1986;155(5):999–1001.

34. Resnik R, Swartz WH, Plumer MH, et al. Amniotic fluid embolism with survival. Obstet Gynecol 1976;47(3):295–8.

35. Balinger KJ, Chu Lam MT, Hon HH, et al. Amniotic fluid embolism: despite progress, challenges remain. Curr Opin Obstet Gynecol 2015;27(6):398–405.

36. Tamura N, Nagai H, Maeda H, et al. Amniotic fluid embolism induces uterine anaphylaxis and atony following cervical laceration. Gynecol Obstet Invest 2014;78(1):65–8.
37. Yang RL, Lang MZ, Li H, et al. Immune storm and coagulation storm in the pathogenesis of amniotic fluid embolism. Eur Rev Med Pharmacol Sci 2021;25(4): 1796–803.
38. Fineschi V, Gambassi R, Gherardi M, et al. The diagnosis of amniotic fluid embolism: an immunohistochemical study for the quantification of pulmonary mast cell tryptase. Int J Legal Med 1998;111(5):238–43.
39. Benson MD, Kobayashi H, Silver RK, et al. Immunologic studies in presumed amniotic fluid embolism. Obstet Gynecol 2001;97(4):510–4.
40. Fineschi V, Riezzo I, Cantatore S, et al. Complement C3a expression and tryptase degranulation as promising histopathological tests for diagnosing fatal amniotic fluid embolism. Virchows Arch 2009;454(3):283–90.
41. Sultan P, Seligman K, Carvalho B. Amniotic fluid embolism: update and review. Curr Opin Anaesthesiol 2016;29(3):288–96.
42. Karetzky M, Ramirez M. Acute respiratory failure in pregnancy. An analysis of 19 cases. Medicine (Baltimore) 1998;77(1):41–9. https://doi.org/10.1097/00005792-.
43. Collins NF, Bloor M, McDonnell NJ. Hyperfibrinolysis diagnosed by rotational thromboelastometry in a case of suspected amniotic fluid embolism. Int J Obstet Anesth 2013;22(1):71–6.
44. Harnett MJ, Hepner DL, Datta S, et al. Effect of amniotic fluid on coagulation and platelet function in pregnancy: an evaluation using thromboelastography. Anaesthesia 2005;60(11):1068–72.
45. Fudaba M, Tachibana D, Misugi T, et al. Excessive fibrinolysis detected with thromboelastography in a case of amniotic fluid embolism: fibrinolysis may precede coagulopathy. J Thromb Thrombolysis 2021;51(3):818–20.
46. Society for Maternal-Fetal Medicine. Electronic address pso, Pacheco LD, Saade G, Hankins GD, Clark SL. Amniotic fluid embolism: diagnosis and management. Am J Obstet Gynecol 2016;215(2):B16–24.
47. Stolte L, van Kessel H, Seelen J, et al. Failure to produce the syndrome of amniotic fluid embolism by infusion of amniotic fluid and meconium into monkeys. Am J Obstet Gynecol 1967;98(5):694–7.
48. Fitzpatrick KE, van den Akker T, Bloemenkamp KWM, et al. Risk factors, management, and outcomes of amniotic fluid embolism: a multicountry, population-based cohort and nested case-control study. PLoS Med 2019;16(11):e1002962.
49. Kaaniche FM, Chaari A, Zekri M, et al. Amniotic fluid embolism complicating medical termination of pregnancy. Can J Anaesth 2016;63(7):871–4. https://doi.org/10.1007/s12630-016-0618-x. Embolie amniotique compliquant une interruption médicale de la grossesse.
50. Ray BK, Vallejo MC, Creinin MD, et al. Amniotic fluid embolism with second trimester pregnancy termination: a case report. Can J Anaesth 2004;51(2): 139–44.
51. Drukker L, Sela HY, Ioscovich A, et al. Amniotic fluid embolism: a rare complication of second-trimester amniocentesis. Fetal Diagn Ther 2017;42(1):77–80.
52. Clark SL, Romero R, Dildy GA, et al. Proposed diagnostic criteria for the case definition of amniotic fluid embolism in research studies. Am J Obstet Gynecol 2016;215(4):408–12.
53. Simard C, Yang S, Koolian M, et al. The role of echocardiography in amniotic fluid embolism: a case series and review of the literature. Can J Anaesth 2021;68(10): 1541–8. https://doi.org/10.1007/s12630-021-02065-4. Le rôle de

l'échocardiographie dans l'embolie de liquide amniotique : une série de cas et une revue de la littérature.

54. O'Shea A, Eappen S. Amniotic fluid embolism. *Int Anesthesiol Clin* Winter 2007; 45(1):17–28.

55. Jeejeebhoy FM, Zelop CM, Lipman S, et al. Cardiac arrest in pregnancy: a scientific statement from the american heart association. Circulation 2015;132(18): 1747–73.

56. Pacheco LD, Clark SL, Klassen M, et al. Amniotic fluid embolism: principles of early clinical management. Am J Obstet Gynecol 2020;222(1):48–52.

57. Gonzalez E, Moore EE, Moore HB, et al. Goal-directed hemostatic resuscitation of trauma-induced coagulopathy: a pragmatic randomized clinical trial comparing a viscoelastic assay to conventional coagulation assays. Ann Surg 2016;263(6): 1051–9.

58. Patient Safety, Quality Committee SfM-FMEasso, Combs CA, Montgomery DM, et al. Society for Maternal-Fetal Medicine Special Statement: Checklist for initial management of amniotic fluid embolism. Am J Obstet Gynecol 2021;224(4): B29–32.

59. Durgam S, Sharma M, Dadhwal R, et al. The role of extra corporeal membrane oxygenation in amniotic fluid embolism: a case report and literature review. Cureus 2021;13(2):e13566.

60. Ogihara T, Morimoto K, Kaneko Y. Continuous hemodiafiltration for potential amniotic fluid embolism: dramatic responses observed during a 10-year period report of three cases. Ther Apher Dial 2012;16(2):195–7.

61. Weksler N, Ovadia L, Stav A, et al. Continuous arteriovenous hemofiltration in the treatment of amniotic fluid embolism. Int J Obstet Anesth 1994;3(2):92–6.

62. Tamura N, Farhana M, Oda T, et al. Amniotic fluid embolism: pathophysiology from the perspective of pathology. J Obstet Gynaecol Res 2017;43(4):627–32.

63. Todo Y, Tamura N, Itoh H, et al. Therapeutic application of C1 esterase inhibitor concentrate for clinical amniotic fluid embolism: a case report. Clin Case Rep 2015;3(7):673–5.

64. Tamura N, Kimura S, Farhana M, et al. C1 esterase inhibitor activity in amniotic fluid embolism. Crit Care Med 2014;42(6):1392–6.

Septic Shock and Cardiac Arrest in Obstetrics
A Practical Simplified Clinical View

Luis D. Pacheco, MD[a,b,*], Megan C. Shepherd, MD[c],
George S. Saade, MD[c]

KEYWORDS

• Septic shock • Pregnancy • Cardiac arrest

KEY POINTS

- Septic shock is a medical emergency that requires immediate resuscitation with intravenous fluids.
- Initial care involves obtaining cultures and serum lactate levels together with broad-spectrum antibiotics and source control.
- Norepinephrine is the preferred vasopressor in pregnant patients with septic shock.
- Cardiac arrest management during pregnancy should follow established guidelines for nonpregnant individuals.
- Left lateral displacement of the uterus and early perimortem cesarean delivery are fundamental aspects when managing cardiac arrest in pregnancy.

INTRODUCTION

Septic shock and cardiac arrest during pregnancy, despite being uncommon, carry a high mortality rate among pregnant individuals. Unfortunately, most residency training programs worldwide provide minimal training in the initial management of these conditions. In this article, we present a simplified management strategy including initial key aspects in the management of septic shock and cardiac arrest in pregnant patients.

[a] Department of Obstetrics & Gynecology, Division of Maternal-Fetal Medicine, and Anesthesiology, The University of Texas Medical Branch at Galveston, 301 University Boulevard, Galveston, TX 77555-0587, USA; [b] Department of Obstetrics & Gynecology, Division of Surgical Critical Care, The University of Texas Medical Branch at Galveston, 301 University Boulevard, Galveston, TX 77555-0587, USA; [c] Department of Obstetrics & Gynecology, Division of Maternal-Fetal Medicine, The University of Texas Medical Branch at Galveston, 301 University Boulevard, Galveston, TX 77555-0587, USA
* Corresponding author.
E-mail address: ldpachec@utmb.edu

Obstet Gynecol Clin N Am 49 (2022) 461–471
https://doi.org/10.1016/j.ogc.2022.02.002
0889-8545/22/© 2022 Elsevier Inc. All rights reserved.

SEPTIC SHOCK
Definition and Diagnosis

Sepsis is defined as the presence of acute organ dysfunction secondary to an excessive inflammatory response due to an infectious process.[1] Organ dysfunction is quantified, for academic purposes, as an acute increase of 2 or more points in the Sequential Organ Failure Assessment (SOFA) score.[1] The score includes involvement of the kidney, liver, brain, lung, coagulation cascade, and blood pressure. The SOFA score is depicted in **Table 1**. Although multiple scoring systems adapted to pregnancy have been developed, all lack sensitivity and specificity, and their effect on clinical outcomes is unknown.

Sepsis-induced organ dysfunction may include virtually any system, resulting in confusion, pulmonary edema, systolic and diastolic heart failure, profound vasodilation due to excessive cytokines, hepatitis, acute kidney injury, bowel hypoperfusion with new-onset distention and/or intolerance to enteral feeds, and inflammation-induced clotting activation (disseminated intravascular coagulation) with diffuse microvasculature occlusion.[2] The last of these worsens widespread tissue ischemia and dysfunction. Clinicians should understand that in the setting of a suspected infection, any organ dysfunction (not limited to the organs included in a specific scoring system) should be considered as organ failure secondary to the suspected infectious process, and as such, aggressive treatment should be started without delay.

Septic shock occurs when hypotension persists despite initial fluid resuscitation requiring the use of vasopressors together with a serum lactate greater than 2 mEq/ L.[1] Septic shock is a distributive form of shock in which profound vasodilation (with decreased systemic vascular resistances induced by cytokines) leads to hypotension resulting in hypoperfusion and organ dysfunction. Inflammatory-induced endothelial injury results in third spacing and relative hypovolemia. Organ hypoperfusion, as discussed previously, is further compromised by diffuse microvascular occlusion because monocytes and neutrophils express tissue factor in their surfaces, activating factor VII.[2] Importantly, the heart is commonly affected (septic cardiomyopathy) with decreased systolic function (induced by cytokines), or in some cases, acute diastolic

Table 1
Sequential Organ Failure Assessment score

SOFA Score	1	2	3	4
Respiration (P/F ratio)	<400	<300	<200 with ventilatory support	<100 with ventilatory support
Coagulation Platelets × 10³/mm³	<150	<100	<50	<20
Liver Bilirubin (mg/dL)	1.2–1.9	2–5.9	6–11.9	>12
Cardiovascular MAP	<70	Need for pressors[a]	Need for pressors[a]	Need for pressors[a]
Central nervous system (Glasgow Coma Scale)	13–14	10–12	6–9	<6
Renal Creatinine (mg/dL)	1.2–1.9	2–3.4	3.5–4.9	>5

Abbreviations: MAP, mean arterial blood pressure; P/F ratio, partial pressure of oxygen (Pao₂) divided by the fraction of inspired oxygen (Fio₂).
[a] Score increases as vasopressor requirements increase.

dysfunction due to left ventricular wall edema secondary to fluid third spacing.[3] Acute diastolic dysfunction will compromise ventricular filling, increasing the risk of cardiogenic pulmonary edema.

Initial Management

Septic shock is a medical emergency; early targeted therapy is of paramount importance. Intravenous (IV) access should be obtained followed by initial fluid resuscitation. Ideally, the latter should be with balanced crystalloids (eg, Plasma-Lyte or lactated Ringer), because the use of normal saline may increase the risk of acute kidney injury due to renal vasoconstriction induced by hyperchloremia.[4] Current guidelines recommend administering 30 mL/kg crystalloid in patients with sepsis with systemic hypotension and/or serum lactate levels greater than 4 mEq/L.[5] Simultaneously, cultures should be obtained as indicated together with serum lactate levels. The latter may be followed every 2 to 4 hours as a marker of resuscitation. Importantly, lactate levels decrease slowly (approximately 10% per hour) despite adequate management.[6] Broad-spectrum antibiotics are indicated within 1 hour of diagnosis, aiming to cover gram-positive, gram-negative, and anaerobic bacteria.[5] Broad-spectrum coverage should be narrowed once microbiology results are available. Although a detailed discussion of antibiotics is out of the scope of this article, broad coverage for many life-threatening infections may be achieved with the combination of a carbapenem (eg, meropenem, imipenem, doripenem) and vancomycin.[7] The commonly used regimen of piperacillin-tazobactam with vancomycin, although very popular, should be avoided for prolonged periods because it increases the risk of acute kidney injury.[7] In individuals with a history of life-threatening allergic reactions to beta-lactams, the combination of levofloxacin (or ciprofloxacin) together with metronidazole also provides initial broad coverage.[7] Importantly, the use of quinolones, if indicated, should not be restricted during pregnancy because recent data suggest their safety during pregnancy.[8]

Limitations with the commonly used combination of ampicillin, gentamycin, and clindamycin include significant nephrotoxicity of aminoglycosides, poor lung penetration, and limited anaerobic coverage (compared with metronidazole) with increased risk of *Clostridium difficile* associated with the use of clindamycin.[7]

Achieving rapid source control is paramount, and this may include delivery in chorioamnionitis, dilation and curettage if infected placental tissue is retained, appendectomy, or drainage of perirenal or abdominopelvic abscesses, among others. The least invasive method of source control is preferred to avoid further excessive inflammation.[5]

Hypotension in septic shock will be resistant to fluid resuscitation; as such, vasopressors will be required to increase the mean arterial blood pressure to the desired target of 65 mm Hg.[5] The first-line vasopressor both in nonpregnant and pregnant individuals with septic shock is norepinephrine.[5,9] Norepinephrine is started at low doses (0.02–0.05 μg/kg/min) and titrated as needed to achieve a prespecified blood pressure (mean arterial blood pressure of 65 mm Hg). Norepinephrine must be delivered through a central line; however, if central access is not immediately available and severe hemodynamic instability is present, it may be administered through a peripheral line until central access is obtained. Vasopressin is a commonly used vasopressor in critical care; it achieves vasoconstriction through stimulation of vascular V1 receptors.[5] Minimal data exist on its use during pregnancy, and concern about oxytocin receptor agonism exists. We suggest avoiding vasopressin during pregnancy until more data are available.

Septic cardiomyopathy is present in more than half of patients with septic shock due to cytokine-induced systolic dysfunction.[3] As such, once norepinephrine is started (it is more an alpha-agonist vasoconstrictor when compared with an inotrope with beta-1 agonism), it may "unmask" this underlying cardiomyopathy, because it increases afterload by favoring peripheral vasoconstriction. Evaluation of cardiac output is mandatory in patients who require increasing doses of norepinephrine to maintain the desired blood pressure target. The latter may be achieved with the use of noninvasive cardiac output monitors, transthoracic echocardiography, or following serial central venous mixed oxygen saturation values. If a decline in cardiac output is noted with the use of norepinephrine, adding an inotrope like dobutamine is indicated to increase myocardial contractility.[10]

Cytokines are known to inhibit cortisol production and secretion, leading to critical illness-related corticosteroid insufficiency. The lack of cortisol results in internalization of catecholamine receptors, rendering the patient with sepsis poorly responsive to catecholamines. The latter is the rationale for glucocorticoid supplementation. The use of steroids in septic shock is a controversial topic; however, recent guidelines recommend their use in the setting of catecholamine-resistant septic shock.[5] A recent randomized clinical trial found that the use of steroids (IV hydrocortisone plus oral fludrocortisone) in patients with septic shock requiring more than 0.25 µg/kg/min of norepinephrine decreased the mortality rate.[11] Accordingly, we recommend that in pregnant patients for whom hypotension persists despite more than 0.25 µg/kg/min of norepinephrine, hydrocortisone be started at a dose of 50 mg IV every 6 hours for 7 days regardless of administration of dexamethasone or betamethasone for lung maturity. The use of fludrocortisone is optional, because the latter doses of hydrocortisone usually provide enough mineralocorticoid activity. If given, the recommended dose is 50 µg orally per day.

The fact that a patient with sepsis is on vasopressors does not mean that she will no longer be fluid responsive. Clinicians should periodically assess if further fluid is required to wean norepinephrine as tolerated; this is usually achieved using dynamic measures of preload. Pulse pressure variation in an arterial waveform greater than 13% (while on controlled mechanical ventilation and sinus rhythm) or an increase in stroke volume greater than 10% with passive leg raising indicates fluid responsiveness, and additional fluid boluses may be administered. Passive leg raising may be nonreliable in late pregnancy because uterine compression of the inferior vena cava may preclude preload augmentation normally achieved with leg raising.[12] Similarly, a collapsed inferior vena cava visualized on bedside transthoracic echocardiography that variates in diameter with the respiratory cycle also indicates fluid responsiveness. A detailed discussion on assessment of fluid responsiveness may be found elsewhere.[13]

Fetal Considerations

If septic shock develops before viability (23–24 weeks), daily fetal tones should suffice. No fetal monitoring is indicated. Once viability is achieved, steroids for fetal lung maturation may be administered; septic shock is not a contraindication.[9]

The decision to perform continuous fetal monitoring with the possibility of an emergent cesarean delivery for nonreassuring fetal status must be clearly discussed with the patient and/or family members and neonatology. If the decision to undergo monitoring is reached, continuous monitoring may be started and continued during the initial resuscitation phase. Importantly, many nonreassuring tracings may be improved with maternal resuscitation with fluids and pressors, as improved mean arterial blood pressure will result in increased uterine perfusion pressure. After the acute phase, once hemodynamic stability has been achieved, daily nonstress fetal testing is a potential option.

Fig. 1 summarizes the initial basic steps in the management of septic shock in pregnant patients.

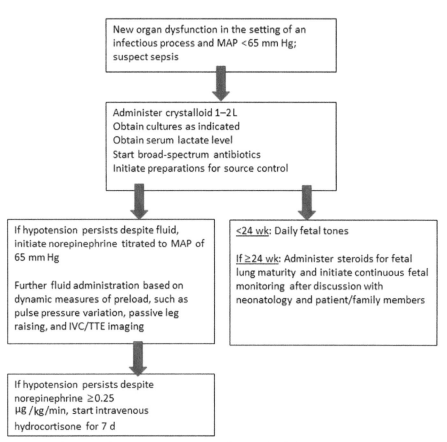

Fig. 1. Initial steps in the acute management of septic shock during pregnancy. IVC, inferior vena cava; MAP, mean arterial blood pressure; TTE, transthoracic echocardiography.

CARDIAC ARREST
Recognition of Cardiac Arrest and Initiation of Cardiopulmonary Resuscitation

Cardiac arrest is a rare occurrence in the obstetric population. Here we provide a basic simplified approach to aid in the immediate management of the pregnant cardiac arrest victim. If a patient is found unresponsive, initial assessment for breathing and carotid pulse should be no longer than 10 seconds.[14] If doubt exists whether there is a pulse or not in a suspected cardiac arrest victim, chest compressions should be started immediately. Once cardiac arrest has been recognized, a code should be called. Typically, a maternal "code blue" team should be multidisciplinary, including obstetricians/maternal-fetal medicine, anesthesia, critical care specialists, neonatologists, and skilled nursing. Early initiation of chest compressions is the single most important immediate action for a patient in cardiac arrest.[14] Chest compressions should be performed like in nonpregnant individuals. The patient should be placed on a firm surface. The heel of one hand of the provider should be placed on the lower half of the sternum, and the heel of the other hand should be placed on top of the first so that the hands are overlapped.[14] Chest compressions should be hard and fast, achieving a depth of at least 2 in (5 cm) and allowing for complete chest recoil at a rate of 100 to 120 compressions per minute. Interruptions of chest compressions should be always minimized.[15] Pregnant patients with an estimated gestational age of 20 weeks or more (fundal height at the umbilicus or higher) should undergo left lateral uterine displacement by an assistant to avoid aortocaval compression by the gravid uterus while maintaining the supine position to optimize efficacy of chest compressions. Although the use of left lateral decubitus is also described, it will jeopardize performance of adequate compressions.[16] Cycles of 30 chest compressions to 2 breaths should be performed if there is no advanced airway in place. Pulse checks (carotid) should be no longer than 10 seconds. Providers performing chest compressions should switch every 2 minutes to avoid fatigue.[17]

Airway Management

Once chest compressions have started, the airway should be opened using the head tilt chin lift technique unless there is trauma to the neck. Endotracheal intubation is not essential to perform adequate basic life support. In the absence of highly trained personnel, ventilation with a bag-mask device (30:2 cycles as discussed previously) should be the preferred method of ventilation. If intubation is considered during active resuscitation efforts, it should be performed with minimal interruptions in chest compressions. A smaller endotracheal tube (6–7 mm) may be needed to accommodate for the edematous airway often seen in pregnant individuals.[16] Once the patient is intubated, or after placement of a supraglottic device (eg, laryngeal mask), one breath should be delivered every 5 to 6 seconds, avoiding excessive ventilation because it may result in air trapping with increased intrathoracic pressure and decreased cardiac preload. Continuous capnography should be used to assess for correct placement of the endotracheal tube, evaluate quality of chest compressions, and identify return of spontaneous circulation (ROSC). Optimal chest compressions should achieve an exhaled partial pressure of carbon dioxide of at least 10 mm Hg and ideally close to 20 mm Hg.[18] Chest compressions should continue at 100 to 120/min while a breath is delivered every 5 to 6 seconds. The 2-handed technique for bag mask ventilation is preferred to create a mask seal and provide sufficient tidal volume to produce visible chest rise.[19] Regardless of the airway present, 100% oxygen should be delivered at a flow of 15 L/min.[16]

Vascular Access

Central venous access is not needed during cardiac arrest, and clinicians should not focus attention on achieving such vascular access. Peripheral IV access suffices and is adequate for administration of all pharmacologic agents indicated during cardiac arrest.[20] If attempts to obtain peripheral vascular access are unsuccessful, rapid intraosseous (IO) access is indicated. IV or IO access should ideally be established above the diaphragm.[17] Fluids, vasopressors, inotropes, and blood products may be safely administered through the IO route.

Providers must understand that the only 2 interventions that improve outcomes in cardiac arrest (high-quality chest compressions and early defibrillation) do not require IV access; as such, extensive periods attempting line placements should be avoided.

Defibrillation

Once defibrillating pads are in place, immediate assessment of cardiac rhythm is the next step. In settings wherein staff have limited heart rhythm recognition skills or where defibrillators are used infrequently, such as on an obstetric floor, the use of an automated external defibrillator should be considered.[21] Electrode pads should be placed on the maternal chest anteriorly below the right clavicle and laterally under the left breast like in nonpregnant individuals. The energy required for defibrillation in the pregnant patient is the same as that in the nonpregnant patient.[22] Although electrocution is theoretic, fetal heart rate monitors should be removed before defibrillation; however, removal of fetal monitors should never delay defibrillation when indicated.[16] Cardiac arrest is due to either shockable rhythms (ventricular fibrillation or pulseless ventricular tachycardia) or nonshockable rhythms (asystole or pulseless electrical activity [PEA]).

Early defibrillation is critical to survival in patients with shockable rhythms.[23,24] Once a shockable rhythm is identified, immediate defibrillation should follow (360 J in monophasic defibrillators and 120–200 J in biphasic defibrillators). After the shock is administered, chest compressions should resume immediately for 2 minutes, after which a pulse may be checked if an organized rhythm is identified. Resuscitation will continue with 2-minute cycles of CPR and evaluation of rhythm and pulse after completion of each cycle. After a second shock is administered, epinephrine 1 mg IV/IO should be started and repeated every 3 to 5 minutes. After a third shock, amiodarone 300 mg IV/IO is indicated with repeated doses of 150 mg IV/IO as needed. This cycle of chest compressions and rhythm assessment is continued every 2 minutes until ROSC or resuscitative efforts are discontinued.[17]

Nonshockable Rhythm

As discussed previously, nonshockable rhythms include asystole and PEA. Early use of epinephrine in asystole and PEA improves ROSC; consequently, epinephrine 1 mg IV/IO every 3 to 5 minutes should be administered early in the resuscitation process together with chest compressions and ventilation as described earlier in the article.[25]

Delivery of Fetus

If resuscitative efforts fail to achieve ROSC in a pregnant patient with a fundal height above the umbilicus, perimortem cesarean delivery (PMCD) may be required to relieve aortocaval compression and ultimately improve the chances of achieving ROSC. Classically, it has been suggested that PMCD should be considered after 4 minutes of CPR; however, this is arbitrary, and clinicians may perform the procedure earlier than 4 minutes into the arrest if indicated. The cesarean delivery should be performed in the same location as the ongoing arrest to avoid delays in care and compromise of the ongoing resuscitative efforts.[26] If available, betadine should be poured over the abdomen. We suggest a midline vertical skin incision because it provides faster and better exposure to the upper abdomen and diaphragm if required. The uterus may be opened through a low transverse or classical incision. The authors commonly perform a classical incision because it may decrease the risk of hysterotomy extensions to the uterine arteries that may not be recognized at the time of the procedure due to minimal blood flow to the uterus. Importantly, chest compressions should be continued throughout the delivery process.[27] **Fig. 2** summarizes the initial management of cardiac arrest during pregnancy.

Postarrest Care

A detailed discussion of post-cardiac arrest is outside of the scope of this article; however, the authors shortly discuss some of the most relevant issues. Post-cardiac arrest patients are often hemodynamically unstable due to ischemia-reperfusion injury leading to systemic vasodilation and cardiac stunning. Vasopressors and inotropes are commonly indicated to achieve a mean arterial blood pressure of 65 mm Hg.[28] Hyperoxia may worsen ischemia-reperfusion injury, so target oxygenation saturation should be 94%.[17] Among comatose survivors of cardiac arrest, targeted temperature

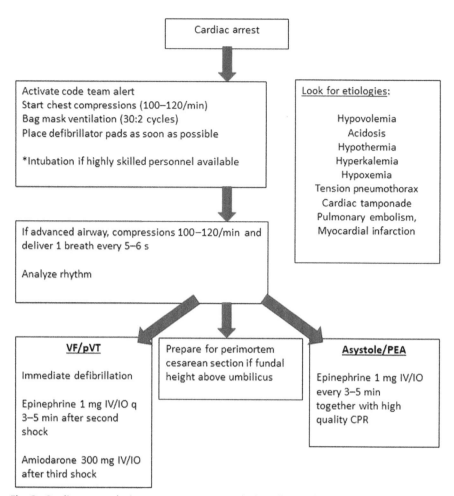

Fig. 2. Cardiac arrest during pregnancy. PEA, pulseless electrical activity; pVT, pulseless ventricular tachycardia; VF, ventricular fibrillation.

management between 32°C and 36°C for 24 hours may improve neurologic outcomes.[17] If used during pregnancy, we suggest targeting a temperature of 36°C (as opposed to 33°C), because it will result in less hypothermia-induced fetal bradycardia.

Glucose control is paramount following cardiac arrest; targeting a blood glucose of 140 to 180 mg/dL is recommended. Hyponatremia should be avoided because it may worsen cerebral edema. Hypotonic solutions, such as PlasmaLyte, lactated Ringers, and dextrose-water should be avoided. We favor the use of normal saline as maintenance fluid following cardiac arrest, because the risk of hyponatremia will be lower. In the absence of seizure activity, prophylactic antiseizure medications are not indicated.[17]

Maternal and neonatal outcomes following cardiac arrest vary significantly depending on the cause and the setting in which the arrest occurs. A recent series reported a maternal survival rate of 58%.[29] Neonatal outcomes depend largely on gestational age, duration of arrest, and timely delivery by operative vaginal delivery or PMCD as indicated.

SUMMARY

Septic shock and cardiac arrest are medical emergencies. The basic concepts of management should not be altered during pregnancy, including early use of fluids, vasopressors, and antibiotics, as well as source control for sepsis. In cases of cardiac arrest during pregnancy, early defibrillation, high-quality cardiopulmonary resuscitation, and use of epinephrine and amiodarone should follow the same recommendations as in nonpregnant individuals. PMCD should be considered in any arrest after 20 weeks' gestation because it may improve resuscitation success.

CLINICS CARE POINTS

- Septic shock is a medical emergency that requires immediate resuscitation with IV fluids.
- Initial care involves obtaining cultures and serum lactate levels together with broad-spectrum antibiotics and source control.
- Norepinephrine is the preferred vasopressor in pregnant patients with septic shock.
- Cardiac arrest management during pregnancy should follow established guidelines for nonpregnant individuals.
- Left lateral displacement of the uterus and early PMCD are fundamental aspects when managing cardiac arrest in pregnancy.

DISCLOSURE

The authors have no conflicts of interest to disclose, and this article was prepared with no external funding source.

REFERENCES

1. Singer M, Deutschman CS, Seymour CW, et al. The Third International Consensus Definitions for Sepsis and Septic Shock (Sepsis-3). JAMA 2016;315:801–10.
2. Marshall JC, Deutschman CS. The multiple organ dysfunction syndrome: Syndrome, metaphor, and unsolved clinical challenge. Crit Care Med 2021;49(9): 1402–13.
3. Daulasim A, Vieillard-Baron A, Geri G. Hemodynamic clinical phenotyping in septic shock. Curr Opin Crit Care 2021;27:290–7.
4. Semler MW, Self WH, Wanderer JP, et al. Balanced crystalloids versus saline in critically ill adults. N Engl J Med 2018;378:829–39.
5. Evans L, Rhodes A, Alhazzani W, et al. Surviving Sepsis Campaign: International guidelines for management of sepsis and septic shock 2021. Crit Care Med 2021. ahead of print.
6. Vincent JL, Bakker J. Blood lactate levels in sepsis: in 8 quiestions. Curr Opin Crit Care 2021;27(3):298–302.
7. Pacheco LD, Saad AF, Saade GR. Practical approach to antibiotic use in critically ill obstetric patients. Obstet Gynecol 2021;138(3):459–65.
8. Yefet E, Schwartz N, Chazan B, et al. The safety of quinolones and fluoroquinolones in pregnancy: a meta-analysis. BJOG 2018;125(9):1069–76.
9. Society for Maternal Fetal Medicine (SMFM), Plante LA, Pacheco LD, et al. SMFM Consult Series #47: Sepsis during pregnancy and the puerperium. Am J Obstet Gynecol 2019;220(4):B2–10.

10. Vincent JL, Joosten AJ, Saugel B. Hemodynamic monitoring and support. Crit Care Med 2021;49(10):1638–50.
11. Annane D, Renault A, Brun-Buisson C, et al. Hydrocortisone plus fludrocortisone for adults with septic shock. N Engl J Med 2018;378(9):809–18.
12. Marques NR, Martinello C, Kramer GC, et al. Passive leg raising during pregnancy. Am J Perinatol 2015;32(4):393–8.
13. Shi R, Monnet X, Teboul JL. Parameters of fluid responsiveness. Curr Opin Crit Care 2020;26(3):319–26.
14. Olasveengen TM, Mancini ME, Perkins GD, et al. on behalf of the Adult Basic Life Support Collaborators. Adult basic life support: 2020 International Consensus on Cardiopulmonary Resuscitation and Emergency Cardiovascular Care Science with Treatment Recommendations. Circulation 2020;142(suppl 1):S41–91.
15. Considine J, Gazmuri RJ, Perkins GD, et al. Chest compression components (rate, depth, chest wall recoil and leaning): A scoping review. Resuscitation 2020;146:188–202.
16. Jeejeebhoy FM, Zelop CM, Lipman S, et al. Cardiac arrest in pregnancy: A scientific statement from the America Heart Association. Circulation 2015;132:1747.
17. Panchal AR, Bartos JA, Cabañas JG, et al. on behalf of the Adult Basic and Advanced Life Support Writing Group. Part 3: adult basic and advanced life support: 2020 American Heart Association Guidelines for Cardiopulmonary Resuscitation and Emergency Cardiovascular Care. Circulation 2020;142(suppl 2):S366–468.
18. Touma O, Davies M. The prognostic value of end tidal carbon dioxide during cardiac arrest: a systematic review. Resuscitation 2013;84:1470–9.
19. Joffe AM, Hetzel S, Liew EC. A two-handed jaw-thrust technique is superior to the one-handed "EC-clamp" technique for mask ventilation in the apneic unconscious person. Anesthesiology 2010;113:873–9.
20. Granfeldt A, Avis SR, Lind PC, et al. Intravenous vs. intraosseous administration of drugs during cardiac arrest: A systematic review. Resuscitation 2020;149:150–7.
21. Link MS, Atkins DL, Passman RS, et al. Part 6: electrical therapies: automated external defibrillators, defibrillation, cardioversion, and pacing: 2010 American Heart Association guidelines for cardiopulmonary resuscitation and emergency cardiovascular care. Circulation 2010;122(suppl 3):S706–19.
22. Nanson J, Elcock D, Williams M, et al. Do physiological changes in pregnancy change defibrillation energy requirements? Br J Anaesth 2001;87:237–9.
23. Bircher NG, Chan PS, Xu Y. American Heart Association's Get With The Guidelines–Resuscitation Investigators. Delays in Cardiopulmonary Resuscitation, Defibrillation, and Epinephrine Administration All Decrease Survival in In-hospital Cardiac Arrest. Anesthesiology 2019;130:414–22.
24. Stiell IG, Walker RG, Nesbitt LP, et al. BIPHASIC Trial: a randomized comparison of fixed lower versus escalating higher energy levels for defibrillation in out-of-hospital cardiac arrest. Circulation 2007;115:1511–7.
25. Holmberg MJ, Issa MS, Moskowitz A, et al. International Liaison Committee on Resuscitation Advanced Life Support Task Force Collaborators. Vasopressors during adult cardiac arrest: A systematic review and meta-analysis. Resuscitation 2019;139:106–21.
26. Lipman SS, Wong JY, Arafeh J, et al. Transport decreases the quality of cardiopulmonary resuscitation during simulated maternal cardiac arrest. Anesth Analg 2013;116:162–7.

27. Einav S, Kaufman N, Sela HY. Maternal cardiac arrest and perimortem caesarean delivery: Evidence or expert-base? Resuscitation 2012;83:1191–200.

28. Nolan JP, Abella BS. Post resuscitation care and prognostication. Curr Opin Crit Care 2021. ahead of print.

29. Beckett VA, Knight M, Sharpe P. The CAPS Study: incidence, management, and outcomes of cardiac arrest in pregnancy in the UK: a prospective descriptive study. BJOG 2017;124(9):1374–81.

Endocrine Emergencies During Pregnancy
Diabetic Ketoacidosis and Thyroid Storm

Odessa P. Hamidi, MD*, Linda A. Barbour, MD, MSPH[1]

KEYWORDS

- Pregnancy • Diabetic ketoacidosis • Euglycemic diabetic ketoacidosis
- Thyroid storm • Endocrine emergencies

KEY POINTS

- The physiologic changes of pregnancy predispose patients to diabetic ketoacidosis (DKA) with a significant fetal mortality rate, especially when it occurs in the late second and third trimester.
- DKA can occur at lower serum glucose levels during pregnancy as low as less than 200 mg/dL (euglycemic DKA), and although is usually seen in Type 1 diabetes, it can occur in Type 2 diabetes or even rarely in insulin-requiring gestational diabetes.
- The management of DKA during pregnancy is similar to that of nonpregnant patients, with the exception of a higher carbohydrate intake requirement due to placental-fetal demands, and includes aggressive intravenous (IV) fluid hydration and IV insulin treatment, as well as close maternal and fetal monitoring.
- Thyroid storm is a life-threatening diagnosis in pregnancy that is most commonly secondary to uncontrolled hyperthyroidism, but can be provoked by several factors.
- Fetal heart rate tracing abnormalities are common in both endocrinological emergencies and usually resolve with treatment of the primary maternal disorder.

DIABETIC KETOACIDOSIS
Introduction, Prevalence, and Pathophysiology

Introduction: Diabetic ketoacidosis (DKA) during pregnancy is a life-threatening medical emergency for both mother and fetus. The incidence of DKA during pregnancy is ~ 3% of diabetic pregnancies, higher with poorly controlled Type 1 diabetes (T1DM), and there remains a high fetal mortality rate (10%–36%) in addition to complications related to possible premature delivery and fetal hypoxia and acidosis.[1–3] Maternal mortality secondary to DKA is also a risk but has significantly decreased over the years to less than 1%.[1,4,5] The risk of DKA is often underappreciated, due to the occurrence

University of Colorado, School of Medicine, Aurora, CO, USA
[1] Present address: 12801 East 17th Avenue, Aurora, CO 80045.
* Corresponding author. 13001 East 17th Place, Aurora, CO 80045.
E-mail address: odessa.hamidi@cuanschutz.edu
Twitter: @Odessa_Hamidi (O.P.H.)

of DKA in pregnancy at lower glucose levels (euglycemic DKA), and often without any clear provocation. Furthermore, due to high placental-fetal glucose demands in the late second trimester and third trimester, inadequate carbohydrate replacement can result in protracted ketosis from starvation ketoacidosis. Despite the known risk of DKA in patients with T1DM, it may be unrecognized in patients with poorly controlled Type 2 diabetes (T2DM) and in insulin-requiring gestational diabetes, especially when provoked by risk factors such as prolonged fasting, infection, or use of corticosteroids.[6–8] Thus, it is increasingly necessary for all obstetric providers to have an understanding of the basic pathophysiology and management of DKA in the context of pregnancy.

Pathophysiology: DKA is typically heralded by significant hyperglycemia that results in a paradoxic lack of glucose at the cellular level in muscle, liver, and adipose tissues.[1,9] The state of perceived hypoglycemia due to the unavailability of adequate insulin to facilitate glucose entering cells results in activation of alternative pathways of energy production. This occurs through the release of counterregulatory hormones (such as glucagon, cortisol, and epinephrine) that activate gluconeogenesis, ketogenesis, and lipolysis pathways.[6] The resultant release of additional glucose into the intravascular space worsens the osmotic gradient that results in glycosuria, profound hypovolemia, and electrolyte derangements. The osmotic diuresis can cause significant sodium abnormalities and profound hypokalemia, which puts patients at risk of seizures, coma, and even death. However, normal or elevated serum potassium levels are frequently encountered in DKA as a lack of insulin results in an inability of potassium to reenter the cells. This puts patients at risk of cardiac arrhythmias and death, including during the treatment of DKA, as potassium is able to reenter the cells. Careful monitoring and treatment of electrolyte abnormalities is a crucial part of managing DKA.

The acidosis that defines DKA is driven by the alternative pathways of energy production that are activated. Lactic acid itself increases because it is a precursor in gluconeogenesis, which is stimulated during DKA. The other major contributor to acidosis is the presence of ketone bodies. These are produced because of the stimulation of lipolysis pathways that release fatty acids that are subsequently oxidized into ketone bodies. β-hydroxybutyric acid and acetoacetic acid are the primary ketone bodies overproduced, with β-hydroxybutyric acid being produced to a much larger extent.[1,10] These ketone bodies dissociate, and the excess hydrogen ions bind up serum bicarbonate resulting in decreased serum bicarbonate levels. The resultant decrease in bicarbonate is what increases the anion gap, measured as $Na^+ - (Cl^- + HCO_3^-)$.

The hyperglycemia in DKA is precipitated by a relative or absolute lack of insulin due to beta cell failure in T1DM and due to marked insulin resistance in T2DM or insulin-requiring gestational diabetes mellitus (GDM), resulting in a relative insulin deficiency. Pregnancy predisposes to DKA due to being a state of insulin resistance associated with a relative insulin deficiency, combined with a decrease in buffering capacity due to the normal respiratory alkalosis of pregnancy, which results in a compensatory metabolic acidosis.[6] The state of relative insulin deficiency from insulin resistance in pregnancy is primarily driven by high levels of human placental lactogen and human placental growth hormone.[1,11–13]

Euglycemic DKA occurs more often in pregnancy due to many reasons. As is the case outside of pregnancy in patients on a sodium-glucose cotransporter-2 inhibitor, pregnancy results in a marked increase in the glomerular filtration of glucose resulting in glycosuria and the lowering of maternal glucose. Glucose is further lowered by the dilutional increase in plasma volume accompanied by pregnancy. Most importantly, continuous glucose utilization and uptake by the fetal-placental unit further lowers glucose given that 80% of the energy demands of the fetus and placenta are met by glucose. Glucose demands by the fetal-placental unit approach 150 g in the third trimester of pregnancy, which result in an early switch from carbohydrate metabolism to lipolysis and fat oxidation, which occurs in pregnant women who have often depleted their glycogen stores after a 12 hour fast. In addition, the maternal metabolic rate increases by ~ 150 to 300 kcal/d in the third trimester, depending on the amount of gestational weight gain in pregnancy.[14] These increased nutritional needs place the mother at risk for ketosis, which occurs much earlier in pregnancy without adequate oral or intravenous (IV) nutrients, frequently referred to as "accelerated starvation of pregnancy." This promotes starvation ketosis, which can greatly contribute to the ketosis in DKA.[15] Due to these predisposing factors, DKA can occur at lower levels of blood glucose during pregnancy (as low as <200 mg/dL) than is typically seen in the nonpregnant state making a high index of suspicion paramount to timely administration of care in cases where "euglycemic DKA" may be encountered.[14,16–18]

Many women with T1DM are now on pump therapy, but disadvantages of insulin pump therapy include a higher risk of DKA as a consequence of rapid acting insulin delivery failure from a kinked catheter or from infusion site problems. Therefore, women on pump therapy should be counseled on becoming vigilant if their glucose level increases for unexpected reasons and do not respond to bolus infusions and should always have both a rapid acting insulin preparation and intermediate or long-acting preparation available that can be given by a syringe or pen.

Patient Evaluation Overview

Patient signs and symptoms: During pregnancy, DKA can present more suddenly than in the nonpregnant state. Any pregnant woman with T1DM who is unable to keep down food or fluids or has persistent severe hyperglycemia should check urine ketones at home. Often the only precipitant for DKA in pregnancy is nausea and vomiting, but other causes such as urinary tract infections should be aggressively investigated. As mentioned, women with T2DM and even women with insulin-requiring GDM can also develop DKA, especially in the context of prolonged fasting, infections, or corticosteroids to promote fetal lung maturity.

Symptoms of DKA can vary but can often present with gastrointestinal symptoms including abdominal pain, nausea and vomiting, and uterine contractions (**Table 1**).[19] Polyuria or polydipsia is common due to the osmotic diuresis and state of dehydration. Dehydration can also lead to sinus tachycardia, hyperventilation/tachypnea, and hypotension. In patients with more advanced DKA, Kussmaul breathing, fruity odor of the breath, and altered mental status may also be seen.[1,19] Kussmaul breathing is characterized by deep long breaths as the body attempts to expel more carbon dioxide and partially reverse the metabolic acidosis.[10] All women with diabetes in pregnancy should be counseled on the signs and symptoms of DKA as well as the risk of DKA occurring with lower glucose levels.

Patient counseling if at risk for DKA: Patients with nausea or vomiting with inadequate oral intake or those experiencing difficulty in lowering their glucoses to less than 200 mg/dL should be instructed to check their urine ketones. If the urine ketones cannot be reduced to a low level with corrections of rapid active insulin and increased oral intake of fluids, the patient should be instructed to seek medical assistance.

Laboratory evaluation: A high index of suspicion should be present especially for any patient with known diabetes affecting pregnancy when presenting with symptoms of infectious illness or protracted nausea and vomiting because these are common precipitating causes of DKA. Prompt laboratory evaluation is needed to quickly establish the

Table 1
Signs and symptoms of DKA in pregnancy

Clinical signs/symptoms	• Abdominal pain • Nausea and vomiting • Polyuria and polydypsia • Uterine contractions • Sinus tachycardia, hypotension • Tachypnea • Hyperventilation/Kussmaul breathing • Fruity odor of the breath • Muscle weakness • Drowsiness/lethargy • Altered mental status
Laboratory findings	• Elevated plasma glucose usually 250 mg/dL or greater (can occur <200 mg/dL in pregnancy) • Elevated anion gap (>12 mEq/L) • Low serum bicarbonate level (<15 mEq/L) • False normal or elevated potassium level • Low serum sodium levels • Arterial pH <7.30 • Elevated base deficit of 4 mEq/L or greater • Elevated serum or urine ketones (β-hydroxybutyric acid > acetoacetic acid) • Elevated blood urea nitrogen and/or creatinine secondary to dehydration
Fetal findings	• Minimal variability • Variable, late, or spontaneous decelerations

diagnosis. Laboratory evaluation should include a complete blood cell count with differential, a complete metabolic panel (including liver function, blood urea nitrogen, creatinine, electrolytes, and glucose), and serum or urine ketones (β-hydroxybutyrate with or without acetoacetate), regardless of a woman's glycemic status. Beta-hydroxybutyrate is the predominant ketoacid in DKA. If the bicarbonate is low (usually less than 15 mEq/L) or an elevated anion gap is present (12 mEq/L or greater), an arterial or venous blood gas should be obtained.[1] Typical symptoms and laboratory findings are shown in **Table 1**. Although DKA is most commonly noted at plasma glucose levels 250 mg/dL or greater, "euglycemic" DKA can occur with glucose levels as low as 200 mg/dL in as many as a third of pregnant women, thus a full laboratory evaluation is still required despite glycemic status.[18] Falsely normal or even high potassium levels are common due to inadequate insulin and acidosis, which shift potassium out of the cell, despite an overall decrease in total body potassium.

Effects on the fetus: A state of maternal acidosis results in fetal acidosis. In addition to ketoacids readily crossing the placenta, there is a decrease in uterine blood flow and thus oxygen delivery to the fetus. Maternal acidosis also decreases 2,3-diphosphoglycerate, which increases maternal hemoglobin affinity for oxygen further worsening oxygen delivery to the fetus.[2] Fetal acidosis and fetal volume depletion from fetal hyperglycemia and fetal osmotic diuresis may occur, jeopardizing the viability of the fetus. Electrolyte abnormalities also pose a risk for a fetal arrhythmia. Due to these changes, a change in fetal heart rate tracing with decreased variability and decelerations are frequently noted. Changes in ultrasound Doppler findings have also been previously reported, but these usually reverse with the treatment of DKA if emergent delivery does not become required.[2,20,21]

Treatment of Diabetic Ketoacidosis

The mainstay of treatment of DKA includes aggressive IV fluid resuscitation, IV insulin therapy, and correction of electrolyte derangements, which often corrects the acidosis. Continuous fetal monitoring and intensive maternal monitoring are required to evaluate response to treatment. A summary of the monitoring and treatment of DKA can be found in **Box 1** and are described in this section.

Fluid replacement: The total fluid deficit in patients with DKA is approximately 6 to 10 L, and thus, an aggressive fluid replacement is needed. On an average, a deficit of 100 mL/kg is noted.[2] A total of 4 to 6 L of replacement is needed within the first 12 hours.[19,22] Initial fluid replacement should be with isotonic (0.9%) saline and hourly monitoring of intake and output should be performed. This also increases insulin responsiveness by lowering the plasma osmolality, reducing vasoconstriction and

---

Box 1
Management of diabetic ketoacidosis during pregnancy

IV Fluids
- Isotonic sodium chloride is used, with total replacement of 4 to 6 L in the first 12 h.
- Insert IV catheters: Maintain hourly flow sheet for fluids and electrolytes, potassium, insulin, and laboratory results.
- Administer normal saline (0.9% NaCl) at 1 to 2 L/h for the first hour.
- Infuse normal saline at 250 to 500 mL/h depending on hydration state (8 h). If corrected serum sodium is elevated, switch to half-normal saline (0.45% NaCl).
- When plasma or serum glucose reaches 200 mg/dL, change to 5% dextrose with NS or 0.45% NS at 150 to 250 mL/h.
- After 8 to 24 hours depending on hydration status, use 5% dextrose with 0.45% NaCl at 125 mL/h. If the patient is unable to keep down oral carbohydrates, consider using 10% dextrose, especially in the late second or third trimester of pregnancy.

Potassium
- Establish adequate renal function (urine output ~50 mL/h).
- If serum potassium is less than 3.3 mEq/L, hold insulin and give 20 to 30 mEq K$^+$/h until K$^+$is more than 3.3 mEq/L or is being corrected.
- If serum K$^+$is more than 3.3 mEq/L but less than 5.3 mEq/L, give 20 to 30 mEq K$^+$in each liter of IV fluid to keep serum K$^+$between 4 and 5 mEq/L.
- If serum K$^+$is more than 5.3 mEq/L, do not give K$^+$but check serum K$^+$every 2 h.

Insulin
- Use regular insulin intravenously.
- Consider a loading dose of 0.1 to 0.2 U/kg as an IV bolus depending on plasma glucose.
- Begin continuous insulin infusion at 0.1 U/kg/h.
- If plasma or serum glucose does not decrease by 50 to 70 mg/dL in the first hour, double the insulin infusion every hour until a steady glucose decline is achieved.
- When plasma or serum glucose reaches 200 mg/dL, reduce insulin infusion to 0.05 to 0.1 U/kg/h.
- Keep plasma or serum glucose between 100 and 150 mg/dL until resolution of DKA.

Bicarbonate
- Assess need and provide based on pH.
- pH > 7.0: No HCO$_3$ is needed.
- pH is 6.9 to 7.0: Dilute NaHCO$_3$ (50 mmol) in 200 mL H$_2$O with 10 mEq KCl and infuse over 1 hour. Repeat NaHCO$_3$ administration every 2 hours until pH is 7.0. Monitor serum K$^+$.
- pH < 6.9 to 7.0: Dilute NaHCO$_3$ (100 mmol) in 400 mL H$_2$O with 20 mEq KCl and infuse for 2 hours. Repeat NaHCO$_3$ administration every 2 hours until pH is 7.0. Monitor serum K$^+$.

Adapted from Elsevier. Obstetrics: Normal and Problem Pregnancies. 8th Edition. Philadelphia (PA): Elsevier; 2021, p. 894; with permission.

improving perfusion, and reducing stress hormone level. The most appropriate IV fluid composition after initial treatment with isotonic saline is determined by the sodium concentration "corrected" for the degree of hyperglycemia. The "corrected" sodium concentration has been estimated to be 1.6 to 2.4 mEq/L for every 100 mg/dL of glucose greater than 100 mg/dL. A reasonable approximation can be made by adding 2 mEq/L to the plasma sodium concentration for each 100 mg/dL of glucose greater than 100 mg/dL. If the sodium level is less than 135 mEq/L, isotonic saline should be continued at a rate of approximately 250 mL/h. If the sodium level is normal or elevated, the IV fluid is generally switched to one-half isotonic saline at a rate of 250 mL/h in order to provide more free water. Tapering of IV fluid administration can then be performed as described in **Box 1** to 250 to 500 mL/h for the next 8 hours and can be modified based on corrected sodium and hydration status as evidenced by urine output and vital sign monitoring. The goal is to correct estimated deficits within the first 24 hours. However, osmolality should not be reduced too rapidly, because this may generate cerebral edema, although much more common in children. When serum glucose reaches 200 mg/dL, 5% dextrose should be added to the fluids (see **Box 1**).[19]

Insulin therapy: The mainstay of treatment of DKA is with IV regular insulin, which has a half-life of only 3 to 7 minutes when given intravenously. Low-dose IV insulin should be administered to all patients with moderate-to-severe DKA who have a serum potassium of 3.3 mEq/L or greater. If the serum potassium is less than 3.3 mEq/L, insulin therapy should be delayed until potassium replacement has begun and the serum potassium concentration has increased. The delay is necessary because insulin will worsen the hypokalemia by driving potassium into the cells, and this could trigger cardiac arrhythmias. With adequate fluid resuscitation, insulin begins to correct the hyperglycemia in addition to inhibit ongoing production of ketoacids. Comparisons have been made with fast-acting insulin analogs; however, they were not found to be superior and regular insulin is more cost-effective, so it remains the preferred choice for an IV insulin drip during the treatment of DKA.[22] Insulin drip doses to decrease the serum glucose concentration by approximately 75 mg/dL per hour are usually targeted and fluids alone will often drop the glucose by 35 to 50 mg/dL per hour. When the bicarbonate level and anion gap have normalized, beta-hydroxybutyrate levels have resolved, and the patient is tolerating PO, weight-based doses of intermediate or long-acting insulin should be resumed in addition to short or rapid insulin if the patient is able to eat. The IV insulin drip should be continued for at least 2 hours after dosing subcutaneous insulin to ensure adequate serum insulin levels before discontinuation and to prevent recurrence of an anion gap. Ultralong-acting insulins such as Degludec (Tresibi) should be avoided due to their duration of action that can be more than 24 hours, which does not allow for frequent dose adjustments.

Serum electrolyte monitoring: Frequent electrolyte monitoring should occur (every 2–3 hours) during the active management of DKA. An average potassium deficit of 5 to 10 mEq/kg body weight occurs in DKA and should be expected even in the setting of a normal or elevated potassium level.[2] Potassium replacement is initiated immediately if the serum potassium is less than 5.3 mEq/L as long as there is adequate urine output (approximately >50 mL/h). Generally, a potassium level of 4 to 5 mEq/L is an optimal goal, and guidelines for replacement and monitoring are shown in **Box 1**. Other electrolyte derangements such as phosphate, magnesium, and calcium have been noted but generally resolve withcorrection of the DKA thus active replacement is not typically required. However, in cases of vomiting or diarrhea that can result in both magnesium and potassium depletion, repletion of cell potassium requires correction of the magnesium deficit. This seems to result from an inability of the cell to maintain the normally high intracellular concentration of potassium, perhaps because of an increase in membrane permeability to potassium and/or inhibition of Na + -K-ATPase. As a result, the cells lose potassium, which is excreted in the urine.[2,14]

Bicarbonate levels will usually correct with the above treatments and suppression of ketoacid production and thus treatment with bicarbonate is rarely required. The treatment of DKA with bicarbonate has remained controversial due to its lack of evidence to improve morbidity and mortality.[2,23] There are also potential risks to its use including a paradoxic effect on cerebral pH and resultant cerebral edema, as well as reducing the rate of reversal of the acidosis and causing hypokalemia.[2,24] It may be considered, however, if severe acidosis with pH < 7.0 is noted.[2,19]

Adequate carbohydrate delivery: Pregnant women unable to take oral nutrients require an additional 100 to 150 g/d of IV glucose to meet the metabolic demands of the fetal-placental unit. Glycogen stores in the liver (on average ~ 100 g) are depleted with fasting in pregnant women much sooner (12–18 hours) than in the nonpregnant state, especially in the second and third trimesters with increasing placental-fetal glucose demands. When glycogen storage in the liver is depleted, stored adipose tissue triglycerides are released into the circulation as fatty acids and glycerol. Ketone bodies are produced by the liver under low carbohydrate and insulin conditions. After correction of the hyperglycemia, acidosis, and volume depletion, women are often maintained on an infusion of D5 ½NS if they are unable to tolerate oral carbohydrates. However, running D5 at 100 cc/h only provides 120 g of glucose in 24 hours and is inadequate for maternal, fetal, and placental glucose demands, especially in the third trimester. To provide adequate carbohydrate availability in a patient unable to eat, often a D10 glucose solution is necessary, otherwise fat will continue to be burned for fuel and the patient in DKA will remain ketotic from a starvation ketosis. The insulin drip rate can simply be increased to cover the higher glucose in D10 if a patient is unable to ingest oral carbohydrate.

Fetal monitoring: Fetal monitoring often demonstrates decreased variability and late decelerations in the setting of contractions, but this typically resolves as DKA is being treated.[19] It is important to maintain a very high threshold for delivery in the setting of nonreassuring fetal status in the setting of maternal DKA as emergent cesarean during a state of critical illness/acidosis could worsen the condition of the mother, and delivery of an acidotic neonate is preferably avoided. The abnormal fetal heart rate tracing typically resolves as the DKA is treated and maternal and fetal acidosis is being reversed. Provider patience and high tolerance of an abnormal fetal heart tracing is required because delivery is rarely, although sometimes, required in this setting. Notably, the fetal heart rate tracing has been reported to take up to 4 to 8 hours to resolve.[20]

Treating underlying causes: Although maternal and fetal stability are being established, investigation into possible precipitating factors should be undertaken. In patients with T1DM, pump failure or malfunction is a common cause that is often unrecognized by the patient. Uncontrolled nausea and vomiting resulting in a starvation state is also a common cause during pregnancy and as such these symptoms should be aggressively managed in pregnant patients with diabetes. Infection is another common trigger for DKA. Infectious sources can be broad, but common causes in pregnancy include urinary tract or respiratory tract infections. Of special note, β-agonists and corticosteroids to induce lung maturity, especially in a patient who is fasting and has correspondingly low insulin levels, can also precipitate DKA and should be avoided and/or discontinued in a patient with DKA.[25]

Prevention

Pregnant patients with pregestational diabetes should be made well aware of the risks of DKA and its warning signs and symptoms.[26,27] During pregnancy, if glucose levels are greater than 200 mg/dL and not coming down with insulin, patients should have access to urine ketone strips and report these results to their providers if urine ketones are moderate or high and do not decrease.[19] Women with DKA are more likely to have complications related to preterm birth, intrauterine fetal demise, and neonatal intensive care unit admissions and measures to avoid this risk should be discussed in detail with the patient.[19]

SUMMARY

DKA is more easily precipitated by the physiologic changes of pregnancy including increasing insulin resistance, decreased buffering capacity, and a rapid switch to fatty acid oxidation with inadequate po intake. These changes also cause DKA to occur at lower levels of serum glucose than in the nonpregnant state. DKA is a significant obstetric and medical emergency that has an up to 35% rate of fetal mortality.[2,28] Prompt evaluation, aggressive IV fluid hydration, and insulin treatment are the mainstays of therapy. A multidisciplinary team is frequently required including critical care and maternal fetal medicine.

CLINICS CARE POINTS

- DKA can occur at lower levels in pregnancy (<200 mg/dL) and can occur in T1DM, T2DM, or insulin-requiring GDM; patients need to be aware of this and have urine ketone strips at home. B-hydroxybutyrate is the predominant ketoacid in DKA.

- IV fluids and IV insulin are the mainstays of treatment of DKA.

- Hourly fluid and glucose level monitoring is needed in addition to q 2 to 4 hour monitoring of electrolytes during the active management of DKA.

- Potassium is typically falsely normal or elevated despite whole body depletion.

- Start intermediate or long-acting insulin (along with short or rapid acting insulin if the patient can eat), at least 2 hours before discontinuing an insulin drip.

- The fetal heart rate tracing may take several hours to recover so one should maintain a high threshold for delivery while medically treating DKA.

THYROID STORM
Introduction/Background/Prevalence

Thyroid storm is another life-threatening endocrine emergency. In the United States survey, 16% of adult inpatients with thyrotoxicosis were diagnosed with storm.[29,30] The incidence of overt hyperthyroidism in pregnancy has been reported at 0.5% to 1% of all pregnancies, with Graves disease accounting for 95% of these cases.[31–33] Most cases of thyroid storm are due to an underlying diagnosis of hyperthyroidism secondary to Graves disease but can also occur in cases of toxic adenomas, multinodular goiters, or an human chorionic gonadotropin (hCG)-secreting hydatidiform mole.[34] Thyroid storm occurs in around 1% to 2% of pregnancies affected by hyperthyroidism and typically occurs in patients with poor disease control and a precipitating factor such as infection, preeclampsia, trauma, surgery, and even labor or cesarean delivery.[30,32,35]

It is uncertain why some patients develop thyroid storm at similar T4 and T3 levels as others who only have uncomplicated thyrotoxicosis. Suspected theories include a rapid rate of increase in serum thyroid hormone (TH) levels, increased responsiveness to catecholamines, or enhanced cellular responses to TH. Often the T4 and T3 concentrations are higher, but other provoking factors or comorbidities may contribute. Pregnancy poses a higher risk for heart failure, and when thyroid storm occurs in pregnancy, there is an elevated (10%) risk of heart failure, highlighting the critical nature of this illness.[32,36] The cardiopulmonary effects of excessive TH are more common in pregnancy. T_4-induced cardiomyopathy or pulmonary hypertension is usually reversible with treatment, unless they have been longstanding. Ultimately, thyroid storm is a clinical diagnosis, and it is paramount to initiate treatment quickly; it should be treated in an ICU setting. Mortality for thyroid storm overall has been reported to be 8% to 25%, even in an ICU setting and much higher if untreated.[34]

Patient Evaluation Overview

Patient signs and symptoms: Thyroid storm is a clinical diagnosis that presents as a hypermetabolic state. Typical clinical signs include significant hyperpyrexia (>103°F), tachycardia (usually >140 bpm), cardiac arrhythmias, and neurologic disturbances including restlessness, altered mental status, and even seizures.[32,37] The clinical Burch-Wartofsky Point Scale scoring system was established to help confirm the clinical diagnosis and evaluate the severity of thyroid storm (**Table 2**).[38] Other possible symptoms include gastrointestinal disturbances such as nausea or vomiting or diarrhea and even hepatic dysfunction and congestive heart failure.[39] Liver function tests are commonly increased but usually less than 3-fold elevated. Congestive heart failure is a more common complication of thyroid storm in pregnancy and has even been noted to occur in up to 9% to 10% of pregnant patients with uncontrolled hyperthyroidism alone.[39–41]

Laboratory evaluation: The thyroid stimulating hormone (TSH) is suppressed in ~20% of women in the first and early second trimesters, and TSH norms are 0.4 uIU/mL lower than the nonpregnant range due to the stimulation of the TSH receptor by high levels of hCG, which shares the same alpha subunit. Furthermore, subclinical hyperthyroidism should never be treated in pregnancy (suppressed TSH with normal T4 and T3 for pregnancy) because it has been shown that maternal–fetal outcomes are just as favorable with a suppressed TSH. Additionally, with overt hypothyroidism (elevated T4 and/or T3 for pregnancy), antithyroid drugs should be titrated to maintain the T4 at the upper limit of the normal pregnancy range to avoid fetal hypothyroidism because antithyroid medications (ATDs) cross more than T4.[30] In thyroid storm, thyroid function tests (TFTs) should demonstrate severe thyrotoxicosis with a completely suppressed TSH and very elevated free T4 or T3 (FT4, FT3) and/or total T4 or T3 (TT4, TT3). The laboratory values are indistinguishable from those of severe uncontrolled hyperthyroidism, with no specific cutoff values indicating thyroid storm. It is clinically important to recognize that the half-life of T4 is 5 to 7 days and T3 is ~1 day for monitoring levels to gauge the effectiveness of treatment.[30] Both T4 and T3 are avidly bound to thyroid binding globulin (TBG) and greater than 99.95% of T4 and 99.5% of T3 in serum are bound to serum proteins such as TBG, transthyretin, albumin, and lipoproteins. With the increase in estrogen-stimulated TBG, TT4 (total T4) and TT3 (total T3) levels significantly increase in pregnancy, rising 1.5 times the nonpregnant reference range by the end of the first trimester (>16 weeks). FT4 and FT3 only represent ~ 0.05% to 0.5% of sampled serum. Indirect analog immunoassays are the most commonly used methods for measuring FT4 and FT3 but accuracy is variable, especially with FT3 due to significantly lower production of T3 than T4 by the

Table 2
Burch-Wartofsky diagnostic criteria for thyroid storm

Thermoregulatory Dysfunction	
Temperature °F	
99–99.9	5
100–100.9	10
101–101.9	15
102–102.9	20
103–103.9	25
≥104.0	30
Central Nervous System Effects	
Absent	0
Mild (Agitation)	10
Moderate (Delirium, psychosis, extreme lethargy)	20
Severe (Seizure, coma)	30
Gastrointestinal-Hepatic Dysfunction	
Absent	0
Moderate (Diarrhea, nausea/vomiting, abdominal pain)	10
Severe (Unexplained jaundice)	20
Cardiovascular Dysfunction	
Tachycardia	
90–109	5
110–119	10
120–129	15
130–130	20
≥140	25
Congestive Heart Failure	
Absent	0
Mild (Pedal edema)	5
Moderate (Bibasilar rales)	10
Severe (Pulmonary edema)	15
Atrial Fibrillation	
Absent	0
Present	10
Precipitant History	
Negative	0
Positive	10

A score of 45 or greater is highly suggestive of thyroid storm; a score of 25–44 is suggestive of impending storm, and a score less than 25 is unlikely to represent thyroid storm.
From Burch HB, Wartofsky L. Life-threatening thyrotoxicosis. Thyroid storm. Endocrinol Metab Clin North Am. 1993;22(2):263-277; with permission.

human thyroid (14:1 T4:T3). Although a FT4 can be used to quantitate the degree of hyperthyroidism, the FT3 immunoassay methods are more inaccurate than FT4. As a result, the TT3 (by adding ∼50% to the upper limit of the pregnancy range by 16 weeks) may be a better indicator of the degree of T3 thyrotoxicosis than an FT3 assay.[30] T3 measured either as TT3 or FT3 may be disproportionately higher in cases of Graves disease with increased peripheral conversion of T_4 to T_3 compared with other causes of hyperthyroidism (toxic multinodular goiter). For purposes of titration of ATDs in the acute setting, it may be easier to follow an FT4 because it is reasonably accurate and pregnancy adjustments for the normal range do not need to be made along with a TT3 (which does require a 50% increase adjustment after 16 weeks gestation). In a patient with a history consistent with thyroid disorder and presenting with signs and symptoms of thyroid storm, prompt treatment should be undertaken.[32,37,39] Additional laboratory abnormalities that often coexist and should be assessed include leukocytosis, hyperglycemia, hypercalcemia, elevated liver enzymes, and electrolyte disturbances.[37]

Fetal evaluation: As with any maternal critical illness, fetal heart rate tracing abnormalities are likely to ensue and deferring delivery if possible is recommended. Because maternal stability is obtained, the fetal status is also likely to improve.[32]

Pharmacologic or Medical Treatment Options

The initial management of thyroid storm includes supportive therapy with administration of fluids, oxygen therapy as needed, and close monitoring and management of electrolyte imbalances. Treatment should occur in an intensive care unit (ICU) setting where this close monitoring is possible. Of note, acetaminophen should be used for the treatment of hyperpyrexia. Acetaminophen is the generally preferred antipyretic in pregnancy but is additionally safer than using aspirin due to the effect of salicylates increasing circulating FT4 by displacing it from binding proteins.[37,39]

There are no prospective studies evaluating the optimal treatment of thyroid storm, but the mainstay of treatment is the use of ATDs such as the thioamides methimazole (MMI) or propylthiouracil (PTU) to block new hormone synthesis. They are usually dosed as MMI 20 mg q 6 hours (total daily dose 80 mg) or PTU with a loading dose of 400 mg followed by 200 mg every 4 to 6 hours (total of 800–1200 mg/d).[30] Both thioamides work quickly (within a few hours) to inhibit TH synthesis, with PTU having the additional benefit of inhibiting peripheral conversion of T4 to T3 and thus is often the preferred agent in managing thyroid storm.[32,37,39] Because of the short half-life of T3, levels of T3 drop by approximately 45% within 24 hours after PTU but only 10% to 15% within 24 hours after MMI. One hour after thioamides are administered, iodine medications should be given to help block further hormonal release. It is important to wait until 1 hour after ATDs have been initiated to avoid the risk of iodine being used as a substrate for further TH synthesis in cases of Graves, toxic adenomas, or multinodular goiters, which would instead worsen thyrotoxicosis. As the cause of thyrotoxicosis is usually due to autonomous function of the thyroid, ATDs should always be given first, followed by iodine medications 1 hour later.[42] Iodine can be administered in the form of Lugol solution, 10 drops po 3 times a day, or potassium iodide 5 drops po 4 times a day. IV forms of iodine are not available in the United States.[37,39]

Additional treatment with high dose glucocorticoid therapy can further reduce peripheral conversion of T4 to T3, promote vasomotor stability, and treat any relative adrenal insufficiency. Hydrocortisone (50–100 mg every 8 hours) is preferred over dexamethasone (2–4 mg every 8 hours). Hydrocortisone is preferable over dexamethasone in pregnancy due to the ability of dexamethasone to cross the placenta and its association with small for gestational age neonates and reduced head circumference with long-term exposure.[43,44] Stress doses of corticosteroids are usually continued for 2 to 3 days, but hyperglycemia due to the insulin resistance of pregnancy needs to be carefully monitored.

Beta-blocker therapy is used to control hyperadrenergic symptoms and can at high doses decrease conversion of T4 to T3. However, they can also reduce myocardial contractility and should be used cautiously, especially in patients in which there are any concerns of cardiac dysfunction. If any degree of cardiac dysfunction is possibly suspected, IV beta blockers with shorter half-lives are safer than oral beta blockers until cardiac function can be assessed by an echocardiogram. Esmolol IV 250 to 500 mcg over a 1-minute loading dose followed by a drip of 50 to 100 mcg/kg/min or metoprolol IV 5 to 10 mg q 2 to 4 hours can be used. If cardiac dysfunction is believed to be highly unlikely, propranolol (60–80 mg po every 6 hours) can be used because at high doses, it inhibits Type 1 deiodinase and decreases conversion of T4 to T3. However, complications of hypotension require careful monitoring in pregnant women who usually have lower blood pressures. Hypotension can also be due to cardiac failure and an echocardiogram to assess cardiac contractility should be considered in most cases. For patients with a history of very mild asthma, metoprolol may be a better choice than propanolol due to its beta-selectivity but must be given very carefully. In patients with a history of moderate-to-severe asthma who cannot tolerate beta blockade, diltiazem IV or po (60–90 mg po q 6–8 hours) can be used. In patients with congestive heart failure, digoxin may also be required. Comanagement with endocrinology or cardiology is recommended. Sometimes, bile acid sequestrants (cholestyramine 4 g p q 6–8 hours) may also be of benefit in severe cases to decrease enterohepatic recycling of THs. A summary of treatment of thyroid storm can be found in **Box 2**. In general, it is recommended to avoid delivery in the presence of thyroid storm as the fetal status may improve because the maternal status is stabilized.

Refractory Cases

Clinical improvement of thyroid storm is typically observed within the first 24 to 48 hours. If this does not occur, or contraindications for ATD therapy exist (such as agranulocytosis), plasma exchange or dialysis may be considered to lower TH concentration as well as circulating levels of thyroid-stimulating hormone receptor antibodies (TRAb).[45,46] In a series of 3 patients who had therapeutic plasma exchange for thyroid storm preoperatively, FT4 levels were reduced on average by 21% after each treatment and by 55% after 4 treatments. In rarer cases where ATDs are contraindicated, surgical intervention with definitive thyroidectomy may be considered after treatment of the hyperthyroidism for several days with plasmapheresis, iodine, beta blockade, hydrocortisone, and bile acid sequestrants. Surgery should not be delayed

---

Box 2
Treatment of thyroid storm

- ICU care
- Aggressive fluid support
- MMI 20 mg q 6 or PTU 200 mg q 4–6h after loading dose of 400 mg
- One hour after PTU or MMI, Lugol solution, 10 drops po 3 times a day, or potassium iodide 5 drops po 4 times a day
- β-Adrenergic blocker therapy (eg, IV esmolol or IV metoprolol if any cardiac dysfunction concerns or po propranolol 60–80 mg q 6 h)
- Glucocorticoids (Hydrocortisone 50–100 mg q 8h)
- Telemetry, possible echocardiogram; consider endocrinology, and/or cardiology consultation

for more than 8 to 10 days because of a phenomenon called escape from the Wolff-Chaikoff effect. Large doses of exogenous iodine inhibit the organification of iodine in the thyroid gland (the Wolff-Chaikoff effect). However, this effect is transient, and the iodide transport system is able to adapt to higher concentrations of iodine, allowing TH synthesis to proceed, with potential exacerbation of thyrotoxicosis (escape of the Wolff-Chaikoff effect). Surgery comes with significantly higher risks during pregnancy, including the risk of inadvertent parathyroidectomy resulting in hypocalcemia due to the highly vascular and enlarged Graves gland and should only be performed by experienced surgeons who specialize in thyroid and parathyroid surgeries.[47,48]

Treatment Follow-Up

Because thyroid storm is more likely in a patient with poorly controlled underlying disease, it is worth briefly mentioning the goals of longer term therapy and therapy monitoring when treating hyperthyroidism in pregnancy. An important principle in managing hyperthyroidism in pregnancy is the knowledge that ATDs cross the placenta more readily than TH, and thus the fetal thyroid can become suppressed, resulting in fetal/neonatal hypothyroidism. Thus, it is recommended to aim for FT4 levels in the upper normal to mildly elevated range. There should be no attempt to normalize the TSH given this results in overtreatment, and it may remain suppressed for months after appropriate lowering of the FT4 to the upper limit of the normal range. In patients with predominant T3 thyrotoxicosis, PTU is preferred due to its effect on decreasing conversion of T4 to T3. T3 crosses the placenta much more poorly than T4, so sometimes, it is necessary to target the maternal T3 at slightly higher levels to avoid lowering the maternal T4 into the mid-normal range, which places the fetus at risk of hypothyroidism from excess ATD treatment. TFTs should be monitored every 2 to 4 weeks after initiation or dose changes. The general rule of thumb is to use PTU TID over MMI BID in the first trimester due to a slightly higher risk for teratogenicity, and then to switch to MMI after the first trimester due to risk of hepatotoxicity with PTU, using a conversion of ~20:1 between PTU and MMI. However, this should be individualized for the patient; for example, PTU is preferred in cases of primary T3 thyrotoxicosis.[32,37,49] With the immunosuppression of pregnancy, PTU and MMI doses usually require active tapering to avoid fetal hypothyroidism as pregnancy progresses.

Hyperthyroidism and Adverse Perinatal Outcomes

In addition to the acute concerns of the critical state of thyroid storm on fetal well-being, it should be noted that untreated overt hyperthyroidism has significant additional risks throughout pregnancy. These include significantly higher rates of miscarriage (~25%), placental abruption, and up to 5 times higher rate of preeclampsia. There are also increased rates of stillbirth (~5-6%), fetal growth restriction, premature delivery (~15%) and fetal and neonatal thyrotoxicosis, and suppression of the fetal pituitary thyrotropes resulting in newborn central hypothyroidism.[37,39,40,49,50] It should also be recalled that elevated Graves antibodies should be measured given they cross the placenta, especially after 18 to 20 weeks. Graves antibodies measured by either a thyroid stimulating immunoglobulin or TRAb assay found to be 3 times higher than the normal range places the fetus at risk for developing fetal or newborn Graves disease. If Graves antibodies are 3 or more times elevated after 18 weeks, serial ultrasounds every 4 weeks are indicated to evaluate the fetal thyroid gland, bone maturation, amniotic fluid volume, evidence of hydrops or fetal cardiac dysfunction, heart rate, and biometry for growth to characterize fetal risk.[30] Enlargement of the fetal thyroid gland is usually due to fetal Graves but can be also caused by transplacental passage of

ATDs causing iatrogenic fetal hypothyroidism, especially if mothers are overtreated. Consultation with maternal–fetal medicine is advised for ongoing management of hyperthyroidism in pregnancy.[49,51]

SUMMARY/DISCUSSION/FUTURE DIRECTIONS

Thyroid storm is a life-threatening medical emergency for mother and fetus. Prompt recognition and treatment is required when thyroid storm is suspected, which is ultimately a clinical diagnosis. Predisposing factors in pregnant patients with uncontrolled hyperthyroidism include infection/sepsis, labor and delivery, preeclampsia, or anemia. Pregnant patients have a stronger likelihood of heart failure and a high rate of mortality. Treatment requires rapid evaluation and multidisciplinary care, which is most appropriately performed in the ICU setting. As with other maternal critical disease states, avoiding delivery if the fetal status allows is strongly preferred.

CLINICS CARE POINTS

- Prompt recognition of thyroid storm can be lifesaving, and the most common symptoms include hyperpyrexia, neuropsychiatric symptoms, and tachycardia. Congestive heart failure and arrhythmias are not uncommon.

- Thyroid storm is a clinical diagnosis and based on the presence of severe and life-threatening symptoms (hyperpyrexia, cardiovascular dysfunction, altered mentation) in a patient with biochemical evidence of marked hyperthyroidism. There are no universally accepted criteria or validated clinical tools for diagnosing thyroid storm and no cutoff TH values but in younger individuals, levels are often more than 4 times elevated.

- Intensive care admission and a multidisciplinary team including endocrinology and cardiology is ideal.

- The mainstay of treatment is ATDs in the form of thioamides and iodine should only be given after antithyroid drug therapy has been started to avoid worsening thyrotoxicosis.

- When following treatment after stabilization and hospital discharge, TSH should not be used to monitor response to ATD therapy; rather FT4 or TT4 should be followed and maintained at the upper limit of the normal trimester range.

- Fetal monitoring may show signs of abnormal heart rate tracing, which are typically reversed with treatment of the maternal condition, and delivery is preferably avoided during thyroid storm.

DISCLOSURE

The authors have nothing to disclose.

REFERENCES

1. Sibai BM, Viteri OA. Diabetic Ketoacidosis in Pregnancy. Obstet Gynecol 2014; 123(1):167–78.
2. Carroll MA, Yeomans ER. Diabetic ketoacidosis in pregnancy. Crit Care Med 2005;33(10):S347–53.
3. Morrison FJR, Movassaghian M, Seely EW, et al. Fetal outcomes after diabetic ketoacidosis during pregnancy. Diabetes Care 2017;40:77–9.
4. Parker JA, Conway DL. Diabetic ketoacidosis in pregnancy. Obstet Gynecol Clin North Am 2007;34:533–43.
5. Eledrisi MS, Beshyah SA, Malik RA. Management of diabetic ketoacidosis in special populations. Diabetes Res Clin Pract 2021;174:1–11.

6. Bryant SN, Herrera CL, Nelson DB, et al. Diabetic ketoacidosis complicating pregnancy. J Neonatal Perinatal Med 2017;10:17–23.
7. Tarif N, Al Badr W. Euglycemic diabetic ketoacidosis in pregnancy. Saudi J Kidney Dis Transpl 2007;18(4):590–3.
8. Pinto ME, Villena JE. Diabetic ketoacidosis during gestational diabetes. A case report. Diabetes Res Clin Pract 2011;93(2):e92–4.
9. Kitabchi A, Miles J, Umpierrez G, et al. Hyperglycemic crises in adult patients with diabetes. Diabetes Care 2009;32(7):1335–43.
10. Chiasson J, Aris-jilwan N, Bélanger R, et al. Diagnosis and treatment of diabetic ketoacidosis and the hyperglycemic hyperosmolar state. CMAJ 2003;168(7): 859–66.
11. Barbour LA, Shao J, Qiao L, et al. Human placental growth hormone increases expression of the P85 regulatory unit of phosphatidylinositol 3- kinase and triggers severe insulin resistance in skeletal muscle. Endocrinology 2004;145(3): 1144–50.
12. Barbour LA, McCurdy CE, Hernandez TL, et al. Cellular mechanisms for insulin resistance in normal pregnancy and gestational diabetes. Diabetes Care 2007; 30(2):S112–9.
13. Barbour LA. Metabolic culprits in obese pregnancies and gestational diabetes mellitus: big babies, big twists, big picture. Diabetes Care 2019;42(5):718–26.
14. Buschur EO, Stetson B, Barbour LA, et al. Diabetes in pregnancy. In: Feingold KR, Anawalt B, Boyce A, et al, editors. Endotext. South Dartmouth, MA: Endotext MDText.com, Inc; 2018.
15. Barbour LA, Hernandez TL, Friedman J. Metabolic changes during normal, obese and GDM pregnancies. In: Reece EA, Coustan DR, editors. Diabetes and obesity in women. Philadelphia, PA: Wolters Kluwer; 2019. p. 140–58.
16. Guo R, Yang L, Li L, et al. Diabetic ketoacidosis in pregnancy tends to occur at lower blood glucose levels : Case – control study and a case report of euglycemic diabetic ketoacidosis in pregnancy. J Obstet Gynaecol Res 2008;34(3): 324–30.
17. Madaan M, Aggarwal K, Sharma R, et al. Diabetic ketoacidosis occurring with lower blood glucose levels in pregnancy: a report of two cases. J Reprod Med 2012;57(9–10):452–5.
18. Dalfrà MG, Burlina S, Sartore G, et al. Ketoacidosis in diabetic pregnancy. J Matern Neonatal Med 2016;29(17):2889–95.
19. American College of Obstetricians and Gynecologists Committee on Practice Bulletins. Pregestational diabetes mellitus. ACOG Pract Bull 2018;132(6):228–48.
20. Hagay ZJ, Weissman A, Lurie S, et al. Reversal of fetal distress following intesive treatment of maternal diabetic ketoacidosis. Am J Perinatol 1994;11(6):430–2.
21. Takahashi Y, Kawabata I, Shinohara A, et al. Transient fetal blood flow redistribution induced by maternal diabetic ketoacidosis diagnosed by Doppler ultrasonography. Prenat Diagn 2000;20:517–25.
22. Mohan M, Mrcog M, Ahmed K, et al. Management of diabetic ketoacidosis in pregnancy. Obstet Gynaecol 2017;19:55–62.
23. Morris L, Murphy M, Kitabchi A. Bicarbonate therapy in severe diabetic ketoacidosis. Ann Intern Med 1986;105(6):836–40.
24. Patel MP, Ahmed A, Gunapalan T, et al. Use of sodium bicarbonate and blood gas monitoring in diabetic ketoacidosis: a review. World J Diabetes 2018;9(11): 199–205.
25. Gabbe SG, Graves CR. Management of diabetes mellitus complicating pregnancy. Am Coll Obstet Gynecol 2003;102(4):857–68.

26. Davidson AJF, Park AL, Berger H, et al. Association of improved periconception hemoglobin A 1c with pregnancy outcomes in women with diabetes. JAMA Netw Open 2021;3(12):1–13.

27. American Diabetes Association. Management of diabetes in pregnancy: standards of medical care in diabetes-2020. Diabetes Cdare 2020;43(Suppl): S183–92.

28. Sibai BM. Management of late preterm and early-term pregnancies complicated by mild gestational hypertension/pre-eclampsia. Semin Perinatol 2011;35(5): 292–6.

29. Galindo RJ, Hurtado CR, Pasquel FJ, et al. National trends in incidence, mortality, and clinical outcomes of patients hospitalized for thyrotoxicosis with and without thyroid storm in the United States, 2004-2013. Thyroid 2019;29(1):36–43.

30. Valent A, Barbour L. Thyroid disease in pregnancy. In: Lockwood CJ, Moore TR, Copel JA, et al, editors. Creasy & Resnik's maternal-fetal medicine: principles and practice. 9th edition. Philadelphia (PA): Elsevier; 2022.

31. Lo JC, Rivkees SA, Chandra M, et al. Gestational thyrotoxicosis, antithyroid drug use and neonatal outcomes within an integrated healthcare delivery system. Thyroid 2015;25(6):698–705.

32. ACOG PRACTICE BULLETIN Clinical Management Guidelines for Obstetrician–Gynecologists Number 223. Thyroid Disease in Pregnancy. Obstet Gynecol Surv 2020;135(6):261–74.

33. Taylor PN, Albrecht D, Scholz A, et al. Global epidemiology of hyperthyroidism and hypothyroidism. Nat Rev Endocrinol 2018;14:301–16.

34. Sarlis NJ, Gourgiotis L. Thyroid emergencies. Rev Endocr Metab Disord 2003;4: 129–36.

35. King JR, Lachica R, Lee RH, et al. Diagnosis and management of hyperthyroidism in pregnancy: a review. Obstet Gynecol Surv 2016;71(11):675–85.

36. Sorah K, Alderson T. Hyperthyroidism in pregnancy. In: StatPearls. Treasure Island (FL): StatPearls Publishing; 2021.

37. Sullivan S, Goodier C, Cuff R. Thyroid and parathyroid diseases in pregnancy. In: Landon M, editor. Obstetrics: normal and problem pregnancies. 8th edition. Philadelphia, PA: Elsevier Inc; 2021. p. 919–44.e9.

38. Burch HB, Wartofsky L. Life-threatening thyrotoxicosis: thyroid storm. Endocrinol Metab Clin North Am 1993;22(2):263–77.

39. Cooper DS, Laurberg P. Hyperthyroidism in pregnancy. Lancet Diabetes Endocrinol 2013;1(3):238–49.

40. Nguyen CT, Sasso EB, Barton L, et al. Graves' hyperthyroidism in pregnancy: a clinical review. Clin Diabetes Endocrinol 2018;4(4):1–9.

41. Sheffield JS, Cunningham FG. Thyrotoxicosis and heart failure that complicate pregnancy. Am J Obstet Gynecol 2004;190:211–7.

42. Nayak B, Burman K. Thyrotoxicosis and thyroid storm. Endocrinol Metab Clin North Am 2006;35(4):663–86, vii.

43. Wapner RJ, Sorokin Y, Thom EA, et al. Single versus weekly courses of antenatal corticosteroids: evaluation of safety and efficacy. Am J Obstet Gynecol 2006;195: 633–42.

44. Murphy KE, Hannah ME, Willan AR, et al. Multiple courses of antenatal corticosteroids for preterm birth (MACS): a randomised controlled trial. Lancet 2008;372: 2143–51.

45. Wyble AJ, Moore SC, Yates SG. Weathering the storm: a case of thyroid storm refractory to conventional treatment benefiting from therapeutic plasma exchange. J Clin Apher 2018;33:678–81.

46. Vyas A, Vyas P, Fillipon NL, et al. Successful treatment of thyroid storm with plasmapharesis in a patient with methimazole-induced agranulocytosis. Endocr Pract 2010;16(4):673–6.
47. Sam S, Molitch M. Timing and special concerns regarding endocrine surgery during pregnancy. Endocrinol Metab Clin North Am 2003;32(2):337–54.
48. Kuy S, Roman SA, Desai R, et al. Outcomes following thyroid and parathyroid surgery in pregnant women. Arch Surg 2009;144(5):399–407.
49. Alexander EK, Pearce EN, Brent GA, et al. 2017 Guidelines of the american thyroid association for the diagnosis and management of thyroid disease during pregnancy and the postpartum. Thyroid 2017;27(3). https://doi.org/10.1089/thy.2016.0457.
50. Männistö T, Mendola P, Grewal J, et al. Thyroid diseases and adverse pregnancy outcomes in a contemporary US Cohort. J Clin Endocrinol Metab 2013;98(7):2725–33.
51. Donnelly MA, Wood C, Casey B, et al. Early severe fetal graves disease in a mother after thyroid ablation and thyroidectomy. Obstet Gynecol 2015;125(5):1059–62.

Shoulder Dystocia
Challenging Basic Assumptions

Suneet P. Chauhan, MD, Hon.D.Sc[a], Robert B. Gherman, MD[b],*

KEYWORDS

- Shoulder dystocia • Neonatal acidemia • Hypoxic-ischemic injury
- Neonatal brachial plexus palsy

KEY POINTS

- The current basis for rapid institution of obstetric maneuvers to alleviate the shoulder dystocia rests on the belief that a reduction in the duration of the shoulder dystocia will mitigate neonatal acidemia and/or hypoxic-ischemic injury. Additional prospective studies are needed to validate the normal head-to-body time, as well as to determine if the "two-step" approach reduces the incidence of shoulder dystocia.
- When describing traction, the goal should be to avoid a subjective assessment of an objective process. We may come to understand that "excessive" force really means a degree of force that is too great for the current situation or above the injury producing threshold of the nerve, rather than being above some arbitrarily defined threshold.
- Until further studies accurately define which patients will experience recurrent shoulder dystocia, we recommend that patients be allowed to make an informed decision, after discussion and documentation of the inherent risks in elective cesarean and attempted vaginal delivery.
- Current strategies to achieve a reduction in neonatal brachial plexus palsy—identification of risk factors, elective cesarean delivery in prespecified conditions, or implementation of shoulder dystocia simulation or drills—are insufficient to reliably decrease the rate of the most common neurologic injury associated with shoulder dystocia.

There are no randomized clinical trials to provide clinical care guidelines for obstetric providers in the management of shoulder dystocia. Most of our knowledge pertaining to this obstetric emergency has emanated from case reports and retrospective studies that have subsequently resulted in empirical management protocols. In this article, we seek to challenge conventional wisdom surrounding current management techniques for shoulder dystocia.

[a] Department of OB/GYN, Division of Maternal/Fetal Medicine, The University of Texas Health Sciences Center at Houston McGovern Medical School, UT Houston, 6431 Fannin, MSB 3.266, Houston, TX 77030, USA; [b] Department of OB/GYN, Division of Maternal/Fetal Medicine, Wellspan Health System York PA, 21636 Ripplemead Drive, Laytonsville, MD 20882, USA
* Corresponding author.
E-mail address: ghermdoc@gmail.com

Obstet Gynecol Clin N Am 49 (2022) 491–500
https://doi.org/10.1016/j.ogc.2022.02.005   obgyn.theclinics.com
0889-8545/22/© 2022 Elsevier Inc. All rights reserved.

CONVENTIONAL ASSUMPTIONS IN SHOULDER DYSTOCIA

- "Two-step" versus "one-step" approach to delivery
- Objective definition of traction
- Shoulder dystocia injury types
  - Future research
- Injury reduction interventions.
  - Ultrasound predictions
  - Cesarean delivery

SHOULD WE ADOPT A "TWO-STEP" APPROACH?

Shoulder dystocia occurs when there is impaction of the anterior fetal shoulder behind the maternal symphysis pubis. It also can occur from impaction of the posterior fetal shoulder on the sacral promontory. As such, the occurrence of shoulder dystocia occurs before the emergence of the fetal head from the maternal vagina. The obstetric provider, therefore, will diagnose shoulder dystocia as a delivery that requires additional obstetric maneuvers following failure of gentle downward traction on the fetal head to effect delivery of the shoulders. Retraction of the delivered fetal head against the maternal perineum (turtle sign) may be present and may assist in the diagnosis. However, one-third of obstetric providers who participated in an online survey responded that the diagnosis of shoulder dystocia is subjective.[1]

The current basis for rapid institution of obstetric maneuvers to alleviate the shoulder dystocia rests on the belief that a reduction in the duration of the shoulder dystocia will mitigate neonatal acidemia and/or hypoxic-ischemic injury. It is currently recommended that a shoulder dystocia occurrence be relieved as soon as possible as the clinician is unable to predict the time required to effect delivery in the face of shoulder dystocia, as well as the inability to determine which shoulder dystocia even will be intractable. This has led to major textbooks to recommend a "one-step" approach, in which delivery of the body is accomplished immediately after delivery of the head. However, the evidence cited by most authors appear to be based on a single study of 22 patients, which suggested a rapid (0.14 U/min) decrease in the umbilical artery pH during the expulsive phase.[2] Studies on the effects of head-to-body interval on neonatal blood gas analysis in the context of shoulder dystocia have not identified a statistically significant relationship.[3,4]

Locatelli and colleagues note that in several institutions outside of the United States, assistance to vaginal delivery uses a "two-step" approach.[5] This method recommends waiting for subsequent contractions to accomplish delivery of the body if the shoulders are not delivered after expulsion of the head. In a prospective study, in which head-to-body interval was timed in 789 deliveries, the mean head-to-body interval was 88 ± 61 seconds. The observed decrease in umbilical artery pH observed in the head-to-body interval was not statistically significant after controlling for the duration of the second stage of labor. In addition, the decrease in umbilical artery pH was only 0.0078 U/min. Zhang[6] recently completed a randomized controlled trial in which 364 women in the study group (delivered by a "two-step" method, in which providers waited for at least one uterine contraction) were compared with 257 cases in the control group (delivery of the shoulder by gentle pressure on the fetal head. The rate of shoulder dystocia was higher in the control group (4/257, 1.55%) as compared with the study group (0/364, 0.00%), $P = .03$. In the one-step group, the mean head-to-shoulder interval was 44.17 seconds, implying that Spong's prior data requires a critical reappraisal.[7]

An infrequently used definition of shoulder dystocia was proposed by Spong in her 1995 article,[7,8] in which 250 deliveries were prospectively timed. The mean intervals in nonmaneuver patients included: head to anterior shoulder 14.8 ± 1.0, anterior to posterior shoulder 3.9 ± 0.6, posterior shoulder to body 54. ± 0.8, and total head-to-body time 24.2 ± 1.3 seconds. The authors arbitrarily proposed defining shoulder dystocia as a prolonged head-to-body delivery time as the mean plus two standard deviations (60 seconds). However, this would have generated an incidence of shoulder dystocia of 11.6% (29/250), which is incongruous with previously reported clinical data. There were only 29 patients with head-to-body delivery intervals ≥ 60 seconds; when maneuvers were used (n = 27), the mean head-to-body time was found to be 82.6 ± 21.5 seconds. Although ancillary obstetric maneuvers were used in 27 of 250 deliveries (10.8%), shoulder dystocia was recognized and recorded by the obstetric attendant in only 16 of these cases. The authors therefore recommended that "further study is needed to confirm the prolonged value of sixty seconds." In a follow-on study, Beall noted 99 deliveries (13.6%) complicated by shoulder dystocia among 725 deliveries, as defined objectively. Among the 99 deliveries, 46 were completed with the assistance of ancillary obstetric maneuvers and 72 had head-to-body times ≥ 60 seconds. The mean head-to-body time was greater among shoulder dystocia cases (67 ± 3 vs 25 ± 1 seconds), but a P value for statistical significance was not generated. At this time, additional prospective studies are needed to validate the normal head-to-body time, as well as to determine if the "two-step" approach reduces the incidence of shoulder dystocia.

TRACTION: IS THERE AN OBJECTIVE DEFINITION?

Older textbooks have sparingly described the subjective direction and degree of traction that should be used during normal vaginal deliveries. In Gabbe's Obstetrics, it is stated that "Once the fetal head is delivered, external rotation (restitution) is allowed; if shoulder dystocia is anticipated, it is appropriate to proceed directly with gentle downward traction of the fetal head before restitution occurs. The anterior shoulder should then be delivered by gentle downward traction in concern with maternal expulsive efforts."[9] Williams Obstetrics likewise notes that "The sides of the head are grasped with two hands, and gentle downward traction is applied until the anterior shoulder appears under the pubic arch. ...With prolonged delay, however, its birth may be hastened by moderate traction on the head and moderate pressure on the uterine fundus."[10]

Neither ACOG Practice Pattern Number 7[11] nor the ACOG Practice Bulletin Number 40[12] mentions the direction in which traction should be used. The Royal College Guideline Number 42 stated that "Routine traction in an axial direction may be employed to diagnose shoulder dystocia."[13,14] However, the word axial is not defined in the RCOG Bulletin and the word "routine" is defined as "that traction required for delivery of the shoulders in a normal vaginal delivery where there is no difficulty with the shoulders."[13] A subsequent edition of the Royal College Bulletin[15] stated that "axial traction is traction in line with the fetal spine (ie, without lateral deviation)," whereas the ACOG 2017 Bulletin defines that "axial traction is applied in alignment with the fetal cervico-thoracic spine and has a downward component typically along a vector estimated to be 25-45 degrees below the horizontal plane when the laboring woman is in a lithotomy position."[16]

A few recent studies have attempted to evaluate force applied during simulated deliveries complicated by shoulder dystocia. Walters makes no mention of any angle of traction in her shoulder dystocia study, where providers rated the amount of force applied as "normal" or "excessive" during both "calm" and "stressed" deliveries.[17]

In addition to the standardly described maneuvers, additional key components for the management of shoulder dystocia include the angle of movement of the fetal head, duration and angle of traction, and time. To semiquantitatively assess the extent to which the fetal head was moved downward, upward, or laterally, Ankumah[18] proposed a visual analog scale. The results of this study revealed that 2 clinicians observing the maximum downward and upward movements of the fetal head could not agree with each other. Although this prospective observational study was limited by small sample size, it identified that the maximum angle the fetal head was moved downward, or upward during vaginal birth was not reproducible (ie, poor interobserver variability).

We believe that additional research endeavors are needed to objectively define the normal degree and direction of traction inherent in all vaginal deliveries. Studies are needed to determine the angle of head movement in an uncomplicated vaginal delivery. Ideally, clinicians delivering or observing the delivery should also be able to reliably estimate the extent to which the head is moved during normal delivery and the extent of traction applied. Rather than using terms such as "gentle," "downward," or "normal," the goal should be to avoid a subjective assessment of an objective process. As criteria are established to assess these parameters, we may come to understand that "excessive" force really means a degree of force that is too great for the current situation or above the injury producing threshold of the nerve, rather than being above some arbitrarily defined threshold.

INJURY AT THE TIME OF SHOULDER DYSTOCIA: FUTURE RESEARCH EFFORTS

Brachial plexus injuries are classically defined as Erb's or Klumpke's palsies. Erb's (upper) type palsy involves cranial nerves C5 and C6. It is recognizable by the characteristic "waiter's tip" arm position caused by muscle imbalance that holds the shoulder in an adducted, internally rotated position with the elbow in extension and forearm in pronation. Klumpke's palsy reflects damage to the lower cervical and upper thoracic nerve roots (C8 and T1). Findings typically associated with Klumpke's palsy are internal rotation of the shoulder, inability to abduct the shoulder, and forearm pronation.

The cause of neonatal brachial plexus palsy (NBPP) associated with shoulder dystocia remains a poorly understood entity, the investigation of which is challenging. Studies have confirmed the inability of obstetricians and midwives to prospectively predict its occurrence. They further reveal that the injury reflects a complex application of internal and external forces that may be applied either antepartum -or intrapartum.[19] Finally, the available evidence suggests that the greatest forces are the result of internal forces outside the control of the accoucheur.

In the past 10 to 15 years, epidemiologic data, case studies, and computer modeling have all provided support to the concept that brachial plexus stretch and injury can result from endogenous forces when the neonate's shoulder presses against the maternal symphysis pubis or sacral promontory.[20] It has been consistently reported that approximately 50% of brachial plexus palsies occur in the absence of clinically recognized shoulder dystocia.[20]

The forces underlying injurious lateral traction may be endogenous (related to maternal and uterine expulsion forces) in the setting of an impacted fetal shoulder, or they may be exogenous (related to the process of delivering the fetal head). This endogenous force can occur without clinician awareness or involvement in the delivery process. The 2014 American College of Obstetrics and Gynecology Task Force Manuscript on Neonatal Brachial Plexus has stated that the existence of brachial plexus palsy does not a priori indicate that exogenous forces were the cause of the injury.[20] When the infant's anterior shoulder impacts against the symphysis pubis, the force resisting delivery is greater on the anterior side of the fetal body as compared with the posterior side. This results in a differential motion between the infant's neck, which continues to advance through the outward maternal force, and the impacted shoulder. Stretching of the brachial plexus occurs because of disproportionate descent, with uterine contractions and maternal pushing providing the necessary intrauterine forces.[21,22] During a posterior shoulder impaction at the level of the sacral promontory, the fetal injury likely precedes expulsion of the fetal head. During descent of the fetus through the maternal pelvis, there is impaction on the sacral promontory and subsequent brachial plexus stretch.

The main challenge remains with regard to how to incorporate the reported risk factors of shoulder dystocia, macrosomia, gestational diabetes, and operative vaginal delivery. These risk factors appear to mediate through fetal birth weight, which is only known after the birth has occurred. Obstetric providers are further hampered by the imprecise nature of clinical and ultrasonographic estimation of weight and an inability to predict exactly which labors will be affected by shoulder dystocia. Moreover, studies of shoulder dystocia simulation have shown no reduction in the incidence of permanent brachial plexus palsy. At this time, no intervention has been identified that will prevent all or even most cases of NBPP. Further research is needed to address[1]: How can obstetric antepartum and intrapartum care be changed to convert these risk factors to modifiable events?[2] Are there specific interventions that may reduce the frequency of NBPP? Only a few studies, from which meaningful conclusions cannot be ascertained, have attempted to address the clinical salient questions pertinent to injury prediction:

1. How does the presence of clavicular fracture influence the rate of neonatal brachial plexus injury associated with shoulder dystocia?[23–25]
2. What factors are associated with neonatal injury following shoulder dystocia?[26–29]
3. Does the use of multiple maneuvers in the management of shoulder dystocia increase the risk of permanent neonatal injury?[23,28,30]
4. Does the length of the 2nd stage impact shoulder dystocia outcomes?[31]
5. Which brachial plexus injuries will resolve and which will become permanent?[28,32–35]

INTERVENTIONS TO DECREASE SHOULDER DYSTOCIA RELATED NEONATAL BRACHIAL PLEXUS PALSY

Traditionally, attempts to decrease the rate of NBPP have focused on 3 strategies related to shoulder dystocia: (1) identification of risk factors for brachial palsy, (2) cesarean delivery for those at high-risk for NBPP, or (3) simulation exercises to manage shoulder dystocia.[36,37] The American College of Obstetricians and Gynecologists Practice Bulletins (PB)[16,38] have identified several factors that are associated with a birth weight of at least 4000 g or with an impacted anterior shoulder (**Table 1**). Thus, it is surmised that awareness of these factors alone can reduce the occurrence of NBPP. There are several shortcomings with this supposition. First, although some of these risk factors are predictable at the first prenatal visit, others are not apparent until the start of labor and some not until the shoulder dystocia (eg, precipitous second stage of labor or macrosomic newborn) has actually occurred. Secondly, it is assumed that the risk factors are additive, though the evidence is lacking in this regard. Third, awareness of a risk factor may increase the likelihood of potentially harmful interventions. Suspected macrosomia, for example, is linked with an increased rate of cesarean delivery without concomitant improvement in neonatal outcomes.[39] Fourth, there

Table 1
Risk factors for macrosomia or shoulder dystocia

	Macrosomia	Shoulder Dystocia
At First Prenatal Visit	Maternal weight at birth > 8 lbs.	
	Grand multiparity	Multiparity
	History of macrosomia	History of shoulder dystocia
	Preexisting diabetes	Preexisting diabetes
	Obesity	
Antepartum Visits	An abnormal value on glucose tolerance test	
	Gestational diabetes	Gestational diabetes
	Excessive gestational weight gain	Excessive gestational weight gain
	Male fetus	
	Estimated fetal weight ≥ 4000 g	AC - BPD
Intrapartum	Gestational age	Oxytocin use
	Estimated fetal weight ≥ 4000 g	Epidural us
		Precipitous second stage of labor
		Prolonged second stage of labor
		Operative vaginal delivery

Abbreviations: AC, abdominal circumference; BPD, biparietal diameter.
Data from ACOG Committee on Practice Bulletins-Gynecology, The American College of Obstetrician and Gynecologists. ACOG practice bulletin clinical management guidelines for obstetrician-gynecologists. Number 40, November 2002. Obstet Gynecol. 2002;100(5 Pt 1):1045-1050. https://doi.org/10.1016/s0029-7844(0202513-9;) and Practice Bulletin No 178: Shoulder Dystocia. Obstet Gynecol. 2017;129(5):e123-e133. https://doi.org/10.1097/AOG.0000000000002043.

is a lack of evidence that foreknowledge of risk factors, combined with clinical acumen, actually decreases the rate of NBPP. Finally, a recent multicenter study found that it is not possible to identify which newborn will or will not experience NBPP after a shoulder dystocia.[40]

The most recent American College of OB/GYN Practice Bulletin[16] recommends that "Elective cesarean delivery should be considered for women without diabetes who are carrying fetuses with suspected macrosomia with an estimated fetal weight of at least 5,000 g and for women with diabetes whose fetuses are estimated to weigh at least 4500 g." The underpinning of the ACOG recommendation appears to be the paper by Rouse and colleagues, published in 1996.[41] First, the recommendation is not based on an observational study or preinterventional and postinterventional trials. Secondly, the study was published over 25 years ago and should be reevaluated based on current estimated fetal weight thresholds. Most newborns with a birth weight over 4500 g are not identified before birth. At a teaching hospital, with over 4100 deliveries in a year, none of the 57 newborns with a weight of 4500 g were identified prenatally.[42] Fourth, the Rouse's cost-effective analysis is based on sonographic estimated fetal weight alone, although it has been recognized that clinical and ultrasonographic assessment of a newborn's weight have similar accuracy.[43] In addition, there is uncertainty about the time interval when sonographic estimated fetal weight needs to be repeated. Some studies have suggested that to identify newborns with a birth weight of at least 4500 g, the sonographic estimated fetal weight should be done weekly.[43,44] Finally, there are significant challenges and limitations of ultrasound to not only accurately predict the estimated fetal weight but to also predict the risk of shoulder dystocia based on specific body-to-head disproportions, such as those seen in diabetics.[45]

A prior history of delivery complicated by shoulder dystocia confers a 6-fold to nearly 30-fold increased risk of shoulder dystocia recurrence in a subsequent vaginal delivery, with most reported rates between 12% and 17%.[46,47] A simplistic conclusion from this statistical might be that all individuals with a history of shoulder dystocia should be offered cesarean delivery with subsequent pregnancies. However, the prior history of shoulder dystocia may not be known to the clinician. Although the birthweight of the newborn who experienced shoulder dystocia is known, the actual weight of the newborn in a subsequent pregnancy is not realistically foreseeable. The risk factors that were present with the shoulder dystocia in prior pregnancies may not be present in the subsequent gestation. Uncommon complications, including maternal death, have been reported in an attempt to avert recurrent shoulder dystocia by elective primary cesarean delivery.[48] At present, there is insufficient evidence that cesarean should be routinely performed to reduce the risk of recurrent shoulder, without increasing maternal morbidity. Until further studies accurately define which patients will experience recurrent shoulder dystocia, we recommend that patients be allowed to make an informed decision, after discussion and documentation of the inherent risks in elective cesarean and attempted vaginal delivery.

The American College of OB/GYN and Royal College of Obstetricians and Gynecologists currently advocate for simulation exercises in an attempt to reduce the complications associated with shoulder dystocia.[15,16] A recent systematic review and Bayesian meta-analysis of all publications on the topic, however, has provided several reasons to question ACOG's level B recommendation.[49] Of the 16 articles that met the study's inclusion criteria, notable variations in shoulder dystocia simulation exercises were noted, including instructor type, whether mannequins were used, the frequency of exercises, and whether attendance was mandatory. Compared with the preimplementation period, implementation of shoulder dystocia interventional exercises significantly increased both the diagnosis of shoulder dystocia and the cesarean delivery rate.[48] No simulation study to date, however, has shown an effect with regard to the rate of persistent brachial plexus palsy, the main area of concern.[49–52] Crofts's time-interrupted series from the United Kingdom did report a reduction in brachial plexus injury at birth, but this decrease in neonatal morbidity was not seen at 6 or 12 months after birth (55). In a study from Ireland, there was no change in the overall rate of NBPP after despite training.[52] In conclusion, current strategies to achieve a reduction in NBPP—identification of risk factors, elective cesarean delivery in prespecified conditions, the infrequent nature of permanent injury, or implementation of shoulder dystocia simulation or drills—are insufficient to reliably decrease the rate of the most common neurologic injury associated with shoulder dystocia.

In summary, this article has identified the existence of large gaps in our clinical knowledge base with regard to the prevention and resolution of shoulder dystocia, as well as its long-term sequelae. Decisions without data are dubious.[48] We have attempted to challenge current recommendations with regard to whether prophylactic cesarean delivery should be performed based on estimated fetal weight alone or a prior history of shoulder dystocia, shoulder dystocia management techniques, what defines "excessive" traction, and the role of simulation training for all clinicians. We hope that this article helps to set the stage for necessary future research to understand and address this incredibly anxiety provoking clinical dilemma.

DISCLOSURE

The authors have nothing to disclose.

REFERENCES

1. Gherman RB, Chauhan SP, Lewis DF. Shoulder dystocia: A survey of Central Association Members about its definition, management, and complications. Obstet Gynecol 2012;119:83–7.
2. Wood C, Ng KH, Hounslow D. Time: an important variable in normal delivery. J Obstet Gynecol Br Commonw 1973;80:295–300.
3. Stallings SP, Edwards RK, Johsnon JWC. Correlation of head-to-body delivery intervals in shoulder dystocia and umbilical artery acidosis. Am J Obstet Gynecol 2001;185:268–74.
4. Allen RH, Rosenbaum TC, Ghidini A, et al. Correlating head-to-body delivery intervals with neonatal depression in vaginal births that result in permanent brachial plexus injury. Am J Obstet Gynecol 2002;187(4):839–42. https://doi.org/10.1067/mob.2002.127128.
5. Locatelli A, Incerti M, Ghidini A, et al. Head-to-body delivery interval using "two step" approach in vaginal deliveries: Effect on umbilical artery pH. J Maternal-fetal Med Neonatal Med 2011;24:799–808.
6. Zhang H, Zhao N, Lu Y, et al. Two-step shoulder delivery method reduces the incidence of shoulder dystocia. Clin Exp Obstet Gynecol 2017;44(3):347–435.
7. Spong CY, Beall M, Rodrigues D, et al. An objective definition of shoulder dystocia: Prolonged head-to-body delivery intervals and/or the use of ancillary obstetric maneuvers. Obstet Gynecol 1995;86:433–6.
8. Beall MH, Spong C, McKay J, et al. Objective definition of shoulder dystocia: A prospective evaluation. Am J Obstet Gynecol 1998;179:934–7.
9. Kilpatrick S, Garrison E. Normal labor and delivery. In: Gabbe SG, Niebyl JR, Simpson JL, editors. Obstetrics: normal and Problem pregnancies. 5th edition. Churchill Livingstone; 2007. p. 303–21.
10. Cunningham FG, Gant NF, Leveno KJ, et al. Conduct of normal labor and delivery. Williams Obstetrics 21st edition. Mc-Graw HIill; 2001. p. 309–29.
11. ACOG practice patterns. Shoulder dystocia. Number 7, October 1997. American College of Obstetricians and Gynecologists. Int J Gynaecol Obstet 1998;60(3):306–13.
12. ACOG Committee on Practice Bulletins-Gynecology. The American College of Obstetrician and Gynecologists. ACOG practice bulletin clinical management guidelines for obstetrician-gynecologists. Number 40, November 2002. Obstet Gynecol 2002;100(5 Pt 1):1045–50. https://doi.org/10.1016/s0029-7844(02)02513-9.
13. Royal College of Obstetricians and Gynaecologists. RCOG Guideline No. 42. 2005. Dec.
14. Chauhan SP, Gherman R, Hendrix NW, et al. Shoulder dystocia: Comparison of the ACOG practice bulletin with another national guideline. Am J Perinatol 2010;27:129–36.
15. Royal College of OB/GYN Guideline Number 42 (2nd edition). Shoulder dystocia. March 2012.
16. Practice Bulletin No 178: Shoulder Dystocia. Obstet Gynecol 2017;129(5):e123–33. https://doi.org/10.1097/AOG.0000000000002043.
17. Walters M, EubanksA, Weissbrod E, et al. Visual estimation of force applied during simulated deliveries complicated by shoulder dystocia. Am J Perinatol Rep 2018;8:e206–2011.

18. Ankumah NE, Chauhan VB, Pedroza C, et al. Angles, traction, and time after delivery of fetal head: Interobserver variation of novel visual analogs. Am J Perinatol 2017;34:1424–514.

19. Dunbar DC, Vilensky JA, Suárez-Quian CA, et al. Risk factors for neonatal brachial plexus palsy attributed to anatomy, physiology, and evolution. Clin Anat 2021;34(6):884–98. https://doi.org/10.1002/ca.23739.

20. Neonatal Brachial Plexus Palsy. acog.org. 2014. Available at. https://www.acog.org/clinical/clinical-guidance/task-force-report/articles/2014/neonatal-brachial-plexus-palsy.

21. Grimm MJ. Maternal endogenous forces and shoulder dystocia. Clin Obstet Gynecol 2016;59:820–9.

22. Wagner SM, Bell CS, Gupta M, et al. Interventions to decrease complications after shoulder dystocia: a systematic review and Bayesian meta-analysis. Am J Obstet Gynecol 2021;225:484–93.

23. Iskender C, Kaymak O, Erkenekli K, et al. Neonatal injury at cephalic vaginal delivery: A retrospective analysis of extent of association with shoulder dystocia. PLOS One 2014;9:1–6.

24. Wall LB, Mills JK, Leveno K, et al. Incidence and prognosis of neonatal brachial plexus palsy with and without clavicular fractures. Obstet Gynecol 2014;123:1288–93.

25. Gandhi RA, DeFrancesco CJ, Shah AS. The association of clavicle fracture with brachial plexus palsy. J Hand Surg Am 2018;1:e1–6.

26. McLaren RA, Chang KW, Ankuma NA, et al. Persistence of neonatal brachial plexus palsy among nulliparous versus parous women. Am J Perinatol Rep 2019;9:1–5.

27. Spain JE, Frey HA, Tuuli MG, et al. Neonatal morbidity associated with shoulder dystocia maneuvers. Am J Obstet Gynecol 2015;212:e1–5.

28. Doty MS, Chauhan SP, Chang KW, et al. Persistence and extent of neonatal brachial plexus palsy: Association with number of maneuvers and duration of shoulder. Am J Perinatol Rep 2020;10:e42–8.

29. Mehta SH, Blackwell SC, Bujold E, et al. What factors are associated with neonatal injury following shoulder dystocia? J Perinatol 2006;26:85–8.

30. Hoffman MK, Bailit JL, Branch DW, et al. A comparison of obstetric maneuvers for the acute management of shoulder dystocia. Obstet Gynecol 2011;117:1272–8.

31. Moragianni VA, Hacker MR, Craparo FJ. The impact of length of second stage of labor on shoulder dystocia outcomes: a retrospective cohort study. J Perinat Med 2012;40:463–5.

32. Gherman RB, Ouzounian JG, Satin AJ, et al. A comparison of shoulder dystocia-associated transient and permanent brachial plexus palsies. Obstet Gynecol 2003;102:544–8.

33. Mollberg M, Lagerkvist AL, Johansson U, et al. Comparison in obstetric management on infants with transient and persistent obstetric brachial plexus palsy. J Child Neurol 2008;23:1424–32.

34. Wilson TJ, Chang KW, Chauhan SP, et al. Peripartum and neonatal factors associated with the persistence of neonatal brachial plexus palsy at one year: A review of 382 cases. J Neurosurg Pediatr 2016;17:618–24.

35. Pondaag W, Allen RH, Malessy MJA. Correlating birthweight with neurological severity of obstetric brachial plexus lesions. BJOG 2011;118:1098–103.

36. Chauhan SP, Rose CH, Gherman RB, et al. Brachial plexus injury: a 23-year experience from a tertiary center. Am J Obstet Gynecol 2005;192:1795–800.

37. Chang KW, Ankumah NA, Wilson TJ, et al. Persistence of Neonatal Brachial Plexus Palsy Associated with Maternally Reported Route of Delivery: Review of 387 Cases. Am J Perinatol 2016;33:765–9.
38. Macrosomia: ACOG Practice Bulletin, Number 216. Obstet Gynecol 2020;135: e18–35.
39. Chauhan SP, Grobman WA, Gherman RA, et al. Suspicion and treatment of the macrosomic fetus: a review. Am J Obstet Gynecol 2005;193:332–46.
40. Narendran LM, Mendez-Figueroa H, Chauhan SP, et al. Predictors of neonatal brachial plexus palsy subsequent to resolution of shoulder dystocia. J Matern Fetal Neonatal Med 2021;1–7.
41. Rouse DJ, Owen J, Goldenberg RL, et al. The effectiveness and costs of elective cesarean delivery for fetal macrosomia diagnosed by ultrasound. JAMA 1996; 276:1480–6.
42. Heywood RE, Magann EF, Rich DL, et al. The detection of macrosomia at a teaching hospital. Am J Perinatol 2009;26:165–8.
43. Chauhan SP, Hendrix NW, Magann EF, et al. A review of sonographic estimate of fetal weight: vagaries of accuracy. J Matern Fetal Neonatal Med 2005;18:211–20.
44. Bicocca MJ, Le TN, Zhang CC, et al. Identification of newborns with birthweight ≥ 4,500g: Ultrasound within one- vs. two weeks of delivery. Eur J Obstet Gynecol Reprod Biol 2020;249:47–53.
45. Doty MS, Al-Hafez L, Chauhan SP. Sonographic Examination of The Fetus Vis-à-Vis Shoulder Dystocia: A Vexing Promise. Clin Obstet Gynecol 2016;59(4): 795–802.
46. Bingham J, Chauhan SP, Hayes E, et al. Recurrent shoulder dystocia: a review. Obstet Gynecol Surv 2010;65:183–8.
47. Recurrent shoulder dystocia: risk factors and counselling. In: Gurewitsch-Allen, editor. Clin Obstet Gynecol 2016;59:803–12.
48. Chauhan RS, Chauhan SP. Montgomery v Lanarkshire Health Board: a paradigm shift. BJOG 2017;124:1152.
49. Wagner SM, Bell CS, Gupta M, et al. Interventions to decrease complications after shoulder dystocia: a systematic review and Bayesian meta-analysis. Am J Obstet Gynecol 2021;225:484.e1–33.
50. Gurewitsch Allen ED, Will SE, Allen RH, et al. Improving shoulder dystocia management and outcomes with a targeted quality assurance program. Am J Perinatol 2017;34:1088–96.
51. Crofts JF, Lenguerrand E, Bentham GL, et al. Prevention of brachial plexus injury-12 years of shoulder dystocia training: an interrupted time-series study. BJOG 2016;123:111–8.
52. Walsh JM, Kandamany N, Ni Shuibhne N, et al. Neonatal brachial plexus injury: comparison of incidence and antecedents between 2 decades. Am J Obstet Gynecol 2011;204:324.e1-6.

Hypertensive Crisis in Pregnancy

Cynthie K. Wautlet, MD, MPH[a],*, Maria C. Hoffman, MD, MSc[a,b,1]

KEYWORDS

- Pregnancy • Hypertension • Hypertensive crisis • Antihypertensive treatment
- Preeclampsia

KEY POINTS

- Hypertensive disorders impact 1 in 10 pregnancies and are a leading cause of preventable maternal morbidity and mortality.
- Current data show a quality gap, with timely pharmacologic treatment (within 30–60 minutes of recognition) being achieved in less than 50% of severe hypertensive episodes.
- Hypertensive disorders during pregnancy are a source of health disparities, with a maternal mortality ratio related to hypertensive disease nearly 4-fold higher among Blacks than Whites.

INTRODUCTION/BACKGROUND/PREVALENCE

Hypertensive disorders in pregnancy are common, affecting up to 1 in 10 pregnancies, and are a leading cause of preventable maternal morbidity and mortality.[1–4] Most medical practitioners will, therefore, encounter pregnant individuals with acute-onset, severely elevated BP who are at risk for end-organ damage and maternal or fetal death. Recognition and timely treatment are crucial to reduce the incidence of serious preventable adverse perinatal outcomes.

Outside of pregnancy, acute severe hypertension (HTN) is defined as a BP > 180/110 to 120 reproducible on 2 occasions as measured by a reliable device.[5] When accompanied by end-organ damage such as stroke, retinal hemorrhages, acute coronary syndrome, or kidney injury, this is deemed "hypertensive emergency," a source of significant short-term morbidity and mortality. Without end-organ damage, acute severe HTN is referred to as "hypertensive urgency" and outpatient management can be undertaken given little association with acute morbidity and a slower goal

[a] Department of Obstetrics and Gynecology, University of Colorado School of Medicine, Denver, CO, USA; [b] Department of Psychiatry, University of Colorado School of Medicine, Denver, CO, USA
[1] Present address: 12631 East 17th Avenue, B-108-1, MFM Division, Academic Office 1, Aurora, CO 80045.
* Corresponding author. 12631 East 17th Avenue, Aurora, CO 80045.
E-mail address: Cynthia.wautlet@cuanschutz.edu
Twitter: @CynthieWautlet (C.K.W.)

Obstet Gynecol Clin N Am 49 (2022) 501–519
https://doi.org/10.1016/j.ogc.2022.02.016
0889-8545/22/© 2022 Elsevier Inc. All rights reserved.

obgyn.theclinics.com

for BP lowering. Together, hypertensive emergency and urgency make up "hypertensive crisis," though agreement on this terminology is not universal. Severe HTN, or "crisis," in pregnancy is defined at a lower BP threshold, leading to potential for under-recognition and delayed inpatient evaluation and management.

Severe HTN in pregnancy is a medical emergency, defined by the American College of Obstetricians and Gynecologists (ACOG) as persistent (consecutive or nonconsecutive) SBP ≥ 160 mm Hg and/or DBP ≥ 110 mm Hg taken 15 minutes up to 4 or more hours apart.[6] Confirmation of severe HTN within 15 minutes can eliminate preventable delay and help ensure timely treatment. ACOG does not define hypertensive "crisis," which includes both hypertensive urgency and emergency in the nonpregnant state. However, ACOG's definition of severe hypertension in pregnancy does encapsulate both hypertensive urgency and emergency due to the lower BP threshold at which pregnant individuals are at risk for end-organ damage, including stroke and death.[7] Recent data published by the California maternal mortality review committee showed that stroke accounted for more than 60% of preeclampsia-related maternal deaths, and nearly all were preceded by SBP greater than 160 mm Hg.[8] This lower BP threshold in pregnancy may be a significant contributor to under-recognition, especially in nonobstetrical health care settings.

When HTN in pregnancy is severe OR is accompanied by any of the following, this is defined as preeclampsia with severe features, regardless of the presence or absence of proteinuria:[6]

- Thrombocytopenia with platelets below 100 x 10^9/L
- Elevated liver function tests to twice the upper limit of normal without alternative etiology
- Persistent right upper quadrant and/or epigastric pain unresponsive to medication
- Renal insufficiency with the doubling of baseline creatinine or creatinine greater than 1.1 mg/dL
- Pulmonary edema
- Headache unresponsive to medication without alternative etiology
- Visual disturbances

Making the diagnosis of preeclampsia with severe features superimposed on pre-existing chronic HTN can be clinically challenging and may warrant specialty consultation. Preeclampsia with severe features carries a 3% to 4% risk of eclampsia,[9] characterized by new-onset seizures in the absence of other causes with associated risk for maternal hypoxia, aspiration pneumonia, and death. Neurologic symptoms such as severe headache, visual changes, and altered mental status warrant particular attention, as up to 83% of eclamptic seizures are preceded by these warning signs,[10] although eclamptic seizures can occur in 20% to 38% of cases without warning.[11]

There are numerous reported medical risk factors for the development of hypertensive pregnancy disorders including chronic kidney disease, chronic HTN, obesity, diabetes, autoimmune disorders such as lupus and antiphospholipid syndrome, obstructive sleep apnea, and advanced maternal age. Obstetric risk factors include nulliparity, multifetal gestation, prior pregnancy complicated by hypertensive disorder or placental insufficiency, and use of assisted reproductive technology. However, most pregnant individuals who develop HTN and preeclampsia are otherwise healthy,[6] making it crucial to recognize and treat severe HTN in all pregnant individuals regardless of identifiable risk factors.

There is a broad spectrum of adverse outcomes that can result from severe HTN during pregnancy.[6] In addition to eclampsia and its associated risks, other adverse outcomes include oliguria, renal failure, coagulopathy, subcapsular liver hematoma, pulmonary edema, stroke, congestive heart failure, and death. Adverse pregnancy outcomes include placental abruption, fetal growth restriction, oligohydramnios, spontaneous and iatrogenic preterm birth, and stillbirth. The pathophysiology underlying these adverse outcomes is only partially understood and is the subject of much ongoing investigation.

Newer evidence has shed light on racial and ethnic disparities in the prevalence of adverse outcomes related to HTN in pregnancy[12] and additionally points to significant quality gaps in the timeliness of treatment.[13,14] Uniform recognition, accurate diagnosis, and timely evidence-based treatment of severe HTN during pregnancy is crucial to eliminate preventable morbidity and mortality and reduce health inequities. This article reviews current recommendations for the evaluation and management of severe HTN episodes in pregnancy.

Patient Evaluation Overview

Blood pressure measurement

Accurate recognition of a severe HTN episode in pregnancy is the first critical element in the pathway to timely treatment and additional risk-reducing measures. BP is frequently measured incorrectly,[15] and should be measured in accordance with well-published guidelines:[6,16]

- Cuff is the appropriate size (bladder width 40% of circumference and encircles 80% of the arm)
- Patient seated or semi-reclined
- Back supported
- Arm at heart's level
- Upper arm bare without restrictive clothing
- Feet flat (not dangling or crossed)
- Measurement preceded by a minimum 10-min rest period
- No tobacco or caffeine use for 30 minutes preceding the measurement

As of Nov 4, 2021, 45 states are enrolled in the Alliance for Innovation on Maternal Health (AIM)[17] and many states are implementing the "Core AIM Patient Safety Bundle – Severe Hypertension in Pregnancy."[18] As a national maternal safety and quality improvement initiative, AIM has published evidence-based safety bundles and eModules designed to align best practices at the hospital, state, and national level[19] with the overarching goal of reducing preventable maternal morbidity and mortality. Included in the severe hypertension bundle, the following eModule (https://safehealthcareforeverywoman.org/eModules/eModule-3-Recognition/presentation_html5.html) summarizes best practices to accurately measure BP and recognize maternal early warning signs.

For patients who are increasingly being asked to monitor BP at home, the Preeclampsia Foundation has developed an online educational resource to facilitate accurate at-home readings.[20] This can serve as a useful resource for both clinicians and patients.

Recognition of a Severe Hypertension Episode

When an acute severe BP episode is noted during pregnancy, regardless of the patient's location or presence of pre-existing chronic HTN, emergent evaluation by a medical provider with knowledge of hypertensive crises in pregnancy is warranted and consideration for hospitalization is advised.

Examples of severe hypertension episodes

Minutes after Onset	-20	-10	0	10	20	30	40	50	60	70	80
Example A			⊘	⊘		⊘		⊘			
Example B			⊘	⊘		⊘	⊘	⊘	⊘		⊘
Example C		⊘	⊘		⊘		⊘		⊘		⊘
Example D			⊘					⊘			
Example E1		⊘	⊘		⊘	⊘		⊘		⊘	
Example E2	⊘		⊘	⊘		⊘		⊘			
Example E3	⊘		⊘	⊘		⊘		⊘			
Example F			⊘								⊘
Example G			⊘							⊘	⊘
Example H		⊘	⊘								

Notes:

Example A: SHTN episode, but not persistent SHTN

Example B: Multiple SHTN observations within 1 hour, none of them persisting more than 10 min

Example C: Persistent SHTN episode, resolved within 20 min

Example D: Persistent SHTN episode, resolved within 50 min

Example E1: Persistent SHTN episode

Example E2: Same observations as E1, shifted left by 20 min (the SHTN at 0 min in D1 is at minus 20 min in D2)
This is not an SHTN episode because the SHTN at 0 min is not the first consecutive SHTN observation.

Example E3: Same observations as E2, but the SHTN at minus 20 min was observed in emergency department.
Episode onset is defined as minute 0, the time of first SHTN on an obstetrical unit.

Example F: Persistent SHTN episode because there is no documentation of a non-SHTN blood pressure
within 15 minutes of episode onset

Example G: Persistent SHTN episode

Example H: Patient Left Against Medical Advice at minute 10. This is a persistent SHTN episode because there
is no documentation of a non-SHTN blood pressure within 15 min.

The definition of an episode does not depend on the treatment given, if any. The *green bar* represents a nonpersistent severe HTN episode; *yellow bars* represent persistent severe HTN episodes; the *blue bar* does not represent an episode because an episode must start with the first consecutive severe HTN measurement; ⊘ (*black*), severe HTN BP measurement; ⊘ (*green*), BP measurement that is not severe HTN, either nonsevere hypertension or normal BP.

BP, blood pressure; min, minute(s); SHTN, severe hypertension.

SMFM *Patient Safety and Quality Committee. Society for Maternal-Fetal Medicine Special Statement: A quality metric for evaluating timely treatment of severe hypertension. Am J Obstet Gynecol 2021.*

Fig. 1. Persistent and nonpersistent severe HTN episodes. (*From* Society for Maternal-Fetal Medicine (SMFM), Combs CA, Allbert JR, et al. Society for Maternal-Fetal Medicine Special Statement: A quality metric for evaluating timely treatment of severe hypertension. Am J Obstet Gynecol. 2022;226(2):B2-B9. https://doi.org/10.1016/j.ajog.2021.10.007;" with permission.)

The Society for Maternal–Fetal Medicine (SMFM) recently proposed a uniform quality metric that provides a clear definition for severe hypertension episodes.[21] In the proposed measure, a severe hypertensive episode begins with the very first severe HTN measurement and ends with the first nonsevere measurement, regardless of episode duration. A severe HTN episode is defined as *nonpersistent* if a nonsevere measurement is recorded within 15 minutes. A severe HTN episode is defined as *persistent* if a nonsevere measurement is not recorded within 15 minutes. To facilitate accurate provider recognition and tracking, SMFM provided examples of both persistent (yellow) and nonpersistent (green) severe HTN episodes, shown in **Fig. 1**.

Maternal and fetal evaluation

In addition to accurate definition and recognition of the severe HTN episode, maternal evaluation includes a thorough history, physical examination, and laboratory evaluation to determine the presence or absence of severe features as defined above. Fetal evaluation includes accurate determination of gestational age, sonographic assessment of the fetal position, estimation of fetal weight, placentation and amniotic fluid volume, and evaluation of the fetal heart rate tracing.

In 2017, the National Partnership for Maternal Safety published a set of best practices for hypertensive crises during pregnancy, known as the "Consensus Bundle on Severe Hypertension During Pregnancy and the Postpartum Period."[22] The bundle is designed to be adapted to local contexts and ensure consistent application of evidence-based practices, including facility-wide guidelines for unit readiness, timely triage, rapid response and immediate medication access for the treatment of severe HTN and eclampsia, and escalation protocols for obtaining consultations and requesting maternal transports when warranted. More recently, the ACOG Safe Motherhood Initiative (SMI) published an example of a brief "Hypertensive Emergency Checklist" (**Fig. 2**)[23] also designed for local adaptation and includes critical elements in the recognition and evaluation of severe HTN in pregnancy.

Finally, the California Maternal Quality Care Collaborative (CMQCC) is well-known nationally for its successes in reducing the state's maternal mortality ratio relative to the rest of the US.[24] The CMQCC has published a "Hypertensive Disorders of Pregnancy Toolkit," which is openly available online[25] and includes a comprehensive diagnostic algorithm based on current evidence-based practices (**Fig. 3**).

Pharmacologic or Medical Treatment Options

Treatment goals
Goals for the treatment of severe HTN in pregnancy are to initiate therapy as soon as feasibly possible, ideally within 30 to 60 minutes after the recognition of an acute severe HTN episode.[6,21] Current data show a significant quality gap, with this goal being achieved in less than 50% of cases.[13,14] In a retrospective cohort study of more than 200 women, factors associated with delays in treatment included the initial BP reading not being in the severe range (lack of recognition), absence of preeclampsia symptoms, severe HTN occurring between 10 PM and 6 AM, and increasing gestational age.[26]

Once recognized, BP should be lowered to achieve goal SBP 130 to 150 and DBP 80 to 100, which reduces the risk for stroke, congestive heart failure, and death, though the ideal rate of BP lowering is not well-defined.[27] Once at goal, further sudden lowering should be avoided given the risk of maternal cerebral or myocardial ischemia/ infarction and risk of reduced uteroplacental perfusion with resulting nonreassuring fetal status.

Medications
Based on a 2013 Cochrane review and a related ACOG Committee Opinion,[28,29] current medication recommendations to treat acute-onset severe HTN in pregnancy include intravenous (IV) labetalol, IV hydralazine, and oral immediate-release nifedipine, all of which have shown similar safety and efficacy. Labetalol is a nonselective beta-blocker with some alpha-blockade, a rapid onset of action, and well-established safety profile.[6,30] Labetalol is often considered first-line therapy for patients with heart rate greater than 100 beats per minute and is contraindicated in the setting of sinus bradycardia or history of asthma. Hydralazine is a direct-acting smooth muscle relaxant with primary vasodilation activity in arterioles. Nifedipine is a calcium channel blocker that produces peripheral arterial vasodilation and is often reserved for situations without IV access. The 2013 Cochrane review concluded that the choice among these agents is guided primarily by timely availability and clinician familiarity and knowledge of the chosen medication, its contraindications, and side effects.

HYPERTENSIVE EMERGENCY:

- Two severe BP values (≥160/110) taken 15-60 minutes apart. Values do not need to be consecutive.
- May treat within 15 minutes if clinically indicated

☐ Call for Assistance

☐ Designate:
  ○ Team leader
  ○ Checklist reader/recorder
  ○ Primary RN

☐ Ensure side rails up

☐ Ensure medications appropriate given patient history

☐ Administer seizure prophylaxis (magnesium sulfate first line agent, unless contraindicated)

☐ Antihypertensive therapy within 1 hour for persistent severe range BP

☐ Place IV; Draw preeclampsia labs

☐ Antenatal corticosteroids (if <34 weeks of gestation)

☐ Re-address VTE prophylaxis requirement

☐ Place indwelling urinary catheter

☐ Brain imaging if unremitting headache or neurological symptoms

☐ Debrief patient, family, and obstetric team

† "Active asthma" is defined as:
Ⓐ symptoms at least once a week, or
Ⓑ use of an inhaler, corticosteroids for asthma during the pregnancy, or
Ⓒ any history of intubation or hospitalization for asthma.

Magnesium Sulfate

Contraindications: Myasthenia gravis; avoid with pulmonary edema, use caution with renal failure

IV access:
☐ Load 4-6 grams 10% magnesium sulfate in 100 mL solution over 20 min
☐ Label magnesium sulfate; Connect to labeled infusion pump
☐ Magnesium sulfate maintenance 1-2 grams/hour

No IV access:
☐ 10 grams of 50% solution IM (5 g in each buttock)

Antihypertensive Medications

For SBP ≥ 160 or DBP ≥ 110
(See SMI algorithms for complete management when necessary to move to another agent after 2 doses.)

☐ **Labetalol** (initial dose: 20mg); **Avoid parenteral labetalol with active asthma, heart disease, or congestive heart failure; use with caution with history of asthma**

☐ **Hydralazine** (5-10 mg IV[a] over 2 min); **May increase risk of maternal hypotension**

☐ **Oral Nifedipine** (10 mg capsules); Capsules should be administered orally, not punctured or otherwise administered sublingually

[a]*Maximum cumulative IV-administered doses should not exceed 220 mg labetalol or 25 mg hydralazine in 24 hours*

Note: *If first line agents unsuccessful, emergency consult with specialist (MFM, internal medicine, OB anesthesiology, critical care) is recommended*

Anticonvulsant Medications

For recurrent seizures or when magnesium sulfate contraindicated

☐ **Lorazepam (Ativan):** 2-4 mg IV x 1, may repeat once after 10-15 min
☐ **Diazepam (Valium):** 5-10 mg IV q 5-10 min to maximum dose 30 mg

Safe Motherhood Initiative

Revised January 2019

Fig. 2. Hypertensive emergency checklist. (*From* ACOG Safe Motherhood Initiative: Example Hypertensive Emergency Checklist. Revised January 2019. Available at: https://www.acog.org/-/media/project/acog/acogorg/files/forms/districts/smi-hypertension-bundle-emergency-checklist.pdf. Accessed December 23, 2021;" with permission.)

ACOG's Practice Bulletin, "Gestational Hypertension and Preeclampsia," includes detailed information about these antihypertensive agents for the urgent treatment of severe HTN episodes in pregnancy, along with dosing recommendations, common side effects, contraindications, and onsets of action (**Table 1**).

The CMQCC toolkit includes an antihypertensive treatment algorithm including magnesium sulfate (**Fig. 4**) and sample order set (**Box 1**) for hypertensive emergencies

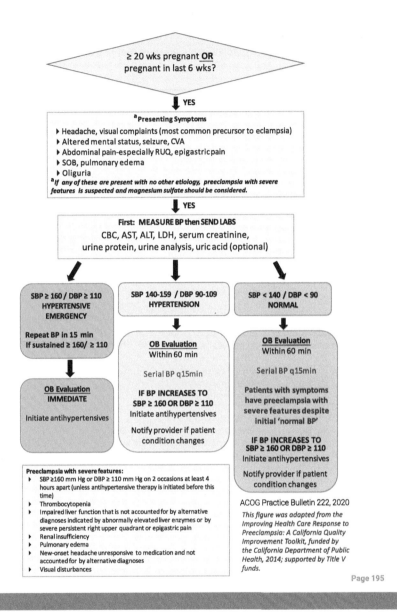

Fig. 3. Acute treatment algorithm. (https://www.cmqcc.org/content/appendix-e-acute-treatment-algorithmFROM: This figure was adapted from the Improving Health Care Response to Preeclampsia: A California QualityImprovement Toolkit, funded by the California Department of Public Health, 2014; supported by Title Vfunds. © Improving Health Care Response to Hypertensive Disorders of Pregnancy, a CMQCC QualityImprovement Toolkit, 2021.)

in pregnancy and includes useful targets for BP lowering as well as recommended BP monitoring intervals once target BP is achieved.

The ACOG SMI "Hypertensive Emergency Checklist" also includes these recommended medication options to treat severe HTN and includes simultaneous

Table 1
Antihypertensive agents used for urgent blood pressure control in pregnancy

Drug	Dose	Comments	Onset of Action
Labetalol	10–20 mg, IV, then 20–80 mg every 10–30 min to a maximum cumulative dosafe of 300 mg; or constant infusion 1–2 mg/min IV	Tachycardia is less common with fewer advise effects. Avoid in women with asthma, preexisting myocardial disease, decompensated cardiac function, and heart block and bradycardia	1–2 min
Hydralazine	5 mg IV or IM, then 5–10 mg IV, every 20–30 min to a maximum cumulative dosage of 20 mg; or constant infusion of 0.5–10 mg/h	Higher or frequent dosage associated with maternal hypotension, headaches, and abnormal fetal heart rate tracings; may be more common than other agents	10–20 min
Nifedipine(immediate release)	10–20 mg orally, repeat in 20 min if needed; then 10–20 mg every 2–6 hrs; maximum daily dose in 180 mg	My observe reflex tachycardia and headaches	5–10 min

Abbreviations: IM, intramuscularly; IV, intravenously.
FROM: Improving Health Care Response to Hypertensive Disorders of Pregnancy Toolkit, A CMQCCQuality Improvement ToolkitThe material used must be cited in the following manner:© Improving Health Care Response to Hypertensive Disorders of Pregnancy, a CMQCC QualityImprovement Toolkit, 2021.

recommendations for the initiation of magnesium sulfate.[23] While magnesium is an appropriate evidence-based medication that reduces the risk for eclamptic seizure, it is not an effective agent for the treatment of HTN and should not be administered for this purpose. The "Core AIM Patient Safety Bundle – Severe Hypertension in Pregnancy" also includes an eModule on optimizing provider response to severe hypertension in pregnancy and can be viewed here https://safehealthcareforeverywoman.org/eModules/eModule-3-Response/presentation_html5.html.

A 2017 systematic review and meta-analysis from the Journal of the American Heart Association demonstrated that the utilization of antihypertensives for pregnant individuals with chronic HTN reduced the risk of developing severe HTN but showed no difference in rates of other adverse perinatal outcomes.[31] Authors found insufficient evidence to guide the choice of antihypertensive agent for those with chronic HTN in pregnancy.

Nonpharmacologic or Surgical/Interventional Treatment Options

There are currently no proven nonpharmacologic options for the treatment of acute-onset, severe episodes of HTN in pregnancy. Watchful waiting, attributing severe HTN to "white coat syndrome" or pain, and failure to remeasure BP at regular intervals

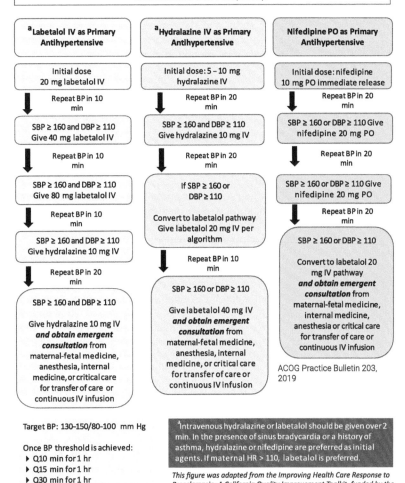

Treatment Recommendations for Sustained Systolic BP ≥ 160 mm Hg or Diastolic BP ≥ 110 mm Hg

[a]Antihypertensive treatment and magnesium sulfate should be administered simultaneously. If concurrent administration is not possible, antihypertensive treatment should be 1st priority.

[a]Labetalol IV as Primary Antihypertensive

Initial dose
20 mg labetalol IV

↓ Repeat BP in 10 min

SBP ≥ 160 and DBP ≥ 110
Give 40 mg labetalol IV

↓ Repeat BP in 10 min

SBP ≥ 160 and DBP ≥ 110
Give 80 mg labetalol IV

↓ Repeat BP in 10 min

SBP ≥ 160 and DBP ≥ 110
Give hydralazine 10 mg IV

↓ Repeat BP in 20 min

SBP ≥ 160 and DBP ≥ 110

Give hydralazine 10 mg IV **and obtain emergent consultation** from maternal-fetal medicine, anesthesia, internal medicine, or critical care for transfer of care or continuous IV infusion

[a]Hydralazine IV as Primary Antihypertensive

Initial dose: 5 – 10 mg hydralazine IV

↓ Repeat BP in 20 min

SBP ≥ 160 and DBP ≥ 110
Give hydralazine 10 mg IV

↓ Repeat BP in 20 min

If SBP ≥ 160 or DBP ≥ 110

Convert to labetalol pathway
Give labetalol 20 mg IV per algorithm

↓ Repeat BP in 10 min

SBP ≥ 160 or DBP ≥ 110

Give labetalol 40 mg IV **and obtain emergent consultation** from maternal-fetal medicine, anesthesia, internal medicine, or critical care for transfer of care or continuous IV infusion

Nifedipine PO as Primary Antihypertensive

Initial dose: nifedipine
10 mg PO immediate release

↓ Repeat BP in 20 min

SBP ≥ 160 or DBP ≥ 110 Give nifedipine 20 mg PO

↓ Repeat BP in 20 min

SBP ≥ 160 or DBP ≥ 110 Give nifedipine 20 mg PO

↓ Repeat BP in 20 min

SBP ≥ 160 or DBP ≥ 110

Convert to labetalol 20 mg IV pathway **and obtain emergent consultation** from maternal-fetal medicine, internal medicine, anesthesia or critical care for transfer of care or continuous IV infusion

ACOG Practice Bulletin 203, 2019

Target BP: 130–150/80–100 mm Hg

Once BP threshold is achieved:
▸ Q10 min for 1 hr
▸ Q15 min for 1 hr
▸ Q30 min for 1 hr
▸ Q1hr for 4 hrs

[a]Intravenous hydralazine or labetalol should be given over 2 min. In the presence of sinus bradycardia or a history of asthma, hydralazine or nifedipine are preferred as initial agents. If maternal HR > 110, labetalol is preferred.

This figure was adapted from the Improving Health Care Response to Preeclampsia: A California Quality Improvement Toolkit, funded by the California Department of Public Health, 2014; supported by Title V funds.

Fig. 4. Antihypertensive treatment algorithm for hypertensive emergencies (https://www.cmqcc.org/content/appendix-e-acute-treatment-algorithmFROM: This figure was adapted from the Improving Health Care Response to Preeclampsia: A California QualityImprovement Toolkit, funded by the California Department of Public Health, 2014; supported by Title Vfunds. © Improving Health Care Response to Hypertensive Disorders of Pregnancy, a CMQCC QualityImprovement Toolkit, 2021)

are not appropriate management strategies and can contribute to significant diagnostic delays and avoidable patient harm.

Bed rest

In a Cochrane review including 4 good quality trials, only one small trial of the 4 concluded that some bed rest was associated with lower rates of severe HTN and preterm birth.[32] However, the side effects and cost implications of bed rest were not adequately addressed by any study and patients showed a preference for greater mobility. Bed rest has not been shown to significantly improve any maternal or fetal outcomes and therefore should not be recommended.

Delivery

Aside from timely pharmacologic treatment, delivery is the only long-term, nonpharmacologic intervention that may reliably improve BP over time. After delivery, though BP may initially worsen until the 3rd to 6th day postpartum,[33] BP can be expected to subsequently trend downward to pregravid levels by the end of the sixth postpartum week.[34] When BP remains elevated after the sixth postpartum week, the diagnosis of CHTN is made and the patient should be referred for antihypertensive management and cardiovascular risk reduction.

A thorough review on selecting the appropriate timing and mode of delivery is beyond the scope of this article; however, cesarean delivery should generally be reserved for typical obstetric indications and preterm delivery delayed until 34 weeks, if possible, based on response to medical management, clinical stability, and ongoing maternal and fetal testing.[6] Regardless of gestational age, delivery should generally not be delayed in the setting of severe features or adverse outcomes such as refractory headache, refractory right upper quadrant or epigastric pain, persistent visual disturbances, stroke, myocardial infarction, eclampsia, pulmonary edema, vaginal bleeding, nonreassuring fetal testing, intrauterine fetal demise or lethal fetal anomaly, or extreme prematurity without expectation for neonatal survival. Delivery should also not be delayed regardless of gestational age in the setting of uncontrollable severe HTN (SBP $\geq$ 160 mm Hg or DBP $\geq$ 110 mm Hg) that is not responsive to medication management.[6]

Combination Therapies

When acute, severe HTN in pregnancy does not respond to the initially chosen antihypertensive agent, a change in therapy or combination of therapies is recommended. According to the CMQCC's "Acute Treatment Algorithm" (see **Fig. 4**), when severe BP does not respond to 3 escalating doses of IV labetalol, additional therapy with IV hydralazine should be administered while simultaneous emergent consultation is sought from maternal–fetal medicine, anesthesia, internal medicine, or critical care. Similarly, when severe HTN does not respond to 2 doses of IV hydralazine, therapy should be converted to IV labetalol per the algorithm while emergent consultation is requested. Finally, when an adequate BP response is not achieved with 3 escalating doses of oral nifedipine, therapy should be converted to IV labetalol and expert consultation and/or transfer of care should be sought.

ACOG also recommends escalating doses of IV labetalol and hydralazine or repeat doses of oral immediate-release nifedipine (see **Table 1**) but does not specifically make a recommendation for selecting secondary therapy in refractory cases. As target BP levels are achieved, oral therapy with labetalol or nifedipine can be added and up-titrated as needed to maintain BP in range during ongoing observation and management. In cases where SBP remains greater than 160, there is increased risk for

Box 1
Sample order set for acute control of hypertensive emergencies

Note: This is a SAMPLE developed by a particular facility and the content is NOT specifically endorsed by the HDP Task Force. The sample is provided as an example to work from. You may need to adjust based on the individual circumstances of your facility.

Medications
Once any of the Preeclampsia Antihypertensive Subphase orders have been administered, the provider should evaluate and discontinue the active subplan when the patient is stabilized and reorder the subplan in case of another hypertensive crisis.

If starting with hydralazine: (hydralazine may be preferred if maternal HR is < 60)

Hydralazine
☐ 10 mg, IV Push, INJ, x1, priority: NOW, Step 1.
Administer slow IV Push at a max rate of 5 mg/min
For systolic greater than or equal to 160 and/or diastolic greater than or equal to 110.
☐ 5 mg, IV Push, INJ, x1, priority: NOW, Step 1.
Administer slow IV Push at a max rate of 5 mg/min
For systolic greater than or equal to 160 and/or diastolic greater than or equal to 110.

Hydralazine
☐ 10 mg, IV Push, INJ, q20 min, PRN Hypertension, Step 2, for 2 Dose/Time
Administer slow IV Push at a max rate of 5 mg/min
If systolic is greater than or equal to 160 and/or diastolic greater than or equal to 110 in 20 minutes, give additional 10 mg.
If no response 20 minutes after last dose, give additional 10 mg.
If no response in 20 minutes give labetalol 20 mg.

Labetalol
20–40 mg, IV Push, q10 min, PRN Hypertension, Step 3, for 2 Dose/Time
IV Push Rate 10 mg/min
Give 20 mg IV Push if adequate response NOT achieved with hydralazine. Repeat BP in 10 minutes. If elevated, administer labetalol 40 mg IV Push and obtain anesthesia consult.

If starting with labetalol:

Labetalol
20 mg, IV Push, INJ, x1, priority: NOW, Step 1
IV Push Rate: 10 mg/min
For systolic greater than or equal to 160 and/or diastolic greater than or equal to 110.

Labetalol
40–80, mg, IV Push, q10 min, PRN Hypertension, Step 2, for 2 Dose/Time
Give 40 mg if systolic greater than or equal to 160 and/or diastolic greater than or equal to 110 10 minutes after initial 20 mg dose.
If no response 10 minutes after 40 mg dose, increase dose to 80 mg.
If 80 mg given and no BP response, give hydralazine 10 mg and notify provider and anesthesia.
20–80, mg, IV Push, q10 min, PRN Hypertension, Step 2, for 3 Dose/Time
If more than 1 hour since initially achieving BP control with 20 mg, and systolic is again greater than or equal to 160 and/or diastolic greater than or equal to 110, give 20 mg labetalol IV Push.
If no response 10 minutes after 20 mg dose, increase dose to 40 mg.
If no response 10 minutes after 40 mg dose, increase dose to 80 mg.
If 80 mg given and no BP response, give hydralazine 10 mg IV Push and notify provider and anesthesia.

Hydralazine
10 mg, IV Push, INJ, x1, PRN Hypertension, Step 3
Administer slow IV Push at a max rate of 5 mg/min
Give if BP still elevated after Step 1 and Step 2 of labetalol.
Repeat BP in 10 minutes, if elevated obtain anesthesia consult.

If using nifedipine as first line

Nifedipine
10 mg, PO, Cap, x1, priority: NOW
For systolic greater than or equal to 160 and/or diastolic greater than or equal to 110.

Nifedipine
10 mg, PO, Cap, q20 min, PRN Hypertension
If systolic greater than or equal to 160 and/or diastolic greater than or equal to 110 in 20 minutes, give additional 10 mg.
If no response 20 minutes after the last dose give additional 10 mg.
Maximum of 5 doses, if not appropriate BP response, notify provider and anesthesia.

From CMQCC Appendix M: Sample Order Set for Acute Control of Hypertensive Emergencies" Available at: https://www.cmqcc.org/content/appendix-m-sample-order-set-acute-control-hypertensive-emergencies. Accessed December 27, 2021; with permission.

maternal stroke, other cerebrovascular complications such as posterior reversible encephalopathy syndrome, or maternal death, making escalation of care an urgent priority.

Treatment Resistance/Complications

In severe cases, BP may not be controllable with parenteral and oral antihypertensive agents recommended above. In such circumstances, clinicians are advised to consult with a specialist in internal medicine, critical care, anesthesia, or maternal–fetal medicine and/or rapidly request maternal transport to higher level of care if this has not already been conducted.

ACOG's summary for the use of antihypertensive agents to urgently control BP (see **Table 1**) includes the option of IV labetalol as a constant infusion of 1 to 2 mg/min. Infusion pump therapy with nicardipine can also be considered in refractory cases. In a small case study, nicardipine produced rapid BP control in patients with severe features and refractory HTN in pregnancy by selectively reducing afterload and reducing mean arterial pressure.[35] Despite evidence of reflex tachycardia and increased cardiac output, there were no other significant changes to maternal or fetal hemodynamics. In select cases, nitroglycerin, esmolol, or nitroprusside can be considered; however, there are minimal data on safety and efficacy in pregnancy and should be utilized in consultation with specialists who have extensive experience with these agents.

Complications of antihypertensive therapies include hypotension, allergic reactions, and bothersome and sometimes dangerous side effects such as bradycardia, asthma exacerbation or heart block (labetalol), reflex tachycardia (nifedipine), or headaches (hydralazine, nifedipine) (see **Table 1**). Complications of rapid BP lowering may include maternal myocardial or cerebral ischemia or infarction or a sudden decrease in uteroplacental perfusion and nonreassuring fetal testing.

Self-Management Strategies

With recent advances in postpartum remote BP monitoring programs and social distancing practices related to the COVID pandemic, patients are increasingly being asked to self-monitor BP at home. A 2018 systematic review published in the journal Hypertension included 41 articles, more than 2000 pregnant individuals, and 28 different BP devices.[36] The used BP measurement device was validated in only 61% of the studies included in the review, and in only 34% of studies where a device was successfully validated was that device used without a protocol violation.

Utilization of validated BP devices and evidence-based patient education on how to accurately self-measure BP is critical in these situations and should be ensured by clinicians and health systems whenever home monitoring is undertaken.

Patients with HTN in pregnancy should be provided with accurate and timely education and instructed to seek immediate care for any of the following symptoms, which can be considered maternal warning signs and/or severe features of HTN in pregnancy:[6]

- Persistent headache unresponsive to medications
- Visual disturbances
- Right upper quadrant or epigastric pain
- Chest pain or shortness of breath
- Confusion
- Seizures

As part of its' quality improvement toolkit, the CMQCC has produced a patient-facing, freely available visual aid for use in emergency room, obstetric triage, and other relevant health care settings (**Fig. 5**). Such visual aids are increasingly being used to provide universal patient education in other settings as well, such as primary care, obstetric offices, and postpartum units.

New Developments

The Chronic Hypertension and Pregnancy (CHAP) Project was a multicenter US randomized trial designed to evaluate the benefits and potential harms of the treatment (with Nifedipine or Labetalol) of CHTN in pregnancy at various BP thresholds.[37] This recently published study showed a reduced risk in the primary composite outcome of preeclampsia with severe features, medically-indicated preterm birth <35 weeks, placental abruption, or fetal or neonatal death amongst pregnant individuals randomized to receive antihypertensive therapy for CHTN at a BP threshold of 140/90 compared to a higher BP threshold group. In response, ACOG released clinical guidance recommending 140/90 as the threshold at which medical therapy for CHTN in pregnancy should be initiated or titrated.[38] These data are currently under review by SMFM.[39]

Maternal Mortality Review Committees (MMRCs) are emerging as increasingly important sources of detailed information regarding maternal deaths.[40,41] These multidisciplinary committees meet regularly, often with support from states and the US Centers for Disease Control and Prevention (CDC), to perform comprehensive reviews of all deaths within their jurisdiction that occur among pregnant individuals and within the first year postpartum. The CDC recently released a brief including data from 14 MMRCs for the years 2008 to 2017 showing that cardiovascular conditions, preeclampsia, and eclampsia were among the leading causes of maternal mortality accounting for more than 22% of deaths, with nearly 66% of all deaths deemed preventable.[12] This report also showed that the leading causes of pregnancy-related deaths vary significantly by race and ethnicity, with the percentage of deaths due to preeclampsia and eclampsia being twice as high among non-Hispanic Blacks (11.4%) compared with non-Hispanic Whites (6.5%). MMRCs continue to improve in their ability to provide timely information about maternal deaths related to HTN and other causes and have recently added a field for reporting whether (based on the committees' determination) discrimination was a contributing factor in the death. These efforts hold great potential to identify areas for targeted quality improvements and to address health disparities.

There has been widespread development and implementation of evidence-based safety bundles aimed at standardizing best practices and promoting continuous

Appendix G: Stop Sign for Patient Information

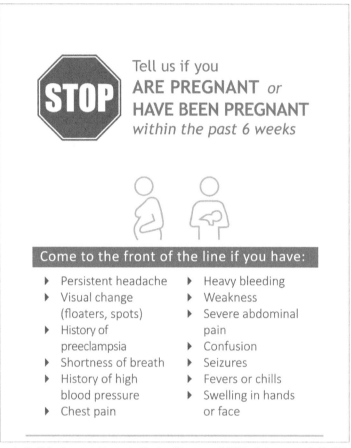

Tell us if you
ARE PREGNANT *or*
HAVE BEEN PREGNANT
within the past 6 weeks

Come to the front of the line if you have:

- Persistent headache
- Visual change (floaters, spots)
- History of preeclampsia
- Shortness of breath
- History of high blood pressure
- Chest pain
- Heavy bleeding
- Weakness
- Severe abdominal pain
- Confusion
- Seizures
- Fevers or chills
- Swelling in hands or face

Improving Health Care Response to Hypertensive Disorders of Pregnancy, a CMQCC Quality Improvement Toolkit, 2021.

Improving Health Care Response to Hypertensive Disorders of Pregnancy
CMQCC Quality Improvement Toolkit   Page 199

Fig. 5. Stop sign for patient information. (https://www.cmqcc.org/content/appendix-g-stop-sign-patient-informationFROM: Improving Health Care Response to Hypertensive Disorders of Pregnancy Toolkit, A CMQCCQuality Improvement ToolkitThe material used must be cited in the following manner:© Improving Health Care Response to Hypertensive Disorders of Pregnancy, a CMQCC QualityImprovement Toolkit, 2021)

quality improvement.[42] Perinatal quality collaboratives (PQCs) like the CMQCC referenced above have made significant strides in advancing patient and provider knowledge regarding hypertensive disorders in pregnancy and the benefits of timely treatment. After the implementation of a maternal HTN quality improvement initiative, the Illinois Perinatal Quality Collaborative sustained significant improvements in the timely treatment (within 60 minutes) of severe HTN.[43]

Postpartum management protocols that rely on outpatient strategies are being increasingly used and studied. Telehealth with remote BP monitoring of postpartum women at risk for severe HTN has been shown to be feasible and associated with high patient satisfaction.[44] When compared with standard care, postpartum remote BP monitoring was associated with a significant reduction in hospital readmissions and may reduce disparities in postpartum HTN care.[45,46]

Data are increasingly emerging on the significant problem of health disparities related to hypertensive disorders in pregnancy, with Black individuals disproportionately impacted. A September 2021 study published in the journal Hypertension analyzed more than 1.5 million live births and 3287 hypertension-related maternal deaths in the US.[47] The maternal mortality ratio related to hypertensive disorders in pregnancy, defined as death during pregnancy or within 42 days postpartum, was nearly 4-fold higher among Black compared with White women. While causes of these disparities remain underexamined, delayed recognition, lack of timely initiation of treatment, and racism in medicine are all important potentially causative factors that warrant urgent investigation.

Evaluation of Outcome and/or Long-Term Recommendations

To evaluate outcomes, SMFM has recommended a standardized quality metric.[21] The denominator includes the total number of pregnant patients with at least one episode of persistent severe HTN, while the numerator includes those from the denominator who received pharmacologic treatment within 60 minutes of the first severe HTN measurement. The metric is intended for use by health care facilities to establish their benchmark and design quality improvement projects. As this quality metric becomes widely adopted, facilities will be able to evaluate the timely treatment of severe HTN episodes in pregnancy and compare performance over time, both within and across institutions.

Prophylactic low dose aspirin (81 mg/d) is the only intervention shown to reduce the incidence of hypertensive disorders during pregnancy and is recommended by ACOG, SMFM, and the US Preventive Services Task Force.[48,49] Low-dose daily aspirin is now recommended ideally starting by 12 to 16 weeks gestational age and continued until delivery for those with one or more factors associated with high risk of preeclampsia (expected preeclampsia incidence roughly 8%), 2 or more moderate risk factors, or one or both of the following 2 moderate risk factors: Black race (as a proxy for racism, not due to underlying biological risk) or low-income (due to environmental and other inequities that shape health). Further description of these risk factors is detailed in the ACOG SMFM 2021 joint Practice Advisory.[50] In some settings where moderate risk factors are common, a universal recommendation to take daily low-dose aspirin is a reasonable approach. Consistent recommendations for prophylactic low-dose aspirin in qualifying pregnant individuals are encouraged and the development of related quality metrics should be considered.

Summary/Discussion/Future Directions

Hypertensive disorders in pregnancy are common and are a leading cause of preventable maternal morbidity and mortality. Most health care providers are, therefore, likely to encounter pregnant individuals with acute severe HTN who are at risk for preventable morbidity or maternal or fetal death. Prompt recognition of acute severe HTN in pregnancy is essential and occurs at a lower BP threshold than that used to define hypertensive crisis outside of pregnancy. The lower BP threshold reflects additional risks, especially for maternal stroke or death at lower BP ranges, but may be a barrier to prompt recognition, especially in nonobstetrical health care settings.

Timely treatment as soon as feasibly possible, at least within 30 to 60 minutes, should be initiated with IV labetalol, IV hydralazine, or oral immediate-release nifedipine. The use of algorithms or institutional evidence-based protocols is recommended to reduce delays and improve the provision of appropriate escalating doses of BP-lowering medications. Simultaneous treatment with magnesium sulfate for seizure prevention is recommended. When target SBP 130 to 150 and DBP 80 to 100 cannot be achieved despite initial medication administration, expert consultation and consideration for maternal transport are recommended.

Despite increasing efforts by perinatal quality collaboratives and local quality improvement initiatives, gaps in recognition are common and treatment delays are frequent. Health care disparities related to hypertensive disorders include a 4-fold increased risk of maternal mortality for Blacks compared with Whites, which warrants urgent investigation and remedy. Adopting standardized quality metrics, such as that recommended by SMFM, holds promise to assist facilities and health systems in establishing current baselines for the timely treatment of severe HTN in pregnancy and tracking improvements within and across institutions over time.

CLINICS CARE POINTS

- Severe hypertension in pregnancy is a medical emergency, defined by persistent (consecutive or nonconsecutive) systolic BP $\geq$ 160 mm Hg and/or diastolic BP $\geq$ 110 mm Hg taken from 15 minutes up to 4 or more hours apart.

- The BP threshold used to define hypertensive crisis in pregnancy is lower than that in nonpregnant individuals, leading to significant potential for under-recognition and delayed treatment.

- BP is frequently measured incorrectly and should be taken according to published protocols.

- Goals for the treatment of severe hypertension in pregnancy are to initiate therapy as soon as feasibly possible, at least within 30 to 60 minutes of recognition of the severe hypertension episode.

- Current medications recommended for the treatment of acute-onset severe HTN in pregnancy are intravenous (IV) labetalol, IV hydralazine, and oral immediate-release nifedipine, all of which have shown similar safety and efficacy. Choice of medical therapy should be based on institutional protocols where possible, timely medication availability, and provider knowledge of the chosen medication.

DISCLOSURE

The authors have nothing to disclose.

REFERENCES

1. Clark SL, Christmas JT, Frye DR, et al. Maternal mortality in the Unites States: predictability and the impact of protocols on fatal postcesarean pulmonary embolism and hyper-related intracranial hemorrhage. Am J Obstet Gynecol 2014;211(1): 32.e1-9.
2. Wallis AB, Saftlas AF, Shia J, et al. Secular trends in the rates of preeclampsia, eclampsia, and gestational hypertension, Unites States, 1978-2004. Am J Hypertens 2008;21:521–6.
3. Kuklina EV, Ayala C, Callaghan WM. Hypertensive disorders and severe obstetric morbidity in the Unites States. Obstet Gynecol 2009;113:1299–306.

4. Petersen EE, Davis NL, Goodman D, et al. Vital signs: pregnancy-related deaths, Unites States, 2011-2015, and strategies for prevention, 13 states, 2013-2017. MMWR Morb Mortal Wkly Rep 2019;68:423–9.

5. Peixoto AJ. Acute severe hypertension. N Engl J Med 2019;381:1843–52.

6. Gestational hypertension and preeclampsia. ACOG Practice Bulletin No. 222. American College of Obstetricians and Gynecologists. Obstet Gynecol 2020; 135:e237–60.

7. Martin JN Jr, Thigpen BD, Moore RC, et al. Stroke and severe preeclampsia and eclampsia: a paradigm shift focusing on systolic blood pressure. Obstet Gynecol 2005;105:246–54.

8. Judy AE, McCain CL, Lawton ES, et al. Systolic hypertension, preeclampsia-related mortality, and stroke in California. Obstet Gynecol 2019;133(6):1151–9.

9. Coetzee EJ, Dommisse J, Anthony J. A randomized controlled trial of intravenous magnesium sulphate versus placebo in the management of women with severe preeclampsia. Br J Obstet Gynaecol 1998;105:300–3.

10. Cooray SD, Edmonds SM, Tong S, et al. Characterization of symptoms immediately preceding eclampsia. Obstet Gynecol 2011;118:995–9.

11. Noraihan MF, Sharda P, Jammal AB. Report of 50 cases of eclampsia. J Obstet Gynaecol Res 2005;31:302–9.

12. Davis NL, Smoots AN, Goodman DA. Pregnancy-Related Deaths: Data from 14 U.S. Maternal Mortality Review Committees, 2008-2017. Atlanta, GA: Centers for Disease Control and Prevention, U.S. Department of Health and Human Services. 2019. Available at: https://www.cdc.gov/reproductivehealth/maternal-mortality/erase-mm/mmr-data-brief.html. Accessed December 15, 2021.

13. Deshmukh US, Lundsberg LS, Culhane JF, et al. Factors associated with appropriate treatment of acute-onset severe obstetrical hypertension. Am J Obstet Gynecol 2021;225(3):329.e1–10.

14. Shields LE, Wiesner S, Klein C, et al. Early standardized treatment of critical blood pressure elevations is associated with a reduction in eclampsia and severe maternal morbidity. Am J Obstet Gynecol 2017;216(4):415.e1–5.

15. Sebo P, Pechère-Bertschi A, Herrmann FR, et al. Blood pressure measurements are unreliable to diagnose hypertension in primary care. J Hypertens 2014; 32(3):509.

16. Whelton PK, Carey RM, Aronow WS, et al. Guideline for the prevention, detection, evaluation, and management of high blood pressure in adults: A report of the American College of Cardiology/American Heart Association Task Force on Clinical Practice Guidelines. Hypertenion 2018;71(6):e13.

17. Alliance for Innovation on Maternal Health: AIM State Participation. Available at: https://safehealthcareforeverywoman.org/aim/about-us/aim-state-participation-2/. Accessed December 23, 2021.

18. Council on Patient Safety in Women's Health Care: Severe Hypertensin in Pregnancy (+AIM). Available at: https://safehealthcareforeverywoman.org/council/patient-safety-bundles/maternal-safety-bundles/severe-hypertension-in-pregnancy-aim/. Accessed December 14, 2021.

19. Alliance for Innovation on Maternal Health: Taking AIM at Maternal Morbidity and Mortality. Available at: https://safehealthcareforeverywoman.org/aim/. Accessed December 14, 2021.

20. Preeclampsia Foundation. Blood Pressure. Check. Know. Share. Available at: https://www.preeclampsia.org/blood-pressure. Accessed December 12, 2021.

21. SMFM Patient Safety and Quality Committee. Society for Maternal-Fetal Medicine Special Statement: A quality metric for evaluating timely treatment of severe

hypertension. Am J Obstet Gynecol 2021. https://doi.org/10.1016/j.ajog.2021.10.007.

22. Bernstein PS, Martin JN Jr, Barton JR, et al. National Partnership for Maternal Safety: Consensus bundle on severe hypertension during pregnancy and the postpartum period. Obstet Gynecol 2017;130(2):347–57.

23. ACOG Safe Motherhood Initiative. Example Hypertensive Emergency Checklist. Revised January 2019. Available at: https://www.acog.org/-/media/project/acog/acogorg/files/forms/districts/smi-hypertension-bundle-emergency-checklist.pdf. Accessed December 23, 2021.

24. California Maternal Quality Care Collaborative. Who We Are. Available at: https://www.cmqcc.org/who-we-are. Accessed December 15, 2021.

25. California Maternal Quality Care Collaborative: Hypertensive Disorders of Pregnancy Toolkit. Available at: https://www.cmqcc.org/resources-tool-kits/toolkits/HDP. Accessed December 23, 2021.

26. Kantarowska A, Heiselman CJ, Halpern TA, et al. Identification of factors associated with delayed treatment of obstetric hypertensive emergencies. Am J Obstet Gynecol 2020;223:250.e1-11.

27. Visintin C, Mugglestone MA, Almerie MQ, et al. Management of hypertensive disorders during pregnancy: Summary of NICE guidance. BMJ 2010;341:c2207.

28. Duley L, Meher S, Jones L. Drugs for treatment of very high blood pressure during pregnancy. Cochrane Database Syst Rev 2013;7:CD001499. Art. No.

29. Emergent therapy for acute-onset, severe hypertension during pregnancy and the postpartum period. ACOG Committee Opinion No. 767. American College of Obstetricians and Gynecologists. Obstet Gynecol 2019;133:e174–80.

30. Peacock WF 4th, Hilleman DE, Levy PD, et al. A systematic review of nicardipine vs labetalol for the management of hypertensive crises. Am J Emerg Med 2012;30(6):981–93.

31. Webster LM, Conti-Ramsden F, Seed PT, et al. Impact of antihypertensive treatment on maternal and perinatal outcomes in pregnancy complicated by chronic hypertension: A systematic review and meta-analysis. J Am Heart Assoc 2017;6(5):e005526.

32. Meher S, Abalos E, Carroli G. Bed rest with or without hospitalization for hypertension during pregnancy. Cochrane Database Syst Rev 2005;4:CD003514.

33. Walters BN, Walters T. Hypertension in the puerperium. Lancet 1987;2(8554):330.

34. Podymow T, August P. Postpartum course of gestational hypertension and pre-eclampsia. Hypertens Pregnancy 2010;29(3):294–300.

35. Cornette J, Buijs EA, Duvekot JJ, et al. Hemodynamic effects of intravenous nicardipine in severely pre-eclamptic women with a hypertensive crisis. Ultrasound Obstet Gynecol 2016;47(1):89–95.

36. Bello NA, Woolley JJ, Cleary KL, et al. Accuracy of blood pressure measurement devices in pregnancy: A systematic review of validation studies. Hypertension 2018;71(2):326–35.

37. Tita A, Szychowski J, Boggess K, et al. Treatment for mild chronic hypertension during pregnancy. N Engl J Med 2022;386(19):1781–92.

38. https://www.acog.org/clinical/clinical-guidance/practice-advisory/articles/2022/04/clinical-guidance-for-the-integration-of-the-findings-of-the-chronic-hypertension-and-pregnancy-chap-study (Accessed 8 April 2022), 2022.

39. https://www.smfm.org/publications/439-smfm-statement-antihypertensive-therapy-for-mild-chronic-hypertension-in-pregnancy-the-chap-trial (Accessed 8 April 2022), 2022.

40. Tita A, Cutter G. A pragmatic multicenter randomized clinical trial (RCT) of anti-hypertensive therapy for mild chronic hypertension during pregnancy: Chronic hypertension and pregnancy (CHAP) project. ClinicalTrials.gov Identifier: NCT02299414. Available at: https://clinicaltrials.gov/ct2/show/NCT02299414. Accessed December 27, 2021.

41. Report from Maternal Mortality Review Committees: A View into Their Critical Role. Available at: https://www.cdcfoundation.org/sites/default/files/upload/pdf/MMRIAReport.pdf. Accessed: December 12, 2021.

42. Henderson ZT, Ernst K, Simpson KR, et al. The National Network of State Perinatal Quality Collaboratives: A Growing Movement to Improve Maternal and Infant Health. J Womens Health (Larchmt) 2018;27(2):123–7.

43. King PL, Keenan-Devlin L, Gordon C, et al. Reducing time to treatment for severe maternal hypertension through statewide quality improvement. Am J Obstet Gynecol Oral Plenary 2018;218(1). Supplement S4.

44. Hoppe KK, Williams M, Thomas N, et al. Telehealth with remote blood pressure monitoring for postpartum hypertension: A prospective single-cohort feasibility study. Pregnancy Hypertens 2019;15:171–6.

45. Hoppe KK, Thomas N, Zernick M, et al. Telehealth with remote blood pressure monitoring compared with standard care for postpartum hypertension. Am J Obstet Gynecol 2020;223(4):585–8.

46. Hirshberg A, Downes K, Srinivas S. Comparing standard office-based follow-up with text-based remote monitoring in the management of postpartum hypertension: a randomized clinical trial. BMJ Qual Saf 2018;27(11):871–7.

47. Ananth CV, Brandt JS, Hill J, et al. Historical and recent changes in maternal mortality due to hypertensive disorders in the United States, 1979 to 2018. Hypertension 2021;78:1414–22.

48. ACOG Committee Opinion No. 743. Low-Dose Aspirin Use During Pregnancy. Obstet Gynecol 2018;132(1):e44–52.

49. Davidson KW, Barry MJ, Mangione CM, et al. Aspirin use to prevent preeclampsia and related morbidity and mortality: US Preventive Services Task Force Recommendation Statement. US Preventive Services Task Force. JAMA 2021; 326:1186–91.

50. Practice Advisory. Low-dose aspirin use for the prevention of preeclampsia and related morbidity and mortality. Available at: https://www.acog.org/clinical/clinical-guidance/practice-advisory/articles/2021/12/low-dose-aspirin-use-for-the-prevention-of-preeclampsia-and-related-morbidity-and-mortality. Accessed December 12, 2021.

Pediatric and Adolescent Gynecologic Emergencies

Stephanie M. Cizek, MD*, Nichole Tyson, MD

KEYWORDS

- Ovarian torsion • Tubal torsion • Straddle injury • Vulvar hematoma • Vulvar ulcers
- Aphthous ulcers

KEY POINTS

- Providers should have a high clinical index of suspicion for adnexal torsion for patients with ovaries with acute abdominal pain and vomiting, even if the patient intermittently has miminal or no pain.
- Ultrasound is the first-line imaging for adnexal torsion, but even with doppler studies cannot definitively diagnose or exclude torsion.
- Vulvar aphthous ulcers may be virally associated (but not are not caused by HSV); the diagnosis is clinical and the management is mainly supportive.
- Vulvar straddle injuries can often be evaluated and repaired in the emergency department if adequate analgesia can be obtained; however, there should be a low threshhold to proceed to the operating room if the lesion is incompletely visualized or extends into the vagina. Force/coercion with exams should be avoided.

INTRODUCTION

Pediatric and adolescent gynecology is currently a Focused Practice Designation by the American Board of Obstetrics and Gynecology. Despite its subspecialty status, many emergency room physicians, general gynecologists, pediatricians, and pediatric surgeons are called upon to care for children and adolescents with gynecologic emergencies. Here, the authors focus on 3 of the most common pediatric and adolescent gynecologic emergencies: (1) adnexal torsion, (2) vulvovaginal lacerations, and (3) nonsexually acquired genital ulcers (aphthous ulcers).

ADNEXAL TORSION

Torsion of adnexal structures involves twisting of the ovary, fallopian tube, or both on their vascular ligaments, compromising blood flow to the affected tissue and resulting

---

Pediatric and Adolescent Gynecology, Department of OB/GYN, Stanford University School of Medicine, Center for Academic Medicine, MC 5317, 453 Quarry Road, Palo Alto, CA 94304, USA
* Corresponding author.
E-mail address: Scizek@stanford.edu

Obstet Gynecol Clin N Am 49 (2022) 521–536
https://doi.org/10.1016/j.ogc.2022.02.017
0889-8545/22/© 2022 Elsevier Inc. All rights reserved.

obgyn.theclinics.com

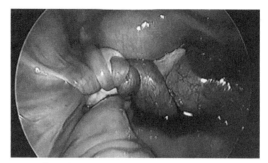

Fig. 1. Adnexal torsion with multiple twists, as seen on laparoscopy. (*Courtesy of* Paula Hillard, MD, Palo Alto, CA.)

in pain and tissue necrosis (**Fig. 1**). It can occur at any age, although it is more likely to occur in people ages 10 years and older.[1,2] It is estimated that torsion affects 5 out of 100,000 people aged 1 to 20 years old.[1] It is the sixth most common pediatric surgical emergency[3] and accounts for 4% of all cases of abdominal pain in the pediatric emergency room.[4]

Key Findings

- *History:*
  - *Acute lower abdominal pain:* Classically, patients with torsion present with acute onset of abdominal pain, usually unilateral (right or left lower quadrant) and often intermittent in nature, either completely resolving between episodes of acutely severe pain or present continuously but waxing and waning in severity, over days or even months.[2]
  - *Nausea and vomiting:* Vomiting may be a good negative predictor of torsion; in 1 study of pediatric torsion, 83% of premenarchal patients and 100% of postmenarchal patients with a confirmed surgical diagnosis of torsion presented with vomiting, in addition to abdominal pain (**Table 1**).[5]
  - *Menstrual history:* Date of last period and an assessment of typical cycle length/pain are useful: severe dysmenorrhea may present as pain with or without vomiting, and hemorrhagic corpus luteum cysts typically present late in cycles and may grow to large sizes during anovulatory cycles.[6]
  - *Sexual history:* Obtain confidentially. Include history of sexual activity, the date of last sexual intercourse, history of sexually transmitted infections, and contraceptive/emergency contraceptive needs.

Table 1
Torsion: presence of vomiting

Presence of Vomiting	Torsion	No Torsion
Premenarchal	$n = 6$ 83% with vomiting (5/6)	$n = 40$ 40% with vomiting
Postmenarchal	$n = 10$ 100% with vomiting (10/10)	$n = 185$ 34% with vomiting

Data from Schwartz BI, Huppert JS, Chen C, Huang B, Reed JL. Creation of a Composite Score to Predict Adnexal Torsion in Children and Adolescents. J Pediatr Adolesc Gynecol. 2018;31(2):132-137. https://doi.org/10.1016/j.jpag.2017.08.007.

- o Other:
  - ▪ Anorexia and flank pain are also associated with torsion.
  - ▪ Diarrhea, dysuria, abnormal vaginal discharge, and vulvovaginal pain/itching are not typically associated with torsion.
  - o *Neonates:* Neonates may present with nonspecific symptoms, such as inconsolability or feeding intolerance, and may have an abdominal mass on examination.[2]
- *Examination:*
  - o *Vital signs*: Vital signs are often normal. Mild temperature elevations may be noted, but true fevers are uncommon.[2] Tachycardia or hypertension may accompany acute pain episodes.
  - o *Abdominal examination:* Note the location and severity of abdominal pain, although there may be minimal pain during the intermittent phase between acute pain episodes. Any masses should be noted. Peritoneal signs may be present.
  - o *Pelvic examination:* Pelvic examinations may be informative for sexually active patients to distinguish pelvic inflammatory disease from torsion (in the latter, pain is typically worst in 1 adnexa, and a mass may be palpable). In all patients, a pelvic examination should be performed judiciously and is *not* necessary to make the diagnosis of torsion[2] (**Box 1**). In young, premenarchal patients, an external examination may be indicated if vulvar pathologic condition or imperforate hymen is suspected.
- Laboratory evaluation
  - o *A pregnancy test* (for postmenarchal patients) and rapid COVID-19 test (required in most operating rooms) should be immediately obtained to facilitate urgent surgery if needed.
  - o *Complete blood count:* Mild leukocytosis is often seen; significant leukocytosis is less common. As the differential includes a ruptured hemorrhagic cyst, a hemoglobin test allows the assessment of significant blood loss.
  - o *Urinalysis*: Urinalysis can help rule out a urinary tract infection causing pain.
  - o *Serum tumor markers:* If imaging reveals an adnexal mass with malignant features (solid and cystic components, large size, increased vascularity within the mass), serum tumor markers should be considered. Even if urgent surgery is performed, baseline tumor markers may guide future tumor surveillance. Young patients are more likely to have a germ or stromal cell tumor and should have a quantitative β-human chorionic gonadotropin, alpha-fetoprotein, lactate dehydrogenase, and inhibin A and B drawn before surgery. All patients (any age) should have a CA-125 test if there is concern for malignancy.[2,7,8]
- Imaging:

Box 1
Clinically indicated pelvic examinations (bimanual/speculum) in the emergency room

Sexually active with:
- Abnormal discharge
- Concern for vaginal trauma, mass, foreign body
- Pelvic or abdominal pain without other clear cause
- Forensic examination for abuse

Everyone, regardless of age or coitarche status:
- Needs to consent to any genital examination
- Consider if examination under sedation ± vaginoscopy is more appropriate

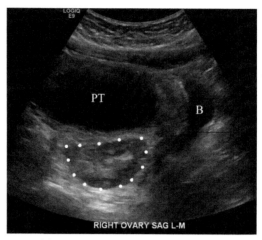

Fig. 2. Peripheralization of follicles (hypoechoic rim) around the edematous stroma of the right ovary (*outlined with dots*). B, bladder; PT, paratubal cyst. This patient had a right paratubal cyst and right adnexal torsion on laparoscopy. (*Courtesy of* Stephanie Cizek, MD, Palo Alto, CA.)

○ Key Findings:
  ■ *Adnexal mass:* The risk of torsion increases in the setting of an adnexal mass greater than 5 cm.[1] However, pediatric and adolescent patients are more likely to have torsion without an ovarian cyst (up to 46%) compared with adults.[1] This is thought to be related to children having relatively longer utero-ovarian ligaments and smaller uterine size, allowing more adnexal mobility.[6]
  ■ *Ovarian stromal edema and peripheralization of follicles:* Stromal edema from venous congestion stretches the ovarian cortex, resulting in follicles being pushed toward the cortex on imaging[1] (**Fig. 2**).
  ■ *Whirlpool sign*: Also called a "swirl" sign, this is visibly twisted adnexal vessels and is a highly specific sign for torsion but is uncommonly detected (**Fig. 3**).

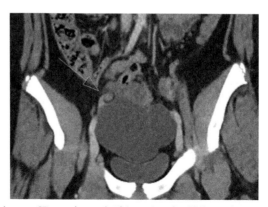

Fig. 3. Whirlpool sign on CT scan (*arrow*). This patient had bilateral paratubal cysts and right adnexal torsion on laparoscopy. (*Courtesy of* Stephanie Cizek, MD, Palo Alto, CA.)

- *Ovarian volume difference*: In the absence of an adnexal mass, the only imaging finding may be volume differences between the torsed and nontorsed ovary, resulting from associated ovarian tissue edema of the torsed ovary.[4] Volume differences in torsion are typically significant (at least 2.5 times greater volume in the torsed ovary).[4]
- *Arterial and venous Doppler imaging:* In a 2020 review, the addition of Doppler imaging to ultrasound slightly improved both sensitivity and specificity for the diagnosis of ovarian torsion, but was not statistically significant.[9] It should be emphasized that the presence of Doppler arterial or venous flow does not rule out a diagnosis of torsion, as patients with normal Dopplers may still have torsion (up to 60% in 1 study).[1,10] Twisting of the adnexa produces either partial or complete vascular obstruction, and lymphatic and venous flow is compromised first (causing ovarian edema, stretching of the ovarian capsule, and pain); therefore, venous or arterial flow may variably appear normal.[11] Ultimately, the diagnosis of ovarian torsion is based on clinical signs and symptoms and not on the presence or absence of Doppler blood flow.
  - Imaging modality:
    - *Pelvic ultrasound:* Ultrasound is considered first line in the assessment of adnexal torsion and should be performed urgently in the emergency department (ED) setting for any patient for whom torsion is considered.[1,9] Transabdominal (rather than transvaginal) ultrasound is typically used in the pediatric and adolescent presexually active population. Transabdominal ultrasound is optimal with a full bladder, although this may not be possible in some patients.
    - *Computed tomography (CT) and MRI*: CT and MRI are considered second-line diagnostic tools. Both have similar sensitivity/specificity compared with ultrasound for the diagnosis of adnexal torsion, may delay evaluation, and may incur higher cost.[1,9] CT involves ionizing radiation and is less preferred in pediatric patients.

Management

- *Surgery is the gold standard:* The definitive diagnosis and management of adnexal torsion is urgent surgery, typically laparoscopy. Approximately 50% of patients taken to the operating room owing to concern for torsion will have torsion found intraoperatively.[1]
  - *Timing of surgery and tissue viability:* There is no time-designated period for duration of symptoms that reliably predicts ovarian viability, and even ovaries with a gross appearance of ischemia are likely still viable. An excellent study by Balasubramaniam and colleagues[12] assessed the degree of apparent ovarian ischemia in 45 salvaged ovaries during detorsion surgery; in follow-up, all of the ovaries had normal sonographic follicular development, including those with black, ischemic-appearing ovaries and despite a range of time from symptom onset to surgery of 1 to 120 days (in fact, 4 patients conceived during follow-up). In another study with a median time of 16 hours (range, 2–144 hours) from symptom onset to surgery, follow-up ultrasound showed normal follicles in 91% of previously torsed ovaries.[13] One study suggests that ovarian tissue appeared less salvageable in patients with multiple twists of torsion.[3] In a comparison of ovarian-to-testicular torsion, patients with ovarian torsion waited 2.5 times longer for imaging and 2.7 times longer for surgery compared with those

with testicular torsion, with a lower gonadal salvage rates (14% for ovaries, 30% for testes).[14]

○ *Oophorectomy is almost never required:* Even a "necrotic"-appearing ovary may retain function, as measured by follicle formation on ultrasound.[2] The concerns for venous thromboembolism with detorsion and risk of infection if necrotic tissue is left in situ have not been demonstrated and are not increased in this population.[2] Although concern for malignancy is often cited as a cause for oophorectomy (approximately 10% of pediatric ovarian masses are malignant), 1 study found only a 1.8% malignancy rate among patients with torsion.[15]

○ *Salpingectomy may be considered:* In contrast to recommendations for ovarian preservation, there are not clear recommendations regarding management of the torsed fallopian tube.[16] Theoretically, a damaged fallopian tube may impair future fertility or increase the future risk of ectopic pregnancy.[16] Fertility rates between patients who had salpingectomy versus salpingostomy for ectopic pregnancy are not significantly different.[17] Judicious removal of an extensively damaged fallopian tube may be considered, with preservation of the tube if feasible.[16]

○ *Paratubal cyst torsion:* Torsion of a paratubal or paraovarian cyst can result in isolated fallopian tube torsion or torsion of the entire adnexa. This is more common in the pediatric population (20.5% of cases in patients <20 years old vs 14.1% in those 20 years to menopause).[18] Patients with obesity or hyperandrogenism may have higher risk of paratubal cysts.[19,20] If the ovary is not involved, it may appear normal on imaging. This is demonstrated in 1 case series of 19 patients with isolated tubal torsion, 14 of whom had a paratubal cyst as the likely cause of the torsion; 18 patients in the series had ultrasound, 78% of these had ipsilateral adnexal pathologic condition, most commonly a simple cyst, and 88% had normal Doppler flow to the ovaries.[21] The bottom line is that in the setting of a simple adnexal cyst and clinical history/signs consistent with torsion, torsion of a paratubal cyst involving the fallopian tube is a very likely diagnosis.

○ *Cystectomy and the role of delayed surgery to improve ovarian salvage:* If a cyst is present, it is ideal to perform cystectomy at the time of detorsion. Surgical planes can be unclear in acute torsion and can prohibit successful cystectomy. In this setting, it is reasonable to detorse the adnexa, followed by observation with imaging to determine if the cyst resolves spontaneously (as expected with a corpus luteum or follicular cyst) and whether a second surgery is needed.[8] If there is high concern for malignancy, in select situations it may be prudent to perform detorsion alone followed by complete oncologic evaluation.[8]

Outcome and Long-Term Recommendations

- *Recurrence rates:* Recurrence of adnexal torsion is approximately 5% to 6%. Patients with initial torsion of a normal ovary have the highest rates of recurrence (15% vs 3% in patients with idiopathic torsion vs torsion in the presence of a mass).[22]

- *Oophoropexy:* The role of oophoropexy in preventing recurrence of torsion is controversial. Oophoropexy aims to reduce torsion risk either by plicating the ovary to a structure in the pelvis or by shortening the utero-ovarian ligament. There are scant data comparing oophoropexy techniques. Torsion rates after oophoropexy are likely between 9% and 17%.[22] Patients at higher risk of recurrence (initial torsion of a normal ovary, bilateral torsion, recurrent torsion, prior oophorectomy, or anatomic risk factors, such as long infundibulopelvic ligaments) may potentially benefit the most from oophoropexy.[22]

Both pediatric and adult patients are at risk for delayed or missed diagnosis of torsion. The presenting symptoms are nonspecific, intermittent, and often ascribed to ruptured or hemorrhagic cysts. Providers may over-rely on imaging to rule out torsion, especially with normal Dopplers. Finally, particularly in young patients, gynecologic causes of pain are often not considered.

Key Points: Adnexal Torsion

- Providers should have a high clinical index of suspicion for adnexal torsion for patients with ovaries with acute abdominal pain and vomiting, even if the patient intermittently has minimal or no pain.
- Ultrasound is first-line imaging. Imaging, including the presence or absence of vascular flow to the ovary, cannot definitively diagnose or exclude torsion.
- Oophorectomy is rarely indicated, even if the ovary appears grossly necrotic.
- Oophoropexy may be beneficial in select situations, but the advantages in most cases of torsion remain unclear.

APHTHOUS ULCERS

Vulvar complaints in children and teens are common and may be a great source of distress for patients and caregivers. Aphthous ulcers, historically known as Lipschutz ulcers, are the most common cause of nonsexually transmissible vulvar ulcers. In fact, these ulcers have become coined "nonsexually acquired genital ulceration (NSGU)."

Evaluation

- *History*: The typical progression of the aphthous ulcer begins with one or more white spots or blood blisters on the vulva that grow into a larger and darker lesion (**Fig. 4**). The crusted area then opens to an ulcerative-appearing lesion, which is associated with erythema, edema, and pain. In an early case series, 19 out of 20 patients with aphthous ulcers reported systemic signs and symptoms that occurred before the development of the ulcer.[23] The prodrome occurred within a mean of 2 days before ulceration and ranged from occurring on the day of ulceration to 2 weeks before the ulcer developed. The top 3 prodromal symptoms

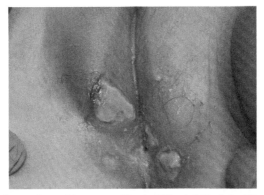

Fig. 4. Vulvar aphthous ulcers. (*Courtesy of* Paula Hillard, MD, Palo Alto, CA.)

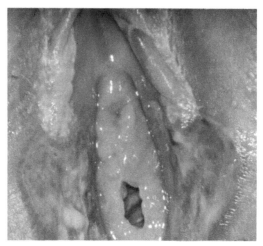

Fig. 5. Vulvar aphthous ulcers with kissing lesions. (*Courtesy of* Paula Hillard, MD, Palo Alto, CA.)

included fever, fatigue, and headache. Patients also reported gastrointestinal symptoms, upper-respiratory symptoms, and about one-third of the time, oral or skin lesions. A typical complaint is dysuria, often mistaken for urinary tract infection; however, this is vulvar pain induced by acidic urine contacting open ulcers.

- *Physical*: Ulcers are exquisitely tender to touch and typically present on the medial aspect of the labia minora. Ulcers may also present on the posterior fourchette, perineal body, and labia majora. They are oval shaped, shallow (approximately 2 mm deep), necrotic lesions that are sharply demarcated, typically greater than 1 cm in diameter, with elevated and red borders. Many patients will have multiple lesions, erosive features, erythema, and edema of the adjacent areas. These ulcers are often labeled "kissing" lesions, as ulcers will mirror each other on each side of the labia minora, perineum, or vagina (**Fig. 5**). Other key physical examination findings include oral lesions (often present in Behcet disease and lichen planus) and lymphadenopathy.
- *Laboratory evaluation*: The diagnosis of vulvar aphthous is a clinical diagnosis of exclusion and involves ruling out sexually transmitted infections. There is no standardized evaluation, and the cause is most commonly idiopathic. Vulvar aphthous ulcers are attributed to a dysregulation of the body's immune

---

Box 2
Conservative management options for vulvar aphthous ulcers

Sitz baths in plain lukewarm/cool water 2 to 3 times a day

Dilute urine by voiding in bathtub or with squirt bottle filled with water

Bland emollients (zinc oxide, petrolatum)

Topical anesthetics (lidocaine jelly)

Nonsteroidal anti-inflammatory drugs (ibuprofen, Naprosyn)

response, most commonly triggered by a viral illness. Aphthous ulcers have been described in case reports associated with Epstein-Barr virus (EBV), cytomegalovirus (CMV), influenza, salmonella, mycoplasma, mumps, recently in COVID-19,[24] and in response to Pfizer COVID-19 vaccine.[25] In the review by Huppert and colleagues[23] of 20 aphthous ulcers, EBV or CMV was identified in 4 out of 20 patients. In another retrospective review, aphthous vulvar ulcers were associated with identified viral syndromes or upper-respiratory infections in 6 of the 10 patients.[26] In a review of 33 aphthous ulcers, a viral diagnosis was identified in 9 (27.3%) patients with 3 cases of CMV and *Mycoplasma pneumoniae* infection, 2 cases of EBV, and 1 case of Parvovirus B19.[27] Viral laboratory test results can be obtained to assess for underlying infection and to rule out other causes, such as for EBV, CMV, Parvovirus B19, or herpes simplex virus (HSV). Biopsy is not indicated routinely but should be considered should the ulcers recur or if there is concern for other pathologic condition.

Management

The key focus of treatment for these patients is symptomatic relief. To date, no consistent protocols have been described. Conservative treatments are reviewed in **Box 2**.

Patients may not respond to conservative treatment, have prolonged ulcers, or experience recurrences requiring additional management (**Box 3**). There have not been case series large enough to permit recommendations of optimal treatment regimens. One small study evaluated the use of topical and oral steroids for acute phase treatment as well as doxycycline for prophylaxis against recurrence.[28] Sixteen (94%) patients achieved rapid pain relief and complete healing of ulcers within 16 days of steroid use, and none of the 14 patients on doxycycline prophylaxis reported any recurrences during a mean follow-up of 18.3 months.

The anti-inflammatory properties of systemic and topical corticosteroids have been useful in treating oral aphthosis. Several regimens that have been prescribed, but not well studied include topical corticosteroids as needed for painful ulcers, prednisolone at 10 to 25 mg per day for recurrent mild to moderate cases, or 40 to 50 mg per day for those with severe cases. The steroid is weaned once the ulcers have healed.[28]

In addition, doxycycline has well-known anti-inflammatory properties. Doxycycline was administered at 50 to 100 mg per day for those who presented with recurrent disease.[28] To date, there are no randomized controlled studies to demonstrate if steroids reduce duration and severity of symptoms or if doxycycline is an effective modality to reduce recurrence risk.

Box 3
Additional management options for vulvar aphthous ulcers nonresponsive to conservative treatment or recurrence

Narcotics (oxycodone)

Place Foley if unable to void

Hospitalization as needed for pain control or nausea/vomiting precludes oral pain medication

Topical corticosteroids, such as clobetasol 0.05% ointment twice a day for 7 days[29]

Oral prednisolone[28] 10 to 25 mg per day (mild to moderate) 40 to 50 mg a day (severe)

Wean with healing of ulcers

Doxycycline 50 to 100 mg per day for recurrence prophylaxis for months to years (liver function test monitoring advised for long-term use)[28]

Outcome and Long-Term Recommendations

Aphthous ulcers generally resolve within 1 to 3 weeks. Approximately one-third of patients will experience recurrences, which are typically less severe.[23,29] Recurrent ulcers should trigger evaluation for other systemic illness, such as Behcet syndrome and Crohn disease. In the former, diagnostic criteria include recurrent oral aphthae plus at least 2 of the following: genital aphthae, synovitis, posterior uveitis, cutaneous pustular vasculitis, or meningoencephalitis. In the latter, patients typically report abdominal pain, diarrhea, rectal bleeding, anorexia, and weight loss. A fecal calprotectin can be a helpful indicator for a gastrointestinal source of the cutaneous manifestation. A more extensive workup including examination under anesthesia and vulvar biopsy may be indicated.

Key Points: Aphthous Ulcers

- Typically present with pain, inability to void, and/or pain with urination
- Lesions are typically larger than those of HSV and often have "kissing" lesions
- Cause is unclear, but thought to be virally associated and often preceded with viral prodromal symptoms
- Symptomatic relief is encouraged with sitz baths, topical analgesics
- May require admission and Foley if unable to void or for pain control
- Consider steroid treatments for recalcitrant ulcers or recurrences
- Vulvar biopsy if diagnosis is in question

STRADDLE INJURIES

Straddle injuries are commonly seen in children following accidental injury leading to trauma to the vulva and vagina. A range of vulvar injuries occurs from superficial abrasions to lacerations and hematomas and often present with vulvovaginal bleeding and pain. These injuries occur in a variety of ways, commonly after falls on bicycles, on playground equipment, in bathtubs, or on furniture. Injuries usually involve the superior vulvar anatomic structures, such as the mons pubis, clitoris, and labia (**Fig. 6**). Nonstraddle blunt genital injuries or penetrating trauma can also occur, such as following motor vehicle collisions or sexual assaults. Most straddle injuries are the results of blunt, nonpenetrating trauma and are amenable to nonoperative management. Studies have demonstrated that failure to identify the extent of these injuries with

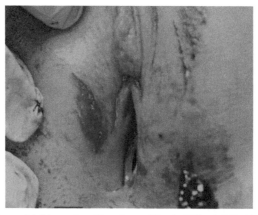

Fig. 6. Straddle injury of labia major. (*Courtesy of* Paula Hillard, MD, Palo Alto, CA.)

timely repair can result in chronic vulvovaginal concerns, such as fissures or stenosis.[30,31]

Patient Evaluation

After a straddle injury, the most common site injured has been reported to be the labia, and less commonly, the hymen and posterior fourchette. Disruption of the hymen and injuries to the posterior fourchette are more frequently seen with sexual trauma. In 1 retrospective review of 358 patients aged 0 to 18 years old who were treated in the ED for genital lacerations, 63% (225/358) had injuries to the labia, 23% (81/358) had injuries to the posterior fourchette or perineum, 10% (36/358) had injuries to the hymen and vagina, and injury to the urethra or anus only occurred 5% of the time (16/358).[32] Nearly 90% experienced laceration, with about 10% experiencing an abrasion or contusion. Approximately 4% experienced a hematoma following their injury. Most of the patients had lacerations less than 3 cm in length.

A thorough evaluation of the injury is often the most critical aspect in the management of straddle injuries in the young patient. This can be challenging because of patient willingness, pain, small size, and bleeding. Some have recommended liberally applying 2% to 5% lidocaine jelly over the injury and irrigating with warm water or saline to optimize examination. Compression with towels or moist cloths can also be helpful in mitigating bleeding.

Most patients can be examined without deep sedation; however, when discomfort prevents an adequate examination, if more extensive injuries are suspected, or if the urethra or rectum may be involved, it is advisable to proceed with conscious sedation or general anesthesia (**Fig. 7**). The highest risk factors associated with the need for examination under anesthesia include those who have penetrating injuries, injuries larger than 3 to 4 cm in size, injuries involving the hymen, vagina, urethra, and anus, injuries that extend beyond the labia, patient unable to tolerate examination, inability to see the full extent of the lesion, and bleeding that cannot be localized (**Fig. 8**). It has been documented that about 10% to 25% of genital injuries require operative intervention in the ER or operating room.[32–34]

Management of Vulvovaginal Lacerations

Optimizing visualization of the lesion is paramount to treatment. Recommending compression with sterile gauze or towels can aid in hemostasis and hematoma

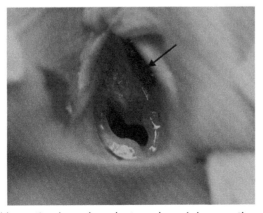

Fig. 7. Periurethral laceration (*arrow*); evaluate and repair in operating room. (*Courtesy of* Paula Hillard, MD, Palo Alto, CA.)

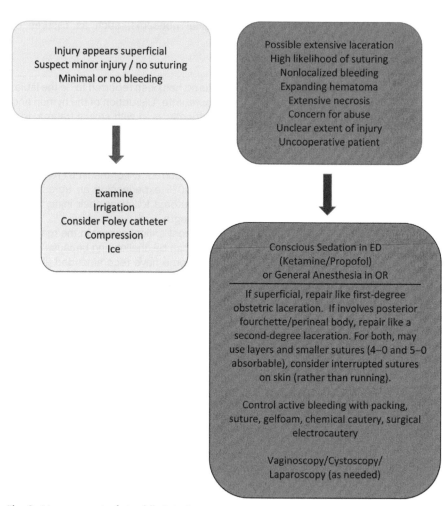

Fig. 8. Management of straddle injuries.

prevention. Applying warm water irrigation can aid with visualizing the laceration. Patient comfort can be aided by Child Life specialists, distraction, and, when needed and if available, sedation administered in the ER. Accessing lighting and equipment to adequately see the extent of the injury is often a hurdle, but a necessity for proper management. Minor bleeding and abrasions are managed conservatively with barrier ointments, ice, and reassurance. More concerning straddle injuries should be thoroughly examined often with deeper sedation or general anesthesia (see **Fig. 8**). Prepubertal girls may also benefit from application of a small amount of estrogen cream twice daily to the injured tissue. It is thought that it may help with healing by promoting granulation tissue and reducing inflammation.[34]

Management of Vulvar Hematomas

Vulvar hematomas develop when the labial branches of the internal pudendal artery are injured (lacerations, perforation) and when the soft tissue and pelvic fascia compress against the pelvic bones (falls, impact). Hematomas can become extensive as blood and edema track along the open planes of the low resistance subcutaneous pelvic fascia.[35] Fortunately, most vulvar hematomas spontaneously resolve over 1 to 5 days with conservative management.[36] Conservative management includes rest, compression, application of ice, and evaluation for injury to adjacent organs, such as urethra, vagina, anus, and bone injury.[37] Adequate analgesia is advised, and a bladder catheter should be placed if there is any concern for voiding difficulties. Surgical intervention is recommended when there is progressive growth, an unstable patient, or pain that is unrelieved.[38] Surgical assessment is traditionally considered when the vulvar hematoma exceeds 4 cm owing to concern for necrosis of the underlying tissue.[39] Appreciating the extent of hematoma can be difficult and may be optimized using transperineal ultrasound.[40]

Surgical approach to controlling hemostasis and evacuating the hematoma starts with an incision over the point of maximum bulge at the mucocutaneous junction or through the vaginal mucosa.[35] Blood clots are evacuated; active bleeding is localized, and hemostasis is achieved with careful tissue handling to avoid additional tissue trauma. Generalized venous oozing is the common finding, as the source of bleeding is often difficult to identify. Hemostatic agents, packing, and a Penrose drain can be placed (at the most inferior region of the hematoma) to diminish the hematoma and reduce the risk of infection.[41] Arterial embolization is also an alternative to surgical management, but its availability may be limited.[42]

Outcome and Long-Term Recommendations

Emergent straddle injuries heal quickly, with abrasions and superficial lacerations typically resolving in 2 to 3 days and deeper lacerations recovering similar to episiotomies with healing time of 6 weeks. If injuries are due to sexual abuse, however, trauma can be longstanding, so recognition and intervention are of the utmost importance.

Key Points: Straddle Injuries

- Remind emergency department to apply pressure to vulvar lacerations with pads or towels with firm leg closure.
- Many lesions can be evaluated in the emergency department if (a) there is complete visualization of the extent of the lesion and (b) lesion does not extend into vagina.
- Always consider and screen for sexual assault.
- Avoid using force/coercion to facilitate examinations, optimize emergency department anesthesia, and have a low threshold to proceed to the operating room.
- Lacerations most commonly involve the labia, and if small/hemostatic, can be managed conservatively with analgesia and close follow-up.
- Vulvar hematomas should be managed conservatively unless expanding rapidly or the patient is hemodynamically unstable.

DISCLOSURE

There are no commercial or financial conflicts of interest for either author, and neither author received funding for this article.

REFERENCES

1. Adnexal torsion in adolescents: ACOG Committee Opinion No. 783. Obstet Gynecol 2019;134(2):e56–63.

2. Childress KJ, Dietrich JE. Pediatric ovarian torsion. Surg Clin North Am 2017; 97(1):209–21.

3. Joudi N, Adams Hillard PJ. Adnexal torsion in a pediatric population: acute presentation with question of chronicity. Eur J Obstet Gynecol Reprod Biol 2021; 268:82–6.

4. Hartman SJ, Prieto JM, Naheedy JH, et al. Ovarian volume ratio is a reliable predictor of ovarian torsion in girls without an adnexal mass. J Pediatr Surg 2021; 56(1):180–2.

5. Schwartz BI, Huppert JS, Chen C, et al. Creation of a composite score to predict adnexal torsion in children and adolescents. J Pediatr Adolesc Gynecol 2018; 31(2):132–7.

6. Brandt ML, Helmrath MA. Ovarian cysts in infants and children. Semin Pediatr Surg 2005;14(2):78–85.

7. Renaud EJ, Sømme S, Islam S, et al. Ovarian masses in the child and adolescent: an American Pediatric Surgical Association Outcomes and Evidence-Based Practice Committee systematic review. J Pediatr Surg 2019;54(3):369–77.

8. Lawrence AE, Minneci PC, Deans KJ. Ovarian masses and torsion: new approaches for ovarian salvage. Adv Pediatr 2020;67:113–21.

9. Wattar B, Rimmer M, Rogozinska E, et al. Accuracy of imaging modalities for adnexal torsion: a systematic review and meta-analysis. BJOG 2021;128(1): 37–44.

10. Ssi-Yan-Kai G, Rivain AL, Trichot C, et al. What every radiologist should know about adnexal torsion. Emerg Radiol 2018;25(1):51–9.

11. Breech LL, Hillard PJA. Adnexal torsion in pediatric and adolescent girls. Curr Opin Obstet Gynecol 2005;17(5):483–9.

12. Balasubramaniam D, Duraisamy KY, Ezhilmani M. Laparoscopic detorsion and fertility preservation in twisted ischemic adnexa - a single-center prospective study. Gynecol Minim Invasive Ther 2020;9(1):24–8.

13. Robertson JJ, Long B, Koyfman A. Myths in the evaluation and management of ovarian torsion. J Emerg Med 2017;52(4):449–56.

14. Piper HG, Oltmann SC, Xu L, et al. Ovarian torsion: diagnosis of inclusion mandates earlier intervention. J Pediatr Surg 2012;47(11):2071–6.

15. Oltmann SC, Fischer A, Barber R, et al. Pediatric ovarian malignancy presenting as ovarian torsion: incidence and relevance. J Pediatr Surg 2010;45(1):135–9.

16. Casey RK, Damle LF, Gomez-Lobo V. Isolated fallopian tube torsion in pediatric and adolescent females: a retrospective review of 15 cases at a single institution. J Pediatr Adolesc Gynecol 2013;26(3):189–92.

17. Mol F, van Mello NM, Strandell A, et al. Salpingotomy versus salpingectomy in women with tubal pregnancy (ESEP study): an open-label, multicentre, randomised controlled trial. Lancet 2014;383(9927):1483–9.

18. Melcer Y, Sarig-Meth T, Maymon R, et al. Similar but different: a comparison of adnexal torsion in pediatric, adolescent, and pregnant and reproductive-age women. J Womens Health (Larchmt) 2016;25(4):391–6.

19. Muolokwu E, Sanchez J, Bercaw JL, et al. Paratubal cysts, obesity, and hyperandrogenism. J Pediatr Surg 2011;46(11):2164–7.

20. Dietrich JE, Adeyemi O, Hakim J, et al. Paratubal cyst size correlates with obesity and dysregulation of the Wnt signaling pathway. J Pediatr Adolesc Gynecol 2017; 30(5):571–7.

21. Webster KW, Scott SM, Huguelet PS. Clinical predictors of isolated tubal torsion: a case series. J Pediatr Adolesc Gynecol 2017;30(5):578–81.

22. Comeau IM, Hubner N, Kives SL, et al. Rates and technique for oophoropexy in pediatric ovarian torsion: a single-institution case series. J Pediatr Adolesc Gynecol 2017;30(3):418–21.
23. Huppert JS, Gerber MA, Deitch HR, et al. Vulvar ulcers in young females: a manifestation of aphthosis. J Pediatr Adolesc Gynecol 2006;19(3):195–204.
24. Christl J, Alaniz VI, Appiah L, et al. Vulvar aphthous ulcer in an adolescent with COVID-19. J Pediatr Adolesc Gynecol 2021;34(3):418–20.
25. Wojcicki AV, O'Flynn O'Brien KL. Vulvar aphthous ulcer in an adolescent after Pfizer-BioNTech (BNT162b2) COVID-19 vaccination. J Pediatr Adolesc Gynecol 2022;35(2):167–70. S1083-3188(21)00304-1.
26. Lehman JS, Bruce AJ, Wetter DA, et al. Reactive nonsexually related acute genital ulcers: review of cases evaluated at Mayo Clinic. J Am Acad Dermatol 2010; 63(1):44–51.
27. Vieira-Baptista P, Lima-Silva J, Beires J, et al. Lipschütz ulcers: should we rethink this? An analysis of 33 cases. Eur J Obstet Gynecol Reprod Biol 2016;198: 149–52.
28. Dixit S, Bradford J, Fischer G. Management of nonsexually acquired genital ulceration using oral and topical corticosteroids followed by doxycycline prophylaxis. J Am Acad Dermatol 2013;68(5):797–802.
29. Rosman IS, Berk DR, Bayliss SJ, et al. Acute genital ulcers in nonsexually active young girls: case series, review of the literature, and evaluation and management recommendations. Pediatr Dermatol 2012;29(2):147–53.
30. Scheidler MG, Schultz BL, Schall L, et al. Mechanisms of blunt perineal injury in female pediatric patients. J Pediatr Surg 2000;35(9):1317–9.
31. Shnorhavorian M, Hidalgo-Tamola J, Koyle MA, et al. Unintentional and sexual abuse-related pediatric female genital trauma: a multiinstitutional study of freestanding pediatric hospitals in the United States. Urology 2012;80(2):417–22.
32. Dowlut-McElroy T, Higgins J, Williams KB, et al. Patterns of treatment of accidental genital trauma in girls. J Pediatr Adolesc Gynecol 2018;31(1):19–22.
33. Iqbal CW, Jrebi NY, Zielinski MD, et al. Patterns of accidental genital trauma in young girls and indications for operative management. J Pediatr Surg 2010; 45(5):930–3.
34. Emans SJ, Laufer MR. Divasta. In: Laufer, Goldstein's Pediatric and Adolescent Gynecology. 7th Edition. Wolters Kluwer; 2020.
35. Hudock JJ, Dupayne N, Mcgeary JA. Traumatic vulvar hematomas; report of six cases and review of the literature. Am J Obstet Gynecol 1955;70(5):1064–73.
36. McCann J, Miyamoto S, Boyle C, et al. Healing of nonhymenal genital injuries in prepubertal and adolescent girls: a descriptive study. Pediatrics 2007;120(5): 1000–11.
37. Jones ISC, O'Connor A. Non-obstetric vulval trauma. Emerg Med Australas 2013; 25(1):36–9.
38. Papoutsis D, Haefner HK. Large vulvar haematoma of traumatic origin. J Clin Diagn Res 2017;11(9):QJ01–2.
39. Hernández-Tiria MC, Navarro-Devia AJ, Osorio-Ruiz AM. Lesión vulvar y perineal secundaria a trauma pelviperineal complejo: presentación de un caso y revisión de la literatura. Rev Colomb Obstet Ginecol 2015;66(4):297.
40. Sherer DM, Stimphil R, Hellmann M, et al. Transperineal sonography of a large vulvar hematoma following blunt perineal trauma. J Clin Ultrasound 2006;34(6): 309–12.

41. Egan E, Dundee P, Lawrentschuk N. Vulvar hematoma secondary to spontaneous rupture of the internal iliac artery: clinical review. Am J Obstet Gynecol 2009; 200(1):e17–8.

42. Machado-Linde F, Capel-Alemán A, Sánchez-Ferrer ML, et al. Major post-traumatic non-obstetric large haematoma: transarterial embolisation. Eur J Obstet Gynecol Reprod Biol 2011;154(1):118–9.

Ectopic Pregnancy

Shawna Tonick, MD*, Christine Conageski, MD, MSc

KEYWORDS

- Ectopic pregnancy • Pregnancy of unknown location • Methotrexate
- Salpingectomy • Salpingostomy

KEY POINTS

- Approximately 2% of pregnancies are considered ectopic. The most common location is the fallopian tube.
- Ectopic pregnancy can be a life-threatening medical emergency and requires prompt evaluation and treatment.
- The most common presenting signs of ectopic pregnancy are pelvic pain and vaginal bleeding.
- Ectopic pregnancy can be treated medically with methotrexate using several different dosing regimens.
- Ectopic pregnancy can be treated surgically with salpingectomy or salpingostomy, typically by laparoscopy.

BACKGROUND

An ectopic pregnancy is any pregnancy in which the developing products of conception implant outside of the endometrial cavity. Approximately 2% of pregnancies are considered ectopic, although the true prevalence is unknown and may be higher because of the lack of standardized reporting systems and available outpatient treatment options.[1] For some, an ectopic pregnancy may represent a life-threatening medical emergency. Ectopic pregnancies are the leading cause of first-trimester mortality and are responsible for approximately 4% of all pregnancy-related mortalities.[2,3]

Over half of ectopic pregnancies occur in patients without known risk factors, stressing the importance of maintaining a high clinical suspicion during the initial evaluation.[4] Risk factors for ectopic pregnancy include history of prior ectopic pregnancy, conditions that lead to fallopian tube damage (such as pelvic infections or pelvic surgeries), smoking, intrauterine device (IUD) use, infertility, and age over 35 years.[5] The most common location of an ectopic pregnancy is the fallopian tube (approximately 90% of cases), but ectopic pregnancies can occur in other locations (interstitial,

Department of OB-GYN, University of Colorado, 12631 East 17th Avenue, AO1, 4th Floor, Aurora, CO 80045, USA
* Corresponding author.
E-mail address: Shawna.tonick@cuanschutz.edu

Obstet Gynecol Clin N Am 49 (2022) 537–549
https://doi.org/10.1016/j.ogc.2022.02.018
0889-8545/22/© 2022 Elsevier Inc. All rights reserved.

ovarian, cesarean scar, abdominal, cervical at approximately 1%–3% each).[6] Within the fallopian tube, the most common location is the ampulla (70%). Less likely tubal locations for ectopic pregnancies are the fimbria (11%) and isthmus (12%).[6] In rare circumstances, an ectopic pregnancy may coexist with an intrauterine pregnancy, as in a heterotopic pregnancy. This risk is greatly increased with advanced reproductive technologies (ART), with an incidence of 1 in 100 for in vitro fertilization versus 1 in 4000 to 30,000 for the general population.[7,8]

EVALUATION

Approximately 20% of patients who present for care in early pregnancy with abdominal pain, vaginal bleeding, or both will have an ectopic pregnancy.[4] The most common presenting symptoms include pelvic pain and bleeding; however, ectopic pregnancies may be asymptomatic.[9] An initial assessment of hemodynamic stability must be included for every patient. Those who present with hemodynamic instability and/or physical examination findings concerning for an acute abdomen should undergo prompt evaluation with point-of-care pregnancy testing and a FAST (focused assessment with sonography for trauma) scan to evaluate for free fluid and the possibility of a ruptured ectopic pregnancy. If a ruptured ectopic pregnancy is suspected, the patient should be managed with emergent surgical intervention.

If the patient is hemodynamically stable, workup begins by obtaining a thorough history and physical examination. Pertinent medical and surgical history includes any previous abdominal, pelvic, or tubal surgeries. Each patient should have a documented gynecologic history, including the date of last menstrual period, history of unprotected intercourse, history of sexually transmitted infections such as gonorrhea or chlamydia, potential current use of contraceptive IUD, any prior gynecologic surgeries or ectopic pregnancies, and recent use of ART. A physical examination includes a thorough abdominal and pelvic examination with both a speculum examination to evaluate for bleeding and a bimanual examination to evaluate for adnexal masses, fullness, or tenderness.

Diagnosis of suspected ectopic pregnancy requires at least laboratory confirmation of pregnancy and pelvic imaging. A urine pregnancy test is typically used as the first-line triage laboratory assessment of pregnancy. Although ectopic pregnancies with a negative urine pregnancy test have been reported, this is an extremely uncommon finding.[10–12] Patients with bleeding should also undergo blood type evaluation to assess for the need for Rh immune globulin if Rh negative. The preferred imaging to evaluate for ectopic pregnancy is transvaginal ultrasound. If the transvaginal ultrasound demonstrates an intrauterine pregnancy, defined as the presence of both a gestational sac and a yolk sac (with possible presence of a fetal pole) within the endometrial cavity, an intrauterine pregnancy has been diagnosed.[13] Although heterotopic pregnancy is possible, it is extremely rare. A gestational sac alone is not diagnostic of an intrauterine pregnancy given the risk of misinterpreting a pseudogestational sac, commonly found in patients with ectopic pregnancies. A pseudogestational sac forms in response to progesterone decidualization of the endometrium and fluid collection.[14] A true gestational sac will typically have findings of a "double decidual sac sign," which appears as 2 concentric echogenic rings surrounding a uniform endometrial fluid collection.[15,16] Conversely, a pseudogestational sac has a single echogenic ring around a more irregularly shaped fluid collection.[17,18]

Ultrasound findings of unilateral adnexal mass and/or pelvic free fluid are suggestive but not diagnostic of ectopic pregnancy. Findings diagnostic of an ectopic pregnancy include a gestational sac with a yolk sac or fetal pole outside of the uterus. More commonly, ectopic pregnancies appear as a unilateral adnexal mass with hypoechoic area, separate from the ovary with peripheral Doppler flow (present in 89% or more of cases).[19,20] Careful diagnosis of an adnexal mass is important, as an ectopic pregnancy can be easily confused with a corpus luteum cyst, which is present in normal intrauterine pregnancies. A large amount of pelvic free fluid should raise suspicion for possible ectopic pregnancy rupture with hemoperitoneum and prompt surgical assessment.

Many patients with a positive pregnancy test will not have ultrasound findings that are diagnostic of either intrauterine or ectopic pregnancy. These patients are diagnosed with pregnancy of unknown anatomic location (PUL) and require ongoing close follow-up starting with an initial serum quantitative beta human chorionic gonadotropin (hCG) level.[13] A single hCG value cannot diagnose the location of a pregnancy. The concept of a "discriminatory zone," an hCG level above which a gestational sac should be seen on a transvaginal ultrasound in a normal intrauterine pregnancy, typically 1500 mIU/mL, has been challenged in recent years.[21,22] Several case series have demonstrated the development of viable intrauterine pregnancies not initially present on ultrasound with hCG levels above the "discriminatory zone."[23,24] In addition, multifetal gestations may present with higher than normal hCG levels.[23] The American College of Obstetricians and Gynecologists therefore recommends that if a discriminatory zone is to be used, providers should use a conservative hCG level cutoff of 3500 mIU/mL.[13] Ultimately, it is likely best to not use a set discriminatory zone and individualize management based on the patient's goals and the hCG trend.

PUL should be seen as a transient stop on the way to a diagnosis, not as a final destination. After initial hCG assessment, serial hCG levels are obtained every 48 hours to evaluate trend over time. It is expected that intrauterine pregnancies will have a more rapid increase of their hCG levels than an abnormal intrauterine or ectopic pregnancy. An increase in hCG level of at least 35% is possibly indicative of a normal intrauterine pregnancy.[25] It is important to keep in mind, however, that higher initial hCG values may be associated with smaller increases than initial hCG levels at lower values, even in patients with normal intrauterine pregnancies. For example, an initial hCG value of 1500 mIU/mL is commonly associated with an average 49% increase, whereas an initial hCG value of greater than 3000 mIU/mL is more commonly associated with a smaller increase, averaging 33%.[26] During serial laboratory assessments, 3 possible scenarios in the hCG level arise, as follows:

- *Increase greater than or equal to 35%:* In normal intrauterine pregnancies, the hCG level is expected to increase 35% every 2 days. In the authors' practice, they trend levels with at least 2 values over 4 days, for a total of 3 values. If the trend remains reassuring, and in the absence of other concerning findings, the authors have these patients return for repeat transvaginal ultrasound within 1 week.
- *Increase less than 35% or plateau:* If the initial trend shows plateau (increase or decrease within 10%) or mild increase that does not meet the 35% threshold, the authors repeat a third hCG level at 48 hours, as long as the patient remains asymptomatic and clinically stable. If the trend continues to be abnormal, they counsel the patient about risk of ectopic pregnancy and offer further diagnosis and management.
- *Decreased initial hCG:* Those patients with an initial decline of their hCG value can be counseled on a narrowed differential diagnosis that includes abnormal intrauterine pregnancy, spontaneous abortion, or ectopic pregnancy. Typically, patients with a spontaneous abortion will show a 48-hour decrease of 21% to

35%.[27] Given the risk of ectopic pregnancy, they follow hCG trends to low levels (<5 mIU/mL) to ensure complete resolution.

Regardless of hCG trend, all patients receive strict return precautions to present to care with severe abdominal pain or heavy vaginal bleeding during monitoring.

Other laboratory tests, such as serum progesterone, have not been proven to help guide definitive clinical decisions. Although values between 3 and 6.2 ng/dL have been associated with abnormal pregnancies, it is not possible to use these values to distinguish between abnormal intrauterine pregnancies and ectopic pregnancies.[28] Progesterone may be helpful in complicated clinical scenarios with an unclear diagnosis; however, it is not diagnostic of an ectopic pregnancy, and a definitive "low-progesterone" value is unknown.

MEDICAL MANAGEMENT

Once an ectopic pregnancy has been diagnosed, patients may be offered 3 management options: surgical, medical, or expectant management. The decision on which option to choose must be individualized for each patient, considering their fertility desires, physical examination findings, medical stability, and patient preference.

Ectopic pregnancy can be medically treated with methotrexate. Methotrexate is a chemotherapeutic drug that competitively inhibits dihydrofolate reductase, an enzyme that participates in the folate pathway. Methotrexate inhibits DNA synthesis in rapidly dividing cells, such as the cells in developing pregnancy tissue.[29] Common adverse effects of methotrexate are gastrointestinal upset (the most common side effect, along with nausea, vomiting, and stomatitis), vaginal spotting, and mild abdominal/pelvic pain.[30] Less common adverse effects are pneumonitis and alopecia.[31] Patients receiving methotrexate should also be counseled about possible risk of birth defects in the setting of an intrauterine pregnancy. For this reason, methotrexate is never an option for patients with a heterotopic pregnancy.

Patients must be carefully selected for medical management. Before administration of methotrexate, patients should undergo an assessment of their medical history and detailed laboratory evaluation, including recent hCG level, complete blood count, liver function tests, and renal function, to determine if any contraindications exist.

Absolute contraindications for methotrexate therapy include hemodynamic instability, suspected ruptured ectopic pregnancy, severe anemia/leukopenia/neutropenia, active pulmonary and/or peptic ulcer disease, clinically significant hepatic and/or renal dysfunction, known sensitivity or allergy to methotrexate, breastfeeding status, and inability to follow-up[13] (**Fig. 1**). Relative contraindications include refusal of blood products, high initial hCG levels (>5000 mIU/mL), embryonic cardiac activity, and ectopic pregnancy greater than 4 cm.[13,32] For patients with relative contraindications, methotrexate may still be attempted after shared decision making with the patient.[32]

Methotrexate may be administered using 1 of 3 available protocols: "single dose," "2 dose," or "multidose" (**Fig. 2**). During any methotrexate protocol, patients should be advised to decrease folic acid intake (including prenatal vitamins and avoiding folate-rich foods) and avoid nonsteroidal anti-inflammatory drugs, as this may interfere with methotrexate's mechanism of action. The authors typically recommend avoiding pregnancy for 3 months after methotrexate administration because of possible risk of teratogenicity, although there is no consensus regarding this recommendation.[33] Overall, resolution of ectopic pregnancy with medical management ranges from 70% to 95%.[34]

Absolute Contraindications

- Intrauterine pregnancy
- Evidence of immunodeficiency
- Moderate to severe anemia, leukopenia, or thrombocytopenia
- Sensitivity to methotrexate
- Active pulmonary disease
- Active peptic ulcer disease
- Clinically important hepatic dysfunction
- Clinically important renal dysfunction
- Breastfeeding
- Ruptured ectopic pregnancy
- Hemodynamically unstable patient
- Inability to participate in follow-up

Relative Contraindications

- Embryonic cardiac activity detected by transvaginal ultrasonography
- High initial hCG concentration
- Ectopic pregnancy greater than 4 cm in size as imaged by transvaginal ultrasonography
- Refusal to accept blood transfusion

Modified from Medical treatment of ectopic pregnancy: a committee opinion. Practice Committee of American Society for Reproductive Medicine. Fertil Steril 2013;100:638–44.

Fig. 1. Contraindications to methotrexate therapy. (*From* American College of Obstetricians and Gynecologists' Committee on Practice Bulletins—Gynecology. ACOG Practice Bulletin No. 193: Tubal Ectopic Pregnancy [published correction appears in Obstet Gynecol. 2019 May;133(5):1059]. Obstet Gynecol. 2018;131(3):e91-e103. https://doi.org/10.1097/AOG. 0000000000002560; with permission)

- *Single-dose protocol*: The patient receives a single dose of methotrexate at a dose of 50 mg/m² on day 1 of treatment. The patient has hCG levels drawn on day 4 and 7. Adequate treatment is considered a decrease in hCG value of at least 15% between day 4 and 7. hCG levels may increase between day 1 and day 4. If an adequate decrease occurs, hCG levels should be followed weekly until negative. If an adequate decrease does not occur, the patient may receive a second dose of methotrexate at 50 mg/m². If an adequate decrease still does not occur after 2 doses, surgical management should be strongly considered.[13,35]
- *Two-dose protocol*: On day 1, the patient receives a single dose of methotrexate at 50 mg/m². The patient then *automatically* receives a second dose of methotrexate at 50 mg/m² on day 4, and hCG is measured this day. hCG is then drawn again on day 7, in which a 15% decrease in hCG is expected. If an adequate decrease occurs, hCG levels are followed weekly until negative. If an adequate decrease does not occur, the patient may receive a third dose of methotrexate 50 mg/m² on day 7, with hCG level checked again on day 11. At least a 15% decrease is anticipated. If the decrease does not occur, a fourth dose of methotrexate 50 mg/m² can be administered on day 11, with hCG level checked again

Single-dose regimen*

- Administer a single dose of methotrexate at a dose of 50 mg/m^2 intramuscularly on d 1
- Measure hCG level on posttreatment d 4 and d 7
  - If the decrease is greater than 15%, measure hCG levels weekly until reaching nonpregnant level
  - If decrease is less than 15%, readminister methotrexate at a dose of 50 mg/m^2 intramuscularly and repeat hCG level
  - If hCG does not decrease after two doses, consider surgical management
- If hCG levels plateau or increase during follow-up, consider administering methotrexate for treatment of a persistent ectopic pregnancy

Two-dose regimen[†]

- Administer methotrexate at a dose of 50 mg/m^2 intramuscularly on d 1
- Administer second dose of methotrexate at a dose of 50 mg/m^2 intramuscularly on d 4
- Measure hCG level on posttreatment d 4 and d 7
  - If the decrease is greater than 15%, measure hCG levels weekly until reaching nonpregnant level
  - If decrease is less than 15%, readminister methotrexate 50 mg/m^2 intramuscularly on d 7   and check hCG levels on d 11
  - If hCG levels decrease 15% between d 7 and d 11   , continue to monitor weekly until reaching nonpregnant levels
  - If the decrease is less than 15% between d 7 and d11, readminister dose of methotrexate 50 mg/m^2 intramuscularly on d 11 and check hCG levels on d 14
  - If hCG does not decrease after four doses, consider surgical management
- If hCG levels plateau or increase during follow-up, consider administering methotrexate for treatment of a persistent ectopic pregnancy

Fixed multiple-dose regimen[‡]

- Administer methotrexate 1 mg/kg intramuscularly on d 1, 3, 5, 7; alternate with folinic acid 0.1 mg/kg intramuscularly on d 2, 4, 6, 8
- Measure hCG levels on methotrexate dose days and continue until hCG has decreased by 15% from its previous measurement
  - If the decrease is greater than 15%, discontinue administration of methotrexate and measure hCG levels weekly until reaching nonpregnant levels (may ultimately need one, two, three, or four doses)
  - If hCG does not decrease after four doses, consider surgical management
- If hCG levels plateau or increase during follow-up, consider administering methotrexate for treatment of a persistent ectopic pregnancy

Abbreviation: hCG, human chorionic gonadotropin.

*Stovall TG, Ling FW. Single-dose methotrexate: an expanded clinical trial. Am J Obstet Gynecol 1993;168:1759-62; discussion 1762–5.

[†]Barnhart K, Hummel AC, Sammel MD, Menon S, Jain J, Chakhtoura N. Use of "2-dose" regimen of methotrexate to treat ectopic pregnancy. Fertil Steril 2007;87:250–6.

[‡]Rodi IA, Sauer MV, Gorrill MJ, Bustillo M, Gunning JE, Marshall JR, et al. The medical treatment of unruptured ectopic pregnancy with methotrexate and citrovorum rescue: preliminary experience. Fertil Steril 1986;46:811–3.

Fig. 2. Methotrexate treatment protocols. (*From* American College of Obstetricians and Gynecologists' Committee on Practice Bulletins—Gynecology. ACOG Practice Bulletin No. 193: Tubal Ectopic Pregnancy [published correction appears in Obstet Gynecol. 2019 May;133(5):1059]. Obstet Gynecol. 2018;131(3):e91-e103. https://doi.org/10.1097/AOG. 0000000000002560; with permission)

on day 14. If a 15% decrease still does not occur, surgical management should be strongly considered.[13,36] Advantages of this protocol include improved efficacy in patients with high initial hCG levels (between 3600 and 5500 mIU/mL) and a shorter resolution to negative hCG levels.[37,38]

- *Multidose protocol*: The multidose regimen differs from the other 2 regimens in that it is a fixed dose and requires frequent injections. The patient receives methotrexate 1 mg/kg intramuscularly on days 1, 3, 5, and 7 of treatment and rescue folinic acid 0.1 mg/kg on days 2, 4, 6, and 8 of treatment to counteract the adverse effects of methotrexate. The patient has hCG levels measured on methotrexate days 1, 3, 5, and 7. If a decrease of 15% is noted, then methotrexate injections can be discontinued, and hCG is measured weekly until negative. If hCG does not decrease the expected amount at the end of treatment, surgical management should be considered.[13,39] Although the multidose protocol may have a higher success rate, it is associated with more adverse side effects than single dose.[40]

SURGICAL MANAGEMENT

Surgical management of ectopic pregnancy is typically performed with the use of laparoscopy. A suspected ruptured ectopic pregnancy should always be treated with surgical management. Other indications for surgical management include failed medical management, need for definitive diagnosis, diagnosis of heterotopic pregnancy, and/or patient preference. Patients with a history of previous ectopic pregnancy may consider surgical management more strongly, given increased risk of recurrence. Surgically, patients typically undergo either salpingectomy or salpingostomy.

Salpingectomy results in complete removal of the fallopian tube. This is commonly performed using a bipolar electrocautery device by ligating the fallopian tube from the uterine cornua, along the mesosalpinx, and out to the fimbriated end. It is important to remove as much fallopian tube tissue at the cornua as possible to prevent the risk of a future interstitial ectopic pregnancy.[41] In certain situations, a salpingostomy may be considered. To perform a salpingostomy, the fallopian tube is incised (typically using monopolar cautery) longitudinally along the fallopian tube, and the pregnancy tissue is removed from the tube. This procedure is technically more challenging, and there is a risk of retained pregnancy tissue. Some surgeons may opt to give methotrexate prophylactically after salpingostomy, which exposes the patient to risks of both surgical and medical management.[42] Theoretically, salpingostomy also leads to tubal damage and may place the patient at increased risk of a future ipsilateral ectopic pregnancy. However, salpingostomy is associated with a higher spontaneous intrauterine pregnancy rate.[43] In certain situations, such as if a patient has 1 remaining tube or the contralateral tube appears damaged, salpingostomy may be preferred. This decision should be made with careful counseling and shared decision making.

COMBINATION THERAPY

Both medical and surgical management may be necessary to treat certain clinical scenarios as in patients with PUL and an abnormal hCG trend. Although a normal intrauterine pregnancy can likely be excluded with an abnormal hCG trend, the location of the pregnancy is still unknown, and there is no expert consensus on treatment in this instance. Options for treatment include the following: administration of methotrexate, dilation and curettage (D&C) before methotrexate, and/or continued expectant management. Administering methotrexate immediately avoids the need for a surgical procedure but does not provide a definitive diagnosis of pregnancy location.

Furthermore, methotrexate poses a teratogenic risk to an intrauterine pregnancy if present (with congenital anomalies, such as craniosynostosis, microcephaly, cardiac defects, and limb defects).[44] A clear abnormal hCG trend must be demonstrated before this treatment option. Immediate methotrexate treatment has not been found to be cost-effective or decrease risks.[45] The other option, D&C, also has risks and benefits. A D&C is a surgical procedure and comes with risks (including the low risk of uterine perforation, anesthesia risks, and discomfort), but it offers avoidance of methotrexate and definitive diagnosis once pathology resulted have been received. Having a definitive diagnosis may be important while counseling patients on the recurrence risk of ectopic pregnancy. It has also been postulated that delaying care while waiting for pathology results may increase the risk of tubal rupture, although this risk is low at 0.03%.[46] In some cases, a patient may be offered continue expectant management but should understand the risks of possible tubal rupture. Clearly, individualized detailed patient counseling is necessary in these scenarios for patients to make informed decisions.

If D&C is chosen as initial management, pathology may provide a definitive diagnosis. If pathology does not demonstrate chorionic villi, it is recommended to obtain an hCG level 12 to 24 hours after the procedure. If there is a 50% drop in hCG level, it can be assumed that an intrauterine pregnancy was present and was simply missed on pathology.[47] hCG should still be trended weekly until negative. If there is a 10% to 15% drop or less (plateau) or an increase in hCG level, there is a higher clinical suspicion for an ectopic pregnancy.[47,48] These patients should be offered management with methotrexate. If the hCG level decreased between 15% and 50%, this creates a clinical conundrum and requires an individualized plan with careful counseling. Although failed intrauterine pregnancy is more common, ectopic pregnancy is still possible.[48,49] These patients should be closely followed and counseled about treatment options and potential of ectopic pregnancy.[13]

TREATMENT RESISTANCE AND COMPLICATIONS

Patients with tubal ectopic pregnancy can be safely managed with either surgical or medical therapies. Medical therapy may fail up to 28% of the time, but can be effectively managed with surgery.[50,51] Failure rate is further affected by initial hCG level greater than 5000 mIU/mL, ectopic size, and presence of pelvic pain or bleeding.[32] Salpingostomy has a 4% to 15% risk of retained pregnancy tissue and may require subsequent medical therapy.[52,53] Salpingectomy is almost always effective at removal of ectopic pregnancy and preventing morbidity from tubal rupture.

Nontubal ectopic pregnancies, such as interstitial, cervical, or cesarean scar ectopic pregnancies, are more challenging to diagnose and manage effectively. These patients often require a multidisciplinary approach with experts from gynecology, interventional radiology, and/or reproductive infertility specialists. Transfer to a tertiary care center may be necessary. More advanced imaging modalities, such as 3-dimensional ultrasound or MRI, may be necessary to make a definitive diagnosis. Furthermore, during treatment, these patients are at increased risk of significant complications, including blood transfusion, need for additional procedures, and/or hysterectomy.[54]

NEW DEVELOPMENTS

For certain patients, expectant management of ectopic pregnancy may be an option. This is becoming more commonplace.[13] However, these patients must be very carefully selected and extensively counseled about the risk of possible rupture, including how this may be life-threatening to the patient and require emergency surgery. It is considered more appropriate to manage patients with low initial hCG levels with signs of resolution (levels with decrease or plateau). Patients with hCG less than 200 show approximately 88% spontaneous resolution of ectopic pregnancy.[55] Patients should also be asymptomatic and able to seek medical care urgently.

As ART rates increase, nontubal ectopic pregnancies are increasing in prevalence.[56] Similar to tubal ectopic pregnancies, hemodynamically unstable patients should be treated with surgical management. For stable patients, clear protocols for treatment are developing, but often there is no clear best treatment. Treatment options range from simple medical therapy with systemic single-dose methotrexate to multimodal therapies that use a combination of surgical and medical therapies. Potassium chloride has been used in these instances as an injection into the ectopic gestation. Surgical procedures vary by type of nontubal ectopic pregnancy. Cesarean scar ectopic pregnancies can be treated with careful D&C, wedge resection, or hysterectomy.[57,58] Interstitial ectopic pregnancies can also be treated surgically with cornual wedge resection or cornuotomy.[59–62] Given the increased prevalence of these cases, clearer protocols may develop as experience with these rare ectopic pregnancies increase. Currently, however, treatment is often driven by expert opinion, small cases series, and local expertise/experience.

EVALUATION OF OUTCOME

Outcomes following ectopic pregnancy vary by patients' desires for future fertility. Patients with a history of ectopic pregnancy are at increased risk for recurrence with an approximately 10% risk.[4,13] Structural abnormalities of the fallopian tubes have been postulated as 1 cause for tubal ectopic pregnancy. Often this injury is bilateral, which increases a patient's risk for recurrence even after unilateral salpingectomy. Patients with a history of ectopic pregnancy should therefore be counseled to seek early care with their subsequent pregnancy.

Patients with history of ectopic pregnancy have successful intrauterine pregnancy rates ranging from 38% to 89%.[53,63] It is important to keep in mind, however, that infertility is a risk factor for ectopic pregnancy, and this factor will affect subsequent pregnancy rates. Patients with a history of salpingostomy have higher rates of intrauterine pregnancy, but also higher rates of repeat ectopic pregnancy.[55] There are no high-quality data to provide guidance on when to conceive after ectopic pregnancy.

SUMMARY

Ectopic pregnancy is a potentially life-threatening medical emergency that most commonly presents with vaginal bleeding and/or pelvic pain. Transvaginal ultrasound is the imaging modality of choice for diagnosis, in which the presence of a gestational sac with a yolk sac is diagnostic. Cases of PUL should be carefully followed with serial hCG levels. When an ectopic pregnancy is diagnosed, hemodynamically unstable patients should proceed directly to surgical management, whereas hemodynamically stable patients may proceed with medical or surgical management. Three methotrexate protocols exist: single dose, 2 dose, and multiple dose. The 2-dose protocol may be more beneficial in cases of high initial hCG level. For surgical management, salpingostomy can be considered if a patient has a damaged contralateral tube or only 1 tube. Salpingostomy may put the patient at risk of future ipsilateral ectopic pregnancy but may also improve future intrauterine pregnancy outcomes. Expectant management may be carefully considered for patients who present with low initial hCG levels and accept the risk of possible ruptured ectopic pregnancy. Further research is needed on the optimal treatment of nontubal ectopic pregnancies.

CLINICS CARE POINTS

- Ectopic pregnancy is a potentially life-threatening medical emergency that presents in approximately 2% of pregnancies, although the true prevalence may be higher. Approximately 18% of patients who present with vaginal bleeding, abdominal pain, or both may have an ectopic pregnancy and should be carefully evaluated with serum testing and imaging.

- Hemodynamically unstable patients should proceed directly to surgical management. Hemodynamically stable patients can be evaluated for medical, surgical, or in some circumstances, expectant management.

- Medical management involves systemic treatment with methotrexate via a single-dose, 2-dose, or multiple-dose protocol.

- Surgical management typically involves laparoscopy with salpingostomy or salpingectomy. Salpingostomy may require further treatment with systemic methotrexate.

- Pregnancy of unknown location is a transient state that should be carefully followed until a diagnosis is made.

DISCLOSURE

The authors have nothing to disclose

REFERENCES

1. Ectopic pregnancy–United States, 1990-1992. MMWR Morb Mortal Wkly Rep 1995;44(3):46–8.
2. Berg CJ, Callaghan WM, Syverson C, et al. Pregnancy-related mortality in the United States, 1998 to 2005. Obstet Gynecol 2010;116(6):1302–9.
3. Creanga AA, Shapiro-Mendoza CK, Bish CL, et al. Trends in ectopic pregnancy mortality in the United States: 1980-2007. Obstet Gynecol 2011;117(4):837–43.
4. Barnhart KT, Sammel MD, Gracia CR, et al. Risk factors for ectopic pregnancy in women with symptomatic first-trimester pregnancies. Fertil Steril 2006;86(1):36–43.
5. Ankum WM, Mol BW, Van der Veen F, et al. Risk factors for ectopic pregnancy: a meta-analysis. Fertil Steril 1996;65(6):1093–9.
6. Bouyer J, Coste J, Fernandez H, et al. Sites of ectopic pregnancy: a 10 year population-based study of 1800 cases. Hum Reprod 2002;17(12):3224–30.
7. Barrenetxea G, Barinaga-Rementeria L, Lopez de Larruzea A, et al. Heterotopic pregnancy: two cases and a comparative review. Fertil Steril 2007;87(2). 417.e9-15.
8. Maymon R, Shulman A. Controversies and problems in the current management of tubal pregnancy. Hum Reprod Update 1996;2(6):541–51.
9. Alkatout I, Honemeyer U, Strauss A, et al. Clinical diagnosis and treatment of ectopic pregnancy. Obstet Gynecol Surv 2013;68(8):571–81.
10. Hughes M, Lupo A, Browning A. Ruptured ectopic pregnancy with a negative urine pregnancy test. Proc (Bayl Univ Med Cent) 2017;30(1):97–8.
11. Sheele JM, Bernstein R, Counselman FL. A ruptured ectopic pregnancy presenting with a negative urine pregnancy test. Case Rep Emerg Med 2016;2016.

12. Kopelman ZA, Keyser EA, Morales KJ. Ectopic pregnancy until proven otherwise... even with a negative serum hCG test: a case report. Case Rep Women's Health 2021;e00288.

13. Obstetricians ACo, Gynecologists. ACOG Practice Bulletin No. 193: tubal ectopic pregnancy. Obstet Gynecol 2018;131(3):e91–103.

14. Dallenbach-Hellweg G. The histopathology of the endometrium. *Histopathology of the Endometrium*. Springer; 1981. p. 89–256.

15. Bradley WG, Fiske CE, Filly RA. The double sac sign of early intrauterine pregnancy: use in exclusion of ectopic pregnancy. *Radiology* 1982;143(1):223–6.

16. Richardson A, Hopkisson J, Campbell B, et al. Use of double decidual sac sign to confirm intrauterine pregnancy location prior to sonographic visualization of embryonic contents. Ultrasound Obstet Gynecol 2017;49(5):643–8.

17. Lazarus E. What's new in first trimester ultrasound. Radiol Clin North Am 2003; 41(4):663–79.

18. Ahmed AA, Tom BD, Calabrese P. Ectopic pregnancy diagnosis and the pseudosac. Fertil Steril 2004;81(5):1225–8.

19. Barnhart KT, Fay CA, Suescum M, et al. Clinical factors affecting the accuracy of ultrasonography in symptomatic first-trimester pregnancy. Obstet Gynecol 2011; 117(2):299–306.

20. Goldstein SR, Snyder JR, Watson C, et al. Very early pregnancy detection with endovaginal ultrasound. Obstet Gynecol 1988;72(2):200–4.

21. Barnhart KT, Simhan H, Kamelle SA. Diagnostic accuracy of ultrasound above and below the beta-hCG discriminatory zone. Obstet Gynecol 1999;94(4):583–7.

22. Ankum WM, Van der Veen F, Hamerlynck JV, et al. Suspected ectopic pregnancy. What to do when human chorionic gonadotropin levels are below the discriminatory zone. J Reprod Med 1995;40(7):525–8.

23. Doubilet PM, Benson CB, Bourne T, et al. Diagnostic criteria for nonviable pregnancy early in the first trimester. N Engl J Med 2013;369(15):1443–51.

24. Doubilet PM, Benson CB. Further evidence against the reliability of the human chorionic gonadotropin discriminatory level. J Ultrasound Med 2011;30(12): 1637–42.

25. Seeber BE, Sammel MD, Guo W, et al. Application of redefined human chorionic gonadotropin curves for the diagnosis of women at risk for ectopic pregnancy. Fertil sterility 2006;86(2):454–9.

26. Barnhart KT, Guo W, Cary MS, et al. Differences in serum human chorionic gonadotropin rise in early pregnancy by race and value at presentation. Obstet Gynecol 2016;128(3):504–11.

27. Barnhart K, Sammel MD, Chung K, et al. Decline of serum human chorionic gonadotropin and spontaneous complete abortion: defining the normal curve. Obstet Gynecol 2004;104(5 Pt 1):975–81.

28. Mol BW, Lijmer JG, Ankum WM, et al. The accuracy of single serum progesterone measurement in the diagnosis of ectopic pregnancy: a meta-analysis. Hum Reprod 1998;13(11):3220–7.

29. Stika CS. Methotrexate: the pharmacology behind medical treatment for ectopic pregnancy. Clin Obstet Gynecol 2012;55(2):433–9.

30. Barnhart K, Coutifaris C, Esposito M. The pharmacology of methotrexate. Expert Opin Pharmacother 2001;2(3):409–17.

31. Horrigan TJ, Fanning J, Marcotte MP. Methotrexate pneumonitis after systemic treatment for ectopic pregnancy. Am J Obstet Gynecol 1997;176(3):714–5.

32. Menon S, Colins J, Barnhart KT. Establishing a human chorionic gonadotropin cutoff to guide methotrexate treatment of ectopic pregnancy: a systematic review. Fertil Steril 2007;87(3):481–4.

33. Hackmon R, Sakaguchi S, Koren G. Effect of methotrexate treatment of ectopic pregnancy on subsequent pregnancy. Can Fam Physician 2011;57(1):37–9.

34. Barnhart KT, Gosman G, Ashby R, et al. The medical management of ectopic pregnancy: a meta-analysis comparing "single dose" and "multidose" regimens. Obstet Gynecol 2003;101(4):778–84.

35. Stovall TG, Ling FW. Single-dose methotrexate: an expanded clinical trial. Am J Obstet Gynecol 1993;168(6 Pt 1):1759–62.

36. Barnhart K, Hummel AC, Sammel MD, et al. Use of "2-dose" regimen of methotrexate to treat ectopic pregnancy. Fertil Steril 2007;87(2):250–6.

37. Song T, Kim MK, Kim ML, et al. Single-dose versus two-dose administration of methotrexate for the treatment of ectopic pregnancy: a randomized controlled trial. Hum Reprod 2016;31(2):332–8.

38. Saadati N, Najafian M, Masihi S, et al. Comparison of two different protocols of methotrexate therapy in medical management of ectopic pregnancy. Iran Red Crescent Med J 2015;17(12):e20147.

39. Rodi IA, Sauer MV, Gorrill MJ, et al. The medical treatment of unruptured ectopic pregnancy with methotrexate and citrovorum rescue: preliminary experience. Fertil Steril 1986;46(5):811–3.

40. Yang C, Cai J, Geng Y, et al. Multiple-dose and double-dose versus single-dose administration of methotrexate for the treatment of ectopic pregnancy: a systematic review and meta-analysis. Reprod Biomed Online 2017;34(4):383–91.

41. Kirschner R, Kimball HW. Interstitial pregnancy following unilateral salpingectomy. A case report. Jama 1961;175:1180–1.

42. Gracia CR, Brown HA, Barnhart KT. Prophylactic methotrexate after linear salpingostomy: a decision analysis. Fertil Steril 2001;76(6):1191–5.

43. Cheng X, Tian X, Yan Z, et al. Comparison of the fertility outcome of salpingotomy and salpingectomy in women with tubal pregnancy: a systematic review and meta-analysis. PLoS One 2016;11(3):e0152343.

44. Verberne EA, de Haan E, van Tintelen JP, et al. Fetal methotrexate syndrome: a systematic review of case reports. Reprod Toxicol 2019;87:125–39.

45. Ailawadi M, Lorch SA, Barnhart KT. Cost-effectiveness of presumptively medically treating women at risk for ectopic pregnancy compared with first performing a dilatation and curettage. Fertil Steril 2005;83(2):376–82.

46. Morse CB, Sammel MD, Shaunik A, et al. Performance of human chorionic gonadotropin curves in women at risk for ectopic pregnancy: exceptions to the rules. Fertil Steril 2012;97(1):101–6.e2.

47. Rivera V, Nguyen PH, Sit A. Change in quantitative human chorionic gonadotropin after manual vacuum aspiration in women with pregnancy of unknown location. Am J Obstet Gynecol 2009;200(5):e56–9.

48. Shaunik A, Kulp J, Appleby DH, et al. Utility of dilation and curettage in the diagnosis of pregnancy of unknown location. Am J Obstet Gynecol 2011;204(2). 130. e1-130. e6.

49. Insogna IG, Farland LV, Missmer SA, et al. Outpatient endometrial aspiration: an alternative to methotrexate for pregnancy of unknown location. Am J Obstet Gynecol 2017;217(2):185.e1–9.

50. Sendy F, AlShehri E, AlAjmi A, et al. Failure rate of single dose methotrexate in managment of ectopic pregnancy. Obstet Gynecol Int 2015;2015:902426. https://doi.org/10.1155/2015/902426.

51. Tawfiq A, Agameya A-F, Claman P. Predictors of treatment failure for ectopic pregnancy treated with single-dose methotrexate. Fertil sterility 2000;74(5): 877–80.
52. Lund C, Nilas L, Bangsgaard N, et al. Persistent ectopic pregnancy after linear salpingotomy: a non-predictable complication to conservative surgery for tubal gestation. Acta Obstet Gynecol Scand 2002;81(11):1053–9.
53. Farquhar CM. Ectopic pregnancy. Lancet 2005;366(9485):583–91.
54. Parker VL, Srinivas M. Non-tubal ectopic pregnancy. Arch Gynecol Obstet 2016; 294(1):19–27.
55. Korhonen J, Stenman UH, Ylöstalo P. Serum human chorionic gonadotropin dynamics during spontaneous resolution of ectopic pregnancy. Fertil Steril 1994; 61(4):632–6.
56. Barrett F, Shaw J, Blakemore JK, et al. Non-tubal ectopic (NTE) pregnancies in assisted reproductive technology (ART): 10-years of experience at a large urban university based fertility center. Fertil Sterility 2021;116(1):e9.
57. Petersen KB, Hoffmann E, Larsen CR, et al. Cesarean scar pregnancy: a systematic review of treatment studies. Fertil Sterility 2016;105(4):958–67.
58. Seow KM, Huang LW, Lin YH, et al. Cesarean scar pregnancy: issues in management. Ultrasound Obstet Gynecol 2004;23(3):247–53.
59. Jermy K, Thomas J, Doo A, et al. The conservative management of interstitial pregnancy. Bjog 2004;111(11):1283–8.
60. Lau S, Tulandi T. Conservative medical and surgical management of interstitial ectopic pregnancy. Fertil Steril 1999;72(2):207–15.
61. Brincat M, Bryant-Smith A, Holland T. The diagnosis and management of interstitial ectopic pregnancies: a review. Gynecol Surg 2019;16(1):1–15.
62. Moawad NS, Mahajan ST, Moniz MH, et al. Current diagnosis and treatment of interstitial pregnancy. Am J Obstet Gynecol 2010;202(1):15–29.
63. Ego A, Subtil D, Cosson M, et al. Survival analysis of fertility after ectopic pregnancy. Fertil Steril 2001;75(3):560–6.

Identification and Treatment of Acute Pelvic Inflammatory Disease and Associated Sequelae

Danielle N. Frock-Welnak, MD, MPH, MS[a,b,]*, Jenny Tam, MD[c]

KEYWORDS

- Pelvic inflammatory disease (PID) • Tubo-ovarian abscess (TOA)
- Sexually transmitted infection (STI) • Acute pelvic pain

KEY POINTS

- Pelvic inflammatory disease (PID) is a clinical diagnosis and often one of exclusion.
- Empiric antibiotic treatment should not be delayed by diagnostic testing when clinical suspicion for PID is high.
- Tubo-ovarian abscesses are a complication of PID. Abscesses greater than 8 cm should be considered for immediate surgical drainage.
- Even with treatment, PID can result in long-term morbidity, including chronic pelvic pain, infertility, and ectopic pregnancy.

INTRODUCTION

Pelvic inflammatory disease (PID) is an ascending infection of the upper female tract that occurs primarily in young, sexually active women.[1,2] Although often associated with sexually transmitted infections (STIs), namely gonorrhea (GC) and chlamydia (CT),[3] PID can also be attributed to native bacteria of the vagina, gastrointestinal, or respiratory tracts.[3–6] Infection of the uterus, fallopian tubes, ovaries, and peritoneal cavity leads to inflammation and long-term consequences in the form of chronic pelvic pain, infertility, or ectopic pregnancy.[7–9]

[a] Division of Academic Specialists in OB/GYN, University of Colorado School of Medicine, Aurora, CO, USA; [b] Obstetrics and Gynecology, School of Medicine, CU Anschutz, Academic Office One, 12631 East 17th Avenue, 4th Floor, Aurora, CO 80045, USA; [c] Division of Academic Specialists in OB/GYN, Department of Obstetrics and Gynecology, University of Colorado, School of Medicine, CU Anschutz, Academic Office One, 12631 East 17th Avenue, 4th Floor, Aurora, CO 80045, USA
* Corresponding author. Division of Academic Specialists in OB/GYN, University of Colorado School of Medicine, Aurora, CO.
E-mail address: danielle.frock-welnak@cuanschutz.edu

Obstet Gynecol Clin N Am 49 (2022) 551–579
https://doi.org/10.1016/j.ogc.2022.02.019
0889-8545/22/© 2022 Elsevier Inc. All rights reserved.

PID Updates Impacting Clinical Practice

- Expiration of the 2015 CDC STD Treatment Guideline Mobile App
- Increased, weight-based dosage for ceftriaxone for outpatient treatment regimen
- Ceftriaxone replaces cefoxitin as first-choice cephalosporin for inpatient treatment regimen
- Recommendation for routine metronidazole use when treating with ceftriaxone and doxycycline
- Recommendation for management of *Mycoplasma genitalis* coinfection
- Recommendation for early surgical interventions for TOA
- Recommendation for management of IUD with PID

Epidemiology

The actual incidence and prevalence of PID are unknown. This is largely due to the lack of public health reporting and absence of unifying diagnostic criteria.[10,11] Data from the 2013 to 2014 NHANES (National Health and Nutrition Examination Survey) suggest that 4.4% of sexually active, reproductive-age women report a history of PID. This equates to ~2.5 million women living with a lifetime diagnosis of PID.[12]

Pathogenesis

PID is a condition in which microorganisms associated with the vagina and cervix migrate cephalad to infect all aspects of the upper female genital tract[13]:

- Uterus (endometritis)
- Fallopian tubes (salpingitis, pyosalpinx)
- Ovaries (tubo-ovarian abscess [TOA])
- Peritoneum (pelvic peritonitis)

This inflammation can extend throughout the peritoneal cavity, leading to liver capsule inflammation and perihepatic adhesions known as Fitz-Hugh-Curtis syndrome or perihepatitis.[14,15] This finding is pathognomonic for PID.

Pathogens

PID is most often associated with pathogens from the female genital tract. This includes sexually transmitted organisms[3] as well as bacteria from the normal vaginal microbiome.[2] Although less common, PID has also been attributed to organisms from respiratory and gastrointestinal sources.[6,16]

Chlamydia trachomatis (CT) and Neisseria gonorrhoeae (GC)

- CT and GC represent the first and second most common STIs in the United States.[17]
- These infections are often asymptomatic. If untreated, the risk of PID increases.
  - Approximately 15% of women with CT will develop PID.[18]
  - Rates for untreated GC are even higher.[19,20]
- Based on 2 large, randomized control trials, GC and CT contribute to approximately 20% to 30% of PID diagnoses.[4,9]

Bacterial vaginosis–associated microbes

- PID is often polymicrobial and includes bacteria from the normal vaginal microbiome.[2]

- These pathogens include strict and facultative anaerobes, such as those associated with bacterial vaginosis (BV): Gardnerella vaginalis, Atopobium vaginae, sneathia, and megasphaera species, and others.[5,8]
- BV is the most common vaginal disorder in reproductive-age women.[21]
- It represents an imbalance in the normal vaginal microbiome. BV is neither infectious nor inflammatory, rather a loss of homeostasis (**Fig. 1**).[22,23]
- The association between BV and PID is well established.[24,25] The presence of BV doubles the risk of PID[8] and greater than 50% of women with PID test positive for BV.[3]
- Routine screening for BV is not recommended. There is no evidence to support that screening results in reduced rates of PID.[26]

Mycoplasma species

- *Mycoplasma genitalium* is an STI associated with urethritis and cervicitis.
  - Similar to BV, its presence doubles the risk of PID[27] and approximately 18% of patients with PID will have *M genitalium*.[3,28]
  - Current PID regimens provide insufficient antimicrobial coverage for *M genitalium*,[29] and its presence is independently associated with PID treatment failure.[30]
  - There are currently no screening recommendations for *M genitalium* at the time of PID diagnosis[28,31]; however, for treatment refractory or recurrent PID, testing can be considered.
- *Ureaplasma urealyticum* and other less common mycoplasma species are commonly identified in the female genital tract.
  - A recent systematic review suggests that the role of *U urealyticum* in PID is limited.[32]
  - Testing and treatment are not recommended.

Actinomyces species

- Many actinomyces species exist as part of the normal vaginal microbiome.
- Pelvic actinomycosis is rare and insidious. It is often confused for gynecologic malignancy or pelvic tuberculosis. A definitive diagnosis is generally determined by surgical pathology.[33]
- Prolonged infection leads to chronic granulomatous disease with profound fibrosis and abscess formation requiring surgical debridement.[34,35]
- Ascending infections are associated with prolonged use of an intrauterine device (IUD).[33,36]
- Nonpathologic actinomyces may be identified on routine cervical cytology. In asymptomatic patients, antibiotic treatment is not recommended; an existing IUD should not be removed.[37]

Gastrointestinal and respiratory pathogens

- Includes gram-negative rods, such as *Escherichia coli* and *Bacteroides fragilis*, as well as a variety of streptococcus and staphylococcus species.[6,16]

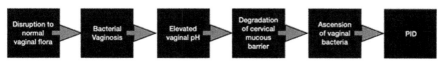

Fig. 1. Association between BV and PID

Mycobacterium tuberculosis

- Pelvic *Mycobacterium tuberculosis* (TB) is an extrapulmonary infection caused by lymphatic or hematogenous dissemination.
- Is more common in developing countries, especially India.[38]
- Results in significant fibrosis of the female genital tract with high rates of endometrial adhesions and tubal factor infertility.[39,40]

A condensed list of PID-associated pathogens can be found in **Table 1**.

DIAGNOSING PELVIC INFLAMMATORY DISEASE
Risk Factors

PID is generally considered to be a condition of sexually active young women; however, the diagnosis should not be overlooked in the absence of risk factors.[1,25] Many risk factors are modifiable and represent opportunities for educational intervention (**Table 2**).[4,10,41]

The Differential Diagnosis for Acute Pelvic Pain

The differential diagnosis for acute pelvic pain is broad and includes genitourinary, gastrointestinal, musculoskeletal, and psychological conditions (**Table 3**).[42,43]

Clinical Presentation

Patients with acute PID present with a variety of nonspecific symptoms and examination findings that can be isolated to the pelvis or may be systemic. The absence of these findings does not eliminate the diagnosis of PID (**Table 4**).[1,44]

Physical examination findings

- Vital signs can be normal. Despite infection, more than two-thirds of patients are afebrile on initial evaluation.[46] Fevers or evidence of systemic inflammatory response syndrome (SIRS) or sepsis occurs in severe cases.[47,48]
- Mild to severe abdominal or pelvic tenderness with or without rebound or guarding.[44]
- Tenderness in the right upper quadrant as in Fitz-Hugh-Curtis syndrome.[15,49]
- Mucopurulent cervical discharge and friability indicating cervicitis.[44]
- Cervical motion tenderness (CMT), uterine, or adnexal tenderness indicating pelvic peritonitis or TOA.[25,50]

Laboratory studies
Patients with PID can have a variety of laboratory findings dependent on disease severity (**Table 5**).

Imaging

Pelvic ultrasound
When PID is suspected or part of the evolving differential diagnosis, a pelvic ultrasound should be performed.

- Transvaginal sonography is superior to transabdominal imaging. In one study, PID-associated findings on transvaginal ultrasound were missed on greater than 70% of transabdominal ultrasounds.[53]
- Ultrasound characteristics most consistent with PID include those associated with tubal inflammation[54–56]:

Table 1
Pelvic inflammatory disease-associated pathogens

	Description	Source	Routine Screening Guidelines	Initial Evaluation for PID	Diagnosis	Treatment	PID-Associated Cases[3]
Neisseria gonorrhoeae	Gram-negative intracellular diplococci	Sexually transmitted	Yes per USPSTF	Yes	NAAT (PCR)	Ceftriaxone	7%
Chlamydia trachomatis	Gram-negative intracellular coccobacillus	Sexually transmitted	Yes per USPSTF	Yes	NAAT (PCR)	Azithromycin Doxycycline	15%
Trichomonas vaginalis	Protozoan parasite	Sexually transmitted	No guidance	No guidance	NAAT (PCR); microscopy	Metronidazole	9%
Gardnerella vaginalis	Facultative anaerobic bacteria	Vaginal flora, associated with bacterial vaginosis	No	Yes	Microscopy	Metronidazole	55%
Mycoplasma genitalium	Mycoplasma, facultative anaerobic parasite	Sexually transmitted, associated with recurrent or treatment refractory PID	No	Only in treatment refractory or recurrent cases	NAAT	Doxycycline + moxifloxacin	18%
Ureaplasma urealyticum	Mycoplasma, facultative anaerobic parasite	Genitourinary, limited association with PID	No	No	NAAT	No treatment recommended	
Actinomyces species	Anaerobic, gram-positive bacillus	Genitourinary, opportunistic bacteria associated	No	Only if clinical suspicion is high	Histopathology	Penicillin G *Do not treat if identified on routine cervical cytology*	

(continued on next page)

Table 1
(continued)

	Description	Source	Routine Screening Guidelines	Initial Evaluation for PID	Diagnosis	Treatment	PID-Associated Cases[3]
		with long-term IUD use					
Mycobacterium tuberculosis	Extrapulmonary manifestation of traditional TB (spirochete)	Respiratory pathogen with extrapulmonary dissemination	Tuberculin skin test in at-risk individuals	Only if clinical suspicion is high	Acid-fast bacilli on microscopy or endometrial biopsy; histopathologic diagnosis of granuloma	Standard treatment: rifampicin, isoniazid (INH), pyrazinamide, ethambutol ×2 mo followed by rifampicin and INH for 4 additional mo. Recommend ID consult to rule out drug resistance in at-risk individuals	
Escherichia coli; Bacteroides fragilis	Anaerobic, gram-negative rod	Intestinal tract	No	No	Culture	Ceftriaxone Ciprofloxacin Gentamicin	
Pepto-streptococcus species	Anaerobic, gram-positive cocci	Intestinal, respiratory, and genital tract	No	No	Culture	Cephalosporins Penicillin G Clindamycin	
H influenzae	Nonencapsulated, gram-negatively coccobacillus	Respiratory tract	No	No	Culture	Cephalosporins	

Table 2
Risk factors for pelvic inflammatory disease

Modifiable Risk Factors		Nonmodifiable Risk Factors
Previous diagnosis of PID	Early age of sexual debut (<15 y)	Black, non-Hispanic (compared with white, non-Hispanic, and Hispanic women)
History of STI(s) including HIV	Lack of contraception, especially barrier	Endometriosis
Greater lifetime number of sexual partners (>10)	Age <25 y	Asymptomatic bacterial vaginosis or *M genitalium* infection[a]
Extended IUD use (postmenopausal women)	Recent oocyte retrieval or pelvic surgery	

[a] Screening not recommended.

○ Tubal edema: Thickening of the fallopian tube walls, generally greater than 5 mm, with or without luminal fluid has up to 100% specificity in diagnosing PID.[54]

○ Cogwheel sign: cross-sectional view of the fallopian tube resulting from tubal wall edema and luminal fluid.

○ Incomplete septations: longitudinal view associated with hydrosalpinx and pyosalpinx.

- Other ultrasound findings are less sensitive and specific but can add support to the diagnosis (**Table 6**).

- Unilateral or bilateral adnexal masses identified as TOAs indicate PID until proven otherwise. This is the only ultrasound finding with acute treatment-specific recommendations.[44]

- Although there are many abnormal ultrasound findings associated with PID, a normal pelvic ultrasound does not exclude PID from the differential diagnosis.

Computed tomographic scan

When patients present to the emergency department with nondescript pelvic pain, a computed tomographic scan of the abdomen and pelvis is generally performed to aid in prompt diagnosis.

- The most specific computed tomographic finding for PID is bilateral tubal thickening (>5 mm) with or without fluid in the tubal lumen (95% specificity).[57]

- Complex fluid collections incorporating the adnexa can represent TOAs; however, abscesses related to appendicitis or diverticulitis should be ruled out.[58]

- PID-associated peritonitis presents as thickening of the uterosacral ligaments, pelvic fat stranding, or obscuring of pelvic fascial planes.[58]

- When considering computed tomographic imaging, intravenous (IV) contrast is preferred. This allows for better evaluation of the uterus and adnexa. The decision to use oral contrast depends on the level of concern for gastrointestinal involvement.[58]

- Refer to **Table 6** for additional computed tomographic findings consistent with PID.

MRI

MRI is not generally used for routine diagnosis of PID. Findings on MRI are similar to those seen during ultrasound or computed tomographic imaging (see **Table 6**).[59]

Table 3
Differential diagnosis of pelvic inflammatory disease

Gynecologic	Urinary	Gastrointestinal	Other
PID, endometritis, or TOA	Acute cystitis	Inflammatory bowel disease or irritable bowel syndrome	Psychosomatic pain
Pelvic congestion syndrome or ovarian vein thrombosis			
Endometriosis	Pyelonephritis	Constipation	Musculoskeletal
Ectopic pregnancy			
IUD migration or partial expulsion	Nephrolithiasis	Diverticulitis or diverticular abscess	Trauma or abuse
GYN malignancy			
Ovarian torsion	Urinary retention	Appendicitis	Malingering
Degenerating leiomyoma			
Hemorrhagic or ruptured ovarian cyst	Interstitial cystitis	Hernia	Narcotic-seeking
Adenomyosis			
Mittelschmerz		Small bowel obstruction or intussusception	Sickle cell crisis
Threatened or spontaneous abortion			

Table 4
Pelvic inflammatory disease–associated symptoms

Common Genitourinary Symptoms[45]	Common Nongenitourinary Symptoms[46]
Pelvic pain	General malaise/fatigue
Abnormal uterine bleeding	Fevers/chills
Postcoital bleeding	Nausea/vomiting
Dyspareunia	Diarrhea
Dysuria	Generalized abdominal pain or right upper quadrant pain (Fitz-Hugh-Curtis syndrome)

- Although MRI is more accurate in diagnosing PID compared with ultrasound (accuracy of 93% vs 80%),[59] ultrasound provides specific diagnostic findings and is more time- and cost-effective.
- MRI is superior in delineating soft tissue structures and can be useful when the diagnosis is unclear.[60]
- MRI is comparable to laparoscopy in differentiating features of PID (fallopian tube dilation and TOAs) from peritoneal inclusion cysts, dermoid cysts, ovarian malignancy, endometriomas, and ovarian torsion.[61]

Procedural Confirmation of Pelvic Inflammatory Disease

Laparoscopy
Historically the gold standard for diagnosis and treatment of PID includes the following[65,66]:

Table 5
Laboratory studies

Serum Studies	
CBC	Generally normal. Patients with leukocytosis are more likely to have severe disease, require hospitalization, or fail initial treatment[48,51]
CMP	Generally normal. Liver and kidney function can be altered in severe sepsis. LFTs are rarely elevated in Fitz-Hugh-Curtis syndrome[52]
ESR/CRP	Normal to elevated. Elevated CRP is associated with antibiotic treatment failure[51]
Vaginal studies	
GC/CT	Positivity rate of 20%–30%[4,9]
BV	Present in >50% of cases[4]
Microscopy	Abundant WBC should be visible on saline microscopy. This finding is nonspecific; however, the negative predictive value is high. The absence of WBCs strongly argues against PID.[46] BV and trichomonas can also be diagnosed on wet prep
Urine studies	
UA with reflex culture	If concern for urinary source, consider catheterization owing to risk for vaginal contamination
UPT	Pregnancy is an indication for inpatient treatment. This can also help to rule out ectopic pregnancy[44]

Abbreviations: CBC, complete blood count; CMP, comprehensive metabolic panel; LFTs, liver function tests; UA, urinalysis; UPT, urine pregnancy test.

- Less frequently used because of improvements in pelvic imaging, antibiotic treatment, and percutaneous drain placement, as well as avoidance of inherent risks associated with anesthesia and surgery.
- As laparoscopy is both diagnostic and therapeutic, indications include the following[65,66]:
  - Diagnostic uncertainty
  - Desire for immediate source control due to sepsis/ruptured TOA
  - Failure of primary treatment regimens when interventional radiology percutaneous drain is not feasible or indicated

Endometrial biopsy

The presence of endometritis confirms the diagnosis of PID; however, pathologic evaluation is time-consuming and should not delay treatment.[44]

- The absence of endometritis does not rule out infection of the adnexa or peritoneum.[67]
- Because of the time required for biopsies and culture to result, endometrial sampling is most useful when evaluating for recurrent or chronic, subacute disease.
- Specimens can be cultured for pathogen and antibiotic sensitivity screening.[67,68]

PID Diagnostic Pearls

- There is no combination of symptoms, physical examination findings, or laboratory values that completely support or refute the diagnosis of PID.

- To assign definitive diagnostic criteria to this condition would risk missing a diagnosis in a patient with mild or atypical symptoms.

- The consequences of inappropriately diagnosing or delaying treatment for PID risks long-term morbidity.

- Clinicians should have a low threshold to diagnose or empirically treat PID when another diagnosis cannot be assigned.

- According to the CDC, PID should be considered a reasonable diagnosis under the following circumstances:

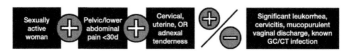

- Significant leukorrhea on wet mount, cervicitis, mucopurulent vaginal discharge, or known GC/CT infection enhances the likelihood of PID but is not required for diagnosis.

- For chronic symptoms or incomplete treatment response, laparoscopy and endometrial biopsy can confirm PID and provide opportunities for targeted therapy in the form of immediate surgical drainage or culture.

Table 7 presents a summary of clinical features associated with PID.

TREATMENT OF PELVIC INFLAMMATORY DISEASE

- Empiric treatment regimens for PID include broad-spectrum antimicrobial coverage against GC, CT, and anaerobic and aerobic bacteria.
- The Centers for Disease Control and Prevention (CDC) publishes regularly updated PID treatment algorithms, which take into account emerging pathogens and antibiotic resistance profiles (**Box 1**).

Table 6
Imaging findings consistent with acute pelvic inflammatory disease

Pelvic Ultrasound[54–56,62,63]	Computed Tomographic Abdomen and Pelvis[58,64]	MRI Abdomen and Pelvis[59–61]
Bilateral adnexal masses with thick walls and separations consistent with TOA Sensitivity 82%; Specificity 83%	Multiseptated or solid-cystic adnexal mass with thick wall consistent with TOA	Complex adnexal masses consistent with TOA
Tubal inflammation evident by thickening of fallopian tube walls with or without fluid in tubal lumen Sensitivity, 85%; Specificity, 100%	Dilated or thickening of the fallopian tube >5 mm (tubal inflammation) Specificity, 95%	Thickened, fluid-filled fallopian tubes
Cogwheel sign indicating tubal inflammation Sensitivity, 0%–86%; Specificity, 95%–99%	Thickening of the uterosacral ligament, pelvic fat stranding, and obscuring of fascial planes (peritoneal inflammation)	Inflammation of the cervix and uterus
Increased Doppler flow within the fallopian tubes (hyperemia indicative of inflammation)	Cervical edema/enlargement (cervicitis)	Polycystic-like ovaries (ovarian edema)
Free fluid in pouch of Douglas (inflammatory or infectious)	Free fluid in pouch of Douglas (inflammatory or infectious)	Free fluid in the pouch of Douglas (inflammatory or infection)
Polycystic-like ovaries (associated with adnexal edema)	Liver capsule inflammation (Fitz-Hugh-Curtis syndrome)	Liver capsule inflammation (Fitz-Hugh Curtis-syndrome)
Incomplete septa (suggesting fluid filled tubal lumen)	Reactive lymphadenopathy, usually para-aortic (inflammation)	

- Last CDC update: July 2021.[44]
- The 2015 CDC STD Treatment Mobile App expired July 2021. As of January 1, 2022, the replacement App had not been released.
- Mobile-friendly guidelines can be found at https://www.cdc.gov/STIapp/.

PID treatment regimens are assigned based on disease severity. Mild to moderate PID can be treated with outpatient therapy, whereas severe disease requires parenteral antibiotics (**Table 8**).[9,44]

First-Line Antibiotic Treatment Regimens

First-line antibiotic treatment regimens include ceftriaxone, doxycycline, and metronidazole (**Table 9**). Alternative regimens are listed in **Fig. 2** and account for antibiotic allergies and microbial resistance patterns.

Table 7
Summary: clinical features associated with pelvic inflammatory disease

Demographic Features or Risk Factors	Symptoms	Examination Findings	Laboratory Findings	Imaging
Sexually active woman	Pelvic or lower abdominal pain for <30 d[a]	CMT, uterine or adnexal tenderness[a]	Leukorrhea on wet mount (increased WBC: squamous cell ratio)[b]	TOA
Age <25 y	Vaginal discharge	Cervicitis/mucopurulent discharge[b]	Bacterial vaginosis on wet mount	Thickened fallopian tube wall/cogwheel sign[b]
History of PID or STI exposure	Nausea/vomiting	Fever >38.3 C/101°F[b]	Leukocytosis	Incomplete septations
Unprotected sexual intercourse	Fever/chills		Elevated CRP, ESR, procalcitonin[b]	Polycystic-like ovaries
Multiple sexual partners			GC/CT positive[b]	Pelvic free fluid

[a] Minimum criteria.
[b] Supporting criteria.

Box 1
2021 changes in pelvic inflammatory disease treatment guidelines

Inpatient treatment: Ceftriaxone replaces cefoxitin as first-line cephalosporin during inpatient admission (Ceftriaxone 1 g IV every 24 hours for a minimum of 2 doses)

Outpatient treatment: Intramuscular (IM) Ceftriaxone increases from 250 mg to 500 mg × 1 dose. The dose increases to 1 g for weight greater than 150 kg (330 lb)

GC resistance to quinolones remains high. Susceptibility testing should be performed before use.

Metronidazole should always be added to ceftriaxone and doxycycline treatment regimen.

M genitalium-associated PID is treated with standard antibiotic regimens + moxifloxacin 400 mg po daily × 14 days

Data from Refs.[3,44,69]

Follow-Up

- *Who:* All patients diagnosed with PID.[17,44]
- *When:*
  - Clinical follow-up: Recommended within 72 hours of diagnosis or hospital discharge.
  - Positive GC/CT: Test for reinfection in 3 months.
- *Why:*
  - To quickly identify cases of treatment failure in order to avoid short- and long-term consequences of inadequately treated PID.
  - Provide education and discuss prevention strategies.

Follow-up rates for PID are low.[71,72] For patients discharged from an emergency department or urgent care, the onus to schedule follow-up appointments is often on the patient. For patients without insurance or an established primary care provider or OB/GYN, timely follow-up might not be feasible. Studies suggest that follow-up rates increase when appointments are scheduled before discharge. Text message reminders can also be effective, especially in adolescents.[73,74]

Follow-up appointments also provide an opportunity for patient education. Patients seen in the emergency department are less likely to receive education on PID, specifically, prevention strategies and risk for future complications. This further highlights the importance of comprehensive follow-up.[75]

Treatment Failure

- *Outpatient treatment*[44]: Failure to achieve clinical improvement after 72 hours of treatment.
  - Indication for hospital admission, parenteral antibiotics, and further evaluation, including clinical examination, laboratory studies, and new or interval imaging.
- *Inpatient treatment*[44]: Failure to demonstrate clinical improvement after 48 to 72 hours of treatment.
  - Indication for prompt reevaluation of the differential diagnosis, including interval imaging to access for growth or development of TOA.

For patients with TOA, approximately 25% will have an inadequate response to antibiotics alone (persistent fevers, pain, leukocytosis). These patients will require procedural intervention.[76] A percutaneous drain can be considered for both source control and culture-specific antibiotic treatment. Drains are generally placed by interventional radiologists using computed tomographic or US guidance and can be inserted trans-abdominally, transvaginally,[77] transgluteally,[78] or even transrectally.[79]

PID Treatment Pearls

- For GC-positive patients, ceftriaxone is the most effective cephalosporin.

- As of July 2021, single-dose IM ceftriaxone increased from 250 mg to 500 mg.

- For weight >136 kg (300 lb), single-dose IM ceftriaxone increases to 1 g.

- For PID, metronidazole should be administered as IV or po. Vaginal metronidazole gel is not sufficiently absorbed to provide adequate systemic coverage.

- The routine addition of metronidazole to ceftriaxone and doxycycline improves PID treatment outcomes

- The bioavailability of po and IV doxycycline and metronidazole is comparable. Patients should be started on, or transitioned to, a po regimen as soon as clinically appropriate.

- Metronidazole should not be combined with alcohol because of severe gastrointestinal upset (disulfiram-like reaction). Advise patients to abstain from alcohol during treatment and for 3 d following completion.

- Penicillin allergies are more likely to cross-react with first-generation cephalosporins and less likely to show cross-reactivity to second-generation (cefoxitin) and third-generation (ceftriaxone) cephalosporins.

- Tetracyclines and fluoroquinolones are contraindicated in pregnancy. For pregnant patients with PID, admission and infectious disease consultation are recommended.

- Consider IR drainage as first-line procedural intervention after TOA antibiotic treatment failure.

- Consider immediate IR drainage of TOA >8 cm.

- For severe sepsis or concerns for ruptured TOA, consider immediate surgical drainage/washout for prompt source control.

TUBO-OVARIAN ABSCESS

TOAs occur in 15% to 35% of patients with PID.[80] TOA is an infectious mass involving the fallopian tubes, ovaries, with or without involvement of adjacent structures, primarily bowel. TOAs are most frequently associated with ascending gynecologic infections but can also result from appendicitis, diverticulitis, or pyelonephritis.[80,81] TOA cultures are generally polymicrobial and include a variety of anaerobic and aerobic species.[48] Common risk factors for TOA development are listed in **Box 2**.

Patients with TOAs can present similarly to those with PID alone; however, they are more likely to be febrile on admission, have leukocytosis, and/or have an elevated C-reactive protein (CRP; >8.2) or procalcitonin. Imaging of the pelvis will demonstrate unilateral or bilateral pelvic or adnexal masses as described above.[85]

TOAs can be treated medically or by surgical intervention. Patients with a TOA or TOAs who are medically stable should be admitted for parenteral antibiotics.[85] First-line treatment is the same as for PID: IV ceftriaxone + IV/oral doxycycline + IV/oral metronidazole.[44] **Fig. 2** provides more details and alternative treatment regimens.

Antibiotic treatment can be effective in 34% to 88% of cases.[76] Treatment failure should be suspected if the patient has new or persistent fevers, worsening pelvic or abdominal pain, persistent or increasing leukocytosis, and/or enlarging pelvic masses

Table 8
Pelvic inflammatory disease classification by severity

	Mild to Moderate PID	Severe PID
Clinical features	Lacks features consistent with severe PID	Fever >38°C or SIRS/sepsis criteria Pregnancy TOA Inability to exclude surgical emergency Inability to tolerate oral medication Failure of outpatient therapy[44]
Treatment regimen	Outcomes are similar for outpatient vs inpatient treatment. There was no significant difference in rates of recurrent PID, chronic pelvic pain, infertility, or ectopic pregnancy (Level 1 Evidence)[9]	Inpatient treatment required[44]
Clinical judgment	In the absence of severe features, clinical judgment alone is reasonable to guide admission (pain control, social barrier to successful OP therapy, and similar).[70] Adolescence is not an indication for inpatient therapy.[44]	

on imaging.[51] Approximately 25% to 30% of women with TOA or TOAs will require surgical drainage following antibiotics.[76,86]

A ruptured TOA has a mortality of 5% to 10%.[80] Patients with severe sepsis and a suspected ruptured TOA should prompt initiation of broad-spectrum antibiotics, fluid resuscitation, and surgical exploration with drainage to improve source control.[87]

There are multiple risk factors associated with antibiotic failure during treatment of PID with TOAs (**Table 10**).

- In one study by Hwang and colleagues,[51] when patients were stratified by risk, the highest risk cohort had a 92% chance of requiring procedural intervention.
  - The risk factors most associated with surgical intervention were age greater than 34.3 years and abscess size greater than 5.9 cm.
  - These patients also exhibited higher white blood cells (WBCs), CRP, and erythrocyte sedimentation rate (ESR).
  - ESR demonstrated a slower response to antibiotic therapy, making it the most reliable marker for medical treatment failure.[51]
- In another study by Fouks and colleagues,[48] in addition to age (>35 years), abscess diameter (≥7 cm), and elevated WBC, bilateral TOAs were found to independently predict antibiotic treatment failure.
- When considering size alone, Reed and colleagues[88] showed that 35% of TOAs 7 to 9 cm in diameter required surgical intervention. The rate increased to 60% in TOAs greater than 9 cm.

Procedural Intervention

Historically, procedural interventions have been used when no clinical improvement is observed within 48 to 72 hours of starting antibiotic therapy. The benefit of earlier surgical intervention is unclear[44]; however, new data suggest that more aggressive surgical management might be beneficial in larger or bilateral TOAs, concurrent leukocytosis, or elevated CRP. In these cases, surgical intervention less than 72 hours from diagnosis has been shown to reduce both acute and chronic morbidity as well as length of hospital

Table 9
First-line treatment

Outpatient Treatment	Inpatient Treatment
First-line treatment: Ceftriaxone 500 mg IM × 1 dose (administer at time of diagnosis) ⊕ Doxycycline 100 mg po bid × 14 d Metronidazole 500 mg po bid × 14 d	First-line treatment: Ceftriaxone 1 g IV every 24 h for 2 doses or more (duration determined by clinical improvement, usually 24–72 h) ⊕ Doxycycline 100 mg po/IV bid × 14 d Metronidazole 500 mg po/IV bid × 14 d
Single-dose ceftriaxone has increased and is now weight based: • <150 kg = 500 mg IM • >150 mg = 1g IM	Doxycycline and metronidazole have similar bioavailability when administered IV vs po • Transition to po when clinically appropriate

To account for antibiotic allergies, alternative regimens are available (see PID Treatment flow sheet).

All treatment regimens provide coverage for GC, CT, and common anaerobic and aerobic bacteria.

stay.[90,91] In one study, immediate surgical intervention for TOAs greater than 8 cm resulted in a significant reduction in length of hospital stay. This parameter alone represents a reasonable cutoff when considering the appropriateness of early surgical intervention.[86] Indications for early surgical intervention are listed in **Box 3**.

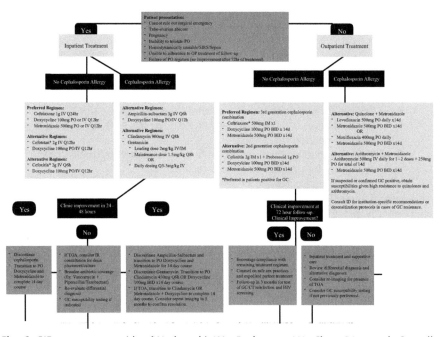

Fig. 2. PID treatment guide. (Workowski KA, Bachmann LH, Chan PA, et al. Sexually Transmitted Infections Treatment Guidelines, 2021. *MMWR Recomm Rep*. 2021;70(4):1-187.) CT, chlamydia; GC, gonorrhea; HIV, human immunodeficiency virus; IM, intramuscular; IV, intravenous; OP outpatient; PO, oral administration; TOA, tubo-ovarian abscess.

Box 2
Risk factors for tubo-ovarian abscess

Immunocompromised state or HIV infection[80,82]

History of TOA[80]

Diabetes mellitus[80]

History of endometriosis[83]

Recent fertility treatment[84]

Procedural intervention includes percutaneous drain placement as well as surgical drainage via laparoscopy or laparotomy. Before broad-spectrum antibiotics, suspected TOAs were treated by laparotomy and often required removal of the uterus, fallopian tubes, and ovaries in order to effectively eradicate the infection.[92] Contemporary treatments favor placement of percutaneous drains when antibiotics have proven ineffective. Drains are generally placed by interventional radiologists under ultrasound or computed tomographic guidance. Drains are often placed transabdominally or transvaginally[77]; however, transgluteal[78] and transrectal[79] placement has also been studied.

Studies have shown IR drainage to be highly effective in the treatment of TOAs with success rates greater than 93% after transvaginal drain placement.[77] When IR drainage is not possible owing to anatomic barriers, lack of a skilled interventional radiologist, or acuity, laparoscopic drainage is preferred over laparotomy.[93] In a 2019 study by Shigemi and colleagues,[94] patients with severe PID treated with laparoscopy compared with laparotomy had shorter operating times, fewer blood transfusions, and shorter length of hospitalization.

Follow-Up

Following treatment of TOA, no clear guidelines exist for interval imaging in asymptomatic patients. The decision to reimage posttreatment is clinician dependent. For patients desiring future fertility, imaging to rule out persistent pathologic condition, such as a hydrosalpinx, is reasonable.

SPECIAL POPULATIONS
Immunocompromised

- Women with compromised immunity (type 2 diabetes, chronic steroid use, malignancy, and so forth) are at an increased risk of PID and are more likely to be GC/CT negative.[95]
- Standard antimicrobial algorithms still apply.[44]
- Patients with HIV are more likely to develop TOAs and may benefit from early surgical drainage for source control and targeted antibiotic therapy.[96,97]

Children and Adolescents

- The age-specific risk for PID is highest in sexually active adolescents. The treatment recommendations, including outpatient treatment for mild/moderate PID, are the same as for adults.[97]
- The decision to admit for inpatient treatment should take into consideration any social barriers exclusive to adolescents that might be improved through inpatient treatment.

Table 10 Tubo-ovarian abscess: features associated with antibiotic failure	
TOA diameter >6 cm	Bilateral TOA
Febrile on admission	Higher parity
Leukocytosis >16 k	Elevated ESR; CP > 14
Age >34 y	Body mass index >26.72

Data from Refs.[51,85,86,89]

- In nonsexually active children and adolescents with PID/TOA, evaluation of genitourinary tract anomalies should be considered.[98]
- Always evaluate for sexual abuse. Abused adolescents are more likely to engage in risky sexual behaviors,[99] which places them at a higher risk for STIs and PID.

Pregnancy

- PID is an uncommon diagnosis in pregnancy because of the physiologic barriers to bacterial ascension. It is rarely described outside of the first trimester.[100,101]
- There should be a careful evaluation of the differential diagnosis, as PID in pregnancy portends a high risk of spontaneous miscarriage, preterm labor, and intrauterine fetal demise.[102]
- For confirmed or strongly suspected PID, patients should be admitted for parenteral antibiotic treatment with guidance from infectious disease specialists.[44]

Intrauterine Device

- The risk of PID with IUD appears highest within the first 4 weeks after insertion.[103]
- At-risk patients, or those who meet screening criteria, should be tested for GC/CT at the time of IUD insertion. If positive, antibiotic treatment should be administered. The IUD does not require removal.[104]
- The presence of asymptomatic GC/CT at the time of IUD insertion does not increase the risk for PID.[104]
- IUDs should not be inserted in patients with mucopurulent cervicitis or known, active GC/CT.[105]
- IUD removal at time of PID diagnosis does not appear to impact treatment response and is not recommended as an initial intervention.[106–108]
- If no clinical improvement after 72 hours of appropriate antimicrobial treatment, IUD removal can be considered.[109]

Tubal Occlusion (Status/Post Tubal Ligation, Salpingectomy, Essure Placement)

- Consider isolated endometritis or persistent tubal patency despite previous occlusive procedure.
- Review the differential diagnosis, carefully considering other sources of PID/TOA not associated with bacterial ascension from the lower genital tract.[110]

Menopause

- These women are less likely to have traditional risk factors and more likely to test GC/CT negative.[111]
- Common risk factors for PID in this population include recent endometrial biopsy and pelvic instrumentation/surgery.[112]
- Other risk factors include being HIV positive or having type 2 diabetes mellitus.[112]

Box 3
Tubo-ovarian abscess: indications for early surgical intervention

Bilateral TOA

TOA >8 cm

Concurrent leukocytosis

Elevated CRP

Data from Refs.[86,90,91]

- The presence or recent removal of a long-standing IUD appears to increase the risk for PID in this population.[113]
- The presence of TOA without obvious explanation should prompt a thorough workup of adnexal pathology, including malignancy.[113] If surgery is required, excised tissue should be sent for frozen pathologic evaluation.[114]

LONG-TERM CONSEQUENCES OF PELVIC INFLAMMATORY DISEASE

PID is seldom life threatening.[7] The risk of mortality is significantly less than 1%.[115] Deaths attributed to PID occur from severe sepsis usually associated with a ruptured TOA or from hemorrhage resulting from a ruptured ectopic pregnancy.[115] The greater impact of PID is attributed to long-term morbidity.

- According to the PEACH trial,[8] during a 3-year follow-up after PID diagnosis:
  - 0.6% of women developed an ectopic pregnancy
  - 18% developed infertility
  - 29% reported chronic pelvic pain
- The risk of ectopic pregnancy doubles after a single episode of PID.[116]
- Recurrent episodes of PID exacerbate these outcomes with the rate of infertility increasing 5× from the first to the third episode.[7]

The PEACH trial represents a cohort of women who received treatment and follow-up for PID. Unfortunately, many women with PID are asymptomatic[10] or develop vague, self-limiting symptoms easily ascribed to more benign processes. As a result, many women with tubal factor infertility will deny a history of PID but will ultimately demonstrate evidence of disease during evaluation (perihepatic adhesions, tubal fibrosis).[37] This further supports the assumption that rates of PID are much higher than reported and places a greater emphasis on the importance of prevention and risk reduction strategies.

PELVIC INFLAMMATORY DISEASE AS A RISK REDUCTION OPPORTUNITY

PID Prevention: Prevention of PID should focus on education and screening.

- The US Preventative Services Task Force (USPSTF) provides screening guidelines for GC/CT[117]:
  - Annual testing for all sexually active women ≤24 years.
  - Annual testing for women ≥25 years with an increased risk of infection.
- *Screening for BV is not recommended.*[118]
- Assess for sexual assault or trafficking.

Table 11
Considerations for additional screening after pelvic inflammatory disease diagnosis

	Type of Screening and When	Test	Additional Considerations
Gonorrhea/Chlamydia	Vaginal or urine screen	NAAT	If positive, follow-up testing for reinfection should be performed in 3 mo
HIV	Serum screening at time of diagnosis	HIV1/HIV2 antibody	The patient should provide consent for screening. Because of the latency period following initial HIV infection, screening should be repeated in 3 mo
Syphilis	Serum screening at the time of diagnosis	RPR/VDRL	If positive, a confirmatory test should be submitted
Hepatitis B	Serum screening at time of diagnosis	Hepatitis B surface antigen	Screen if not vaccinated (series of 3 vaccinations usually administered in childhood)
Hepatitis C	Serum screening at the time of diagnosis	Hepatitis C antibody	Less likely to be sexually transmitted compared with hepatitis B
Trichomonas vaginalis	Vaginal or urine screen	NAAT, microscopy	If trichomonas is present, standard PID antibiotic regimens with metronidazole should provide adequate treatment
Herpes simplex virus	Sample from lesion	PCR	Obtain if cutaneous lesions are present. In the absence of lesions or prodromal symptoms, serum screening is not recommended
HPV	Cervical cytology ± HPV testing at time of diagnosis (outpatient) or at follow-up (ED/urgent care)	Cytology, PCR	Patient should be advised of cervical cancer screening recommendations based on age and risk. Screening should be performed at the recommended interval

			Recommend Gardasil vaccination series if not yet obtained
Bacterial vaginosis	Vaginal sample	Microscopy	Screening not recommended. PID treatment regimens will include coverage for BV (metronidazole)
M genitalium	Vaginal sample	PCR	Consider testing if recurrent or refractory PID. Current treatment regimens do not provide sufficient coverage
Pregnancy	Urine or serum screen	ELISA; quantitative bHCG	A standard urine pregnancy will be positive approximately 10 d after conception. If testing is negative at the time of PID diagnosis, the patient should be encouraged to retest if her menstrual cycle is delayed If appropriate, offer emergency contraception If appropriate, offer contraceptive counseling
Sexual abuse or assault	Validated screening tools: HITS, WAST, HARK[119]	Questionnaire	Perform before examination. If sexual assault was recent/ongoing, forensic nurse will collect specimens per legal protocol

Abbreviations: bHCG, human chorionic gonadotropin; ELISA, enzyme-linked immunosorbent assay; HARK, humiliation, afraid, rape, kick; HITS, hurt, insult, threaten, and scream; NAAT, nucleic acid amplification test; PCR, polymerase chain reaction; WAST, Woman abuse screening tool.

Box 4
Considerations for post–pelvic inflammatory disease anticipatory guidance

Postdiagnosis counseling and actionable recommendations
  Counseling on symptoms associated with recurrent PID/TOA and when to return to the office/hospital for evaluation of chronic/recurrent symptoms.
  Counseling on long-term consequences of PID, including infertility, ectopic pregnancy, and chronic pelvic pain
  Counseling on transmission of STIs and prevention strategies:
  • Consistent condom use
  • Regular screening
  Patients should be aware that many people with STIs are asymptomatic and have no knowledge of their infection.
  Counseling on the importance of partner treatment to prevent reinfection.
  • Per CDC Guidelines, all sexual partners within 60 days of PID symptom onset should be offered testing and treatment.
  • If last sexual intercourse was greater than 60 days from symptom onset, the last sexual partner should be offered testing and treatment.
  • Expedited partner treatment (providing treatment without otherwise evaluating the patient) is supported by the CDC and most state health departments.
  Review recommendations for safe resumption of unprotected intercourse after treatment.
  • Patient and partner or partners should complete their entire treatment regimen and be asymptomatic before engaging in unprotected intercourse.
  • Patients should be aware that they can be reinfected with GC/CT (or other STI) if treatment course is not completed before unprotected intercourse.

Screening Opportunity

At the time of PID diagnosis, GC/CT testing is routinely performed; however, the patient should be offered additional screening (**Table 11**) and anticipatory guidance (**Box 4**) pertinent to STIs, including evaluation for sexual assault.

SUMMARY AND RECOMMENDATIONS

PID is often associated with young, sexually active women but can occur throughout the life course in the absence of identifiable risk factors. A diagnosis of PID can be prompted by high clinical suspicion. Per CDC guidelines, broad-spectrum antibiotics should be initiated empirically and without delay. Patients with mild to moderate symptoms who can tolerate oral antibiotics can be treated on an outpatient basis and should follow up with a provider to evaluate clinical response 72 hours after starting treatment. Patients with severe PID, which includes concurrent pregnancy or TOA, should be admitted to the hospital for parenteral antibiotics and procedural intervention if indicated. Patients with TOA are more likely to require surgical intervention if they are older, are overweight, or have an abscess greater than 6 cm in diameter, leukocytosis, or elevated CRP. When patients with TOA fail initial antibiotic treatment, IR drain placement is an effective method for obtaining source control and should be used when available. For TOAs measuring greater than 8 cm, immediate surgical drainage should be considered. Patients diagnosed with PID should be screened for pregnancy, STIs, and, if indicated, domestic violence or abuse. Patients should be counseled on prevention strategies, treatment compliance, and long-term complications associated with PID, including infertility, ectopic pregnancy, and chronic pelvic pain.

CLINICS CARE POINTS

Do	Do Not
Empirically treat for pelvic inflammatory disease based on clinical symptoms	Fail to diagnose pelvic inflammatory disease because a patient does not have obvious risk factors
Consider immediate IR consultation for drainage of a tubo-ovarian abscess ≥8 cm	Delay treatment for suspected pelvic inflammatory disease while awaiting gonorrhea/chlamydia testing or imaging
Proceed to surgical drainage in patients with suspected ruptured tubo-ovarian abscess or sepsis	Fail to screen for pregnancy during pelvic inflammatory disease evaluation
Encourage consistent condom use for generalized sexually transmitted infection prevention	Discharge patients without arranging for 72-hour follow-up in patients receiving outpatient treatment for pelvic inflammatory disease
Routine screening for gonorrhea/chlamydia per guidelines. If positive test, perform a test for reinfection in 3 mo	Routinely screen for bacterial vaginosis or *M genitalium* in the absence of symptoms
Expedited partner treatment for patients positive for gonorrhea/chlamydia	Immediately remove an intrauterine device if a patient is diagnosed with pelvic inflammatory disease or tests positive for gonorrhea or chlamydia
Educate patients on the causes and consequences of pelvic inflammatory disease. Encourage early evaluation for concerning symptoms or signs of recurrent disease	Miss an opportunity to screen for sexually transmitted infections including HIV and syphilis
Screen for abuse or sexual assault	

DISCLOSURES

The authors have nothing to disclose.

REFERENCES

1. Ness RB, Smith KJ, Chang C-CH, et al. Gynecologic Infection Follow-Through, GIFT, Investigators. Prediction of pelvic inflammatory disease among young, single, sexually active women. Sex Transm Dis 2006;33(3):137–42.
2. Paavonen J, Westrom L, Eschenbach D. Pelvic inflammatory disease. In: Holmes KK, Sparling PF, Stamm WE, et al, editors. Sexually Transmitted Diseases. 4th edition. New York, NY: McGraw-Hill; 2008. p. 1017–50.
3. Wiesenfeld HC, Meyn LA, Darville T, et al. A randomized controlled trial of ceftriaxone and doxycycline, with or without metronidazole, for the treatment of acute pelvic inflammatory disease. Clin Infect Dis 2021;72(7):1181–9.
4. Kreisel KM, Llata E, Haderxhanaj L, et al. The burden of and trends in pelvic inflammatory disease in the United States, 2006-2016. J Infect Dis 2021;224(12 Suppl 2):S103–12.
5. Haggerty CL, Totten PA, Tang G, et al. Identification of novel microbes associated with pelvic inflammatory disease and infertility. Sex Transm Infect 2016; 92(6):441–6.
6. King AL, Stamatopoulos N. Concurrent Escherichia coli tubo-ovarian abscess and Campylobacter jejuni gastroenteritis: a case report. Case Rep Womens Health 2020;26:e00192.

7. Weström L, Joesoef R, Reynolds G, et al. Pelvic inflammatory disease and fertility. A cohort study of 1,844 women with laparoscopically verified disease and 657 control women with normal laparoscopic results. Sex Transm Dis 1992;19(4):185–92.

8. Ness RB, Trautmann G, Richter HE, et al. Effectiveness of treatment strategies of some women with pelvic inflammatory disease: a randomized trial. Obstet Gynecol 2005;106(3):573–80.

9. Ness RB, Soper DE, Holley RL, et al. Effectiveness of inpatient and outpatient treatment strategies for women with pelvic inflammatory disease: results from the Pelvic Inflammatory Disease Evaluation and Clinical Health (PEACH) Randomized Trial. Am J Obstet Gynecol 2002;186(5):929–37.

10. Chappell CA, Wiesenfeld HC. Pathogenesis, diagnosis, and management of severe pelvic inflammatory disease and tuboovarian abscess. Clin Obstet Gynecol 2012;55(4):893–903.

11. Simms I, Stephenson JM. Pelvic inflammatory disease epidemiology: what do we know and what do we need to know? Sex Transm Infect 2000;76(2):80–7.

12. Kreisel K, Torrone E, Bernstein K, et al. Prevalence of pelvic inflammatory disease in sexually experienced women of reproductive age - United States, 2013-2014. MMWR Morb Mortal Wkly Rep 2017;66(3):80–3.

13. Pelvic Inflammatory Disease (PID). The American College of Obstetrics and Gynecology. 2020. Available at: https://www.acog.org/womens-health/faqs/pelvic-inflammatory-disease. Accessed December 2021.

14. Grigoriadis G, Green J, Amin A, et al. Fitz-hugh-curtis syndrome: an incidental diagnostic finding during laparoscopic sterilization. Cureus 2020;12(9):e10304.

15. Fitz-Hugh JT. Acute gonococcal peritonitis of the right upper quadrant in women. J Am Med Assoc 1934;102(25):2094–6.

16. Brunham RC, Gottlieb SL, Paavonen J. Pelvic inflammatory disease. N Engl J Med 2015;372(21):2039–48.

17. National overview - sexually transmitted disease surveillance. Centers for Disease Control and Prevention; 2019–2021. Available at: https://www.cdc.gov/std/statistics/2019/overview.htm#Chlamydia. Accessed December 2021.

18. Haggerty CL, Gottlieb SL, Taylor BD, et al. Risk of sequelae after Chlamydia trachomatis genital infection in women. J Infect Dis 2010;201(Suppl 2):S134–55.

19. Reekie J, Donovan B, Guy R, et al. Risk of pelvic inflammatory disease in relation to chlamydia and gonorrhea testing, repeat testing, and positivity: a population-based cohort study. Clin Infect Dis 2018;66(3):437–43.

20. Price MJ, Ades AE, De Angelis D, et al. Risk of pelvic inflammatory disease following Chlamydia trachomatis infection: analysis of prospective studies with a multistate model. Am J Epidemiol 2013;178(3):484–92.

21. Allsworth JE, Peipert JF. Prevalence of bacterial vaginosis: 2001-2004 National Health and Nutrition Examination Survey data. Obstet Gynecol 2007;109(1):114–20.

22. Nasioudis D, Linhares IM, Ledger WJ, et al. Bacterial vaginosis: a critical analysis of current knowledge. BJOG 2017;124(1):61–9.

23. Horner PJ, Flanagan H, Horne AW. Is there a hidden burden of disease as a result of epigenetic epithelial-to-mesenchymal transition following chlamydia trachomatis genital tract infection? J Infect Dis 2021;224(12 Suppl 2):S128–36.

24. Taylor BD, Darville T, Haggerty CL. Does bacterial vaginosis cause pelvic inflammatory disease? Sex Transm Dis 2013;40(2):117–22.

25. Haggerty CL, Hillier SL, Bass DC, et al. PID Evaluation and Clinical Health study investigators. Bacterial vaginosis and anaerobic bacteria are associated with endometritis. Clin Infect Dis 2004;39(7):990–5.
26. Workowski KA, Bolan GA, Centers for Disease Control and Prevention. Sexually transmitted diseases treatment guidelines, 2015. MMWR Recomm Rep 2015; 64(RR-03):1–137.
27. Rajkumari N, Kaur H, Roy A, et al. Association of mycoplasma genitalium with infertility in north indian women. Indian J Sex Transm Dis AIDS 2015;36(2): 144–8.
28. Simms I, Eastick K, Mallinson H, et al. Associations between Mycoplasma genitalium, Chlamydia trachomatis, and pelvic inflammatory disease. Sex Transm Infect 2003;79(2):154–6.
29. Latimer RL, Read TRH, Vodstrcil LA, et al. Clinical features and therapeutic response in women meeting criteria for presumptive treatment for pelvic inflammatory disease associated with mycoplasma genitalium. Sex Transm Dis 2019; 46(2):73–9.
30. Haggerty CL, Totten PA, Astete SG, et al. Failure of cefoxitin and doxycycline to eradicate endometrial Mycoplasma genitalium and the consequence for clinical cure of pelvic inflammatory disease. Sex Transm Infect 2008;84(5):338–42.
31. Sethi S, Rajkumari N, Dhaliwal L, et al. P3.294 Association of mycoplasma genitalium with cervicitis in north indian women attending gynecologic clinics. Sex Transm Infect 2013;89(Suppl 1):A240.
32. Kletzel HH, Rotem R, Barg M, et al. Ureaplasma urealyticum: the Role as a Pathogen in Women's Health, a Systematic Review. Curr Infect Dis Rep 2018; 20(9):33.
33. Ferjaoui MA, Arfaoui R, Khedhri S, et al. Pelvic actinomycosis: a confusing diagnosis. Int J Surg Case Rep 2021;86:106387.
34. Valour F, Sénéchal A, Dupieux C, et al. Actinomycosis: etiology, clinical features, diagnosis, treatment, and management. Infect Drug Resist 2014;7:183–97.
35. García-García A, Ramírez-Durán N, Sandoval-Trujillo H, et al. Pelvic Actinomycosis. Can J Infect Dis Med Microbiol 2017;2017:9428650.
36. Kelly J, Aaron J. Pelvic actinomycosis and usage of intrauterine contraceptive devices. Yale J Biol Med 1982;55(5–6):453–61.
37. Sehnal B, Beneš J, Kolářová Z, et al. Pelvic actinomycosis and IUD. Ceska Gynekol 2018;83(5):386–90.
38. Gupta N, Sharma JB, Mittal S, et al. Genital tuberculosis in Indian infertility patients. Int J Gynaecol Obstet 2007;97(2):135–8.
39. Sharma JB, Sharma E, Sharma S, et al. Female genital tuberculosis: Revisited. Indian J Med Res 2018;148(Suppl):S71–83.
40. Parikh FR, Nadkarni SG, Kamat SA, et al. Genital tuberculosis–a major pelvic factor causing infertility in Indian women. Fertil Steril 1997;67(3):497–500.
41. Clarizia R, Capezzuoli T, Ceccarello M, et al. Inflammation calls for more: Severe pelvic inflammatory disease with or without endometriosis. Outcomes on 311 laparoscopically treated women. J Gynecol Obstet Hum Reprod 2021;50(3): 101811.
42. Kruszka PS, Kruszka SJ. Evaluation of acute pelvic pain in women. Am Fam Physician 2010;82(2):141–7.
43. Basta Nikolic M, Spasic A, Hadnadjev Simonji D, et al. Imaging of acute pelvic pain. Br J Radiol 2021;94(1127):20210281.
44. Workowski KA, Bachmann LH, Chan PA, et al. Sexually transmitted infections treatment guidelines, 2021. MMWR Recomm Rep 2021;70(4):1–187.

45. Eschenbach DA, Wölner-Hanssen P, Hawes SE, et al. Acute pelvic inflammatory disease: associations of clinical and laboratory findings with laparoscopic findings. Obstet Gynecol 1997;89(2):184–92.

46. Soper DE. Pelvic inflammatory disease. Obstet Gynecol 2010;116(2 Pt 1): 419–28.

47. Dulin JD, Akers MC. Pelvic inflammatory disease and sepsis. Crit Care Nurs Clin North Am 2003;15(1):63–70.

48. Fouks Y, Cohen A, Shapira U, et al. Surgical intervention in patients with tubo-ovarian abscess: clinical predictors and a simple risk score. J Minim Invasive Gynecol 2019;26(3):535–43.

49. Sánchez-Oro R, Jara-Díaz AM, Martínez-Sanz G. Fitz-hugh-curtis syndrome: a cause of right upper quadrant abdominal pain. Med Clin 2020;154(11):447–52.

50. Cortes EG, Adamski JJ. Chandelier sign. In: StatPearls. Treasure Island, FL: StatPearls Publishing; 2022.

51. Hwang JH, Kim BW, Kim SR, et al. The prediction of surgical intervention in patients with tubo-ovarian abscess. J Obstet Gynaecol 2021;25:1–10.

52. Gina S. Sucato and Pamela J. Murray. Pediatric and Adolescent Gynecology. In: Zitelli B, McIntire S, Nowalk A, editors. Atlas of pediatric physical diagnosis. 7th edition. Philadelphia, PA: Elsevier; 2018. p. 658–90.

53. Bulas DI, Ahlstrom PA, Sivit CJ, et al. Pelvic inflammatory disease in the adolescent: comparison of transabdominal and transvaginal sonographic evaluation. Radiology 1992;183(2):435–9.

54. Romosan G, Valentin L. The sensitivity and specificity of transvaginal ultrasound with regard to acute pelvic inflammatory disease: a review of the literature. Arch Gynecol Obstet 2014;289(4):705–14.

55. Cacciatore B, Leminen A, Ingman-Friberg S, et al. Transvaginal sonographic findings in ambulatory patients with suspected pelvic inflammatory disease. Obstet Gynecol 1992;80(6):912–6.

56. Timor-Tritsch IE, Lerner JP, Monteagudo A, et al. Transvaginal sonographic markers of tubal inflammatory disease. Ultrasound Obstet Gynecol 1998; 12(1):56–66.

57. Jung SI, Kim YJ, Park HS, et al. Acute pelvic inflammatory disease: diagnostic performance of CT. J Obstet Gynaecol Res 2011;37(3):228–35.

58. Revzin MV, Mathur M, Dave HB, et al. Pelvic Inflammatory Disease: Multimodality Imaging Approach with Clinical-Pathologic Correlation. Radiographics 2016; 36(5):1579–96.

59. Tukeva TA, Aronen HJ, Karjalainen PT, et al. MR imaging in pelvic inflammatory disease: comparison with laparoscopy and US. Radiology 1999;210(1):209–16.

60. Ha HK, Lim GY, Cha ES, et al. MR imaging of tubo-ovarian abscess. Acta Radiol 1995;36(5):510–4.

61. Rezvani M, Shaaban AM. Fallopian tube disease in the nonpregnant patient. Radiographics 2011;31(2):527–48.

62. Romosan G, Bjartling C, Skoog L, et al. Ultrasound for diagnosing acute salpingitis: a prospective observational diagnostic study. Hum Reprod 2013;28(6): 1569–79.

63. Birnbaum BA, Jeffrey RB Jr. CT and sonographic evaluation of acute right lower quadrant abdominal pain. AJR Am J Roentgenol 1998;170(2):361–71.

64. Lee MH, Moon MH, Sung CK, et al. CT findings of acute pelvic inflammatory disease. Abdom Imaging 2014;39(6):1350–5.

65. Morcos R, Frost N, Hnat M, et al. Laparoscopic versus clinical diagnosis of acute pelvic inflammatory disease. J Reprod Med 1993;38(1):53–6.

66. Charvériat A, Fritel X. [Diagnosis of pelvic inflammatory disease: Clinical, para-clinical, imaging and laparoscopy criteria. CNGOF and SPILF Pelvic Inflammatory Diseases Guidelines]. Gynecol Obstet Fertil Senol 2019;47(5):404–8.

67. Hillier SL, Kiviat NB, Hawes SE, et al. Role of bacterial vaginosis-associated microorganisms in endometritis. Am J Obstet Gynecol 1996;175(2):435–41.

68. Petrina MAB, Cosentino LA, Wiesenfeld HC, et al. Susceptibility of endometrial isolates recovered from women with clinical pelvic inflammatory disease or histological endometritis to antimicrobial agents. Anaerobe 2019;56:61–5.

69. St Cyr S, Barbee L, Workowski KA, et al. Update to CDC's treatment guidelines for gonococcal infection, 2020. MMWR Morb Mortal Wkly Rep 2020;69(50):1911–6.

70. Workowski KA, Berman S, Centers for Disease Control and Prevention (CDC). Sexually transmitted diseases treatment guidelines, 2010. MMWR Recomm Rep 2010;59(RR-12):1–110.

71. Trent M, Chung S-E, Burke M, et al. Results of a randomized controlled trial of a brief behavioral intervention for pelvic inflammatory disease in adolescents. J Pediatr Adolesc Gynecol 2010;23(2):96–101.

72. Butz AM, Gaydos C, Chung S-E, et al. Care-seeking behavior after notification among young women with recurrent sexually transmitted infections after pelvic inflammatory disease. Clin Pediatr 2016;55(12):1107–12.

73. Arora S, Burner E, Terp S, et al. Improving attendance at post-emergency department follow-up via automated text message appointment reminders: a randomized controlled trial. Acad Emerg Med 2014;22(1):31–7.

74. Wolff M, Balamuth F, Sampayo E, et al. Improving adolescent pelvic inflammatory disease follow-up from the emergency department: randomized controlled trial with text messages. Ann Emerg Med 2016;67(5):602–9.e3.

75. Rhodes KV, Bisgaier J, Becker N, et al. Emergency care of urban women with sexually transmitted infections: time to address deficiencies. Sex Transm Dis 2009;36(1):51–7.

76. Granberg S, Gjelland K, Ekerhovd E. The management of pelvic abscess. Best Pract Res Clin Obstet Gynaecol 2009;23(5):667–78.

77. Gjelland K, Ekerhovd E, Granberg S. Transvaginal ultrasound-guided aspiration for treatment of tubo-ovarian abscess: a study of 302 cases. Am J Obstet Gynecol 2005;193(4):1323–30.

78. Harisinghani MG, Gervais DA, Hahn PF, et al. CT-guided transgluteal drainage of deep pelvic abscesses: indications, technique, procedure-related complications, and clinical outcome. Radiographics 2002;22(6):1353–67.

79. Shah RN, West S, Sweeney KM, et al. Transrectal endoscopic ultrasound-guided drainage of a tubo-ovarian abscess via a lumen-apposing metal stent. ACG Case Rep J 2020;7(12):e00486.

80. Munro K, Gharaibeh A, Nagabushanam S, et al. Diagnosis and management of tubo-ovarian abscesses. The Obstetrician & Gynaecologist 2018;20(1):11–9.

81. Rubino C, Barbati F, Regoli M, et al. Recurrent bilateral salpingitis in a sexually inactive adolescent: don't forget about the appendix. J Pediatr Adolesc Gynecol 2021;34(2):217–9.

82. Kamenga MC, De Cock KM, St Louis ME, et al. The impact of human immunodeficiency virus infection on pelvic inflammatory disease: a case-control study in Abidjan, Ivory Coast. Am J Obstet Gynecol 1995;172(3):919–25.

83. Gao Y, Qu P, Zhou Y, et al. Risk factors for the development of tubo-ovarian abscesses in women with ovarian endometriosis: a retrospective matched case-control study. BMC Womens Health 2021;21(1):43.

84. Fouks Y, Cohen Y, Tulandi T, et al. Complicated clinical course and poor reproductive outcomes of women with tubo-ovarian abscess after fertility treatments. J Minim Invasive Gynecol 2019;26(1):162–8.

85. Mollen CJ, Pletcher JR, Bellah RD, et al. Prevalence of tubo-ovarian abscess in adolescents diagnosed with pelvic inflammatory disease in a pediatric emergency department. Pediatr Emerg Care 2006;22(9):621–5.

86. Dewitt J, Reining A, Allsworth JE, et al. Tuboovarian abscesses: is size associated with duration of hospitalization & complications? Obstet Gynecol Int 2010; 2010:847041.

87. Rosen M, Breitkopf D, Waud K. Tubo-ovarian abscess management options for women who desire fertility. Obstet Gynecol Surv 2009;64(10):681–9.

88. Reed SD, Landers DV, Sweet RL. Antibiotic treatment of tuboovarian abscess: comparison of broad-spectrum beta-lactam agents versus clindamycin-containing regimens. Am J Obstet Gynecol 1991;164(6 Pt 1):1556–61 [discussion: 1561-1562].

89. Kinay T, Unlubilgin E, Cirik DA, et al. The value of ultrasonographic tubo-ovarian abscess morphology in predicting whether patients will require surgical treatment. Int J Gynaecol Obstet 2016;135(1):77–81.

90. Chu L, Ma H, Liang J, et al. Effectiveness and adverse events of early laparoscopic therapy versus conservative treatment for tubo-ovarian or pelvic abscess: a single-center retrospective cohort study. Gynecol Obstet Invest 2019;84(4):334–42.

91. Zhu S, Ballard E, Khalil A, et al. Impact of early surgical management on tubo-ovarian abscesses. J Obstet Gynaecol 2021;41(7):1097–101.

92. Pedowitz P, Bloomfield RD. Ruptured adnexal abscess (tuboovarian) with generalized peritonitis. Am J Obstet Gynecol 1964;88:721–9.

93. Carlson S, Batra S, Billow M, et al. Perioperative complications of laparoscopic versus open surgery for pelvic inflammatory disease. J Minim Invasive Gynecol 2021;28(5):1060–5.

94. Shigemi D, Matsui H, Fushimi K, et al. Laparoscopic compared with open surgery for severe pelvic inflammatory disease and tubo-ovarian abscess. Obstet Gynecol 2019;133(6):1224–30.

95. Hida M, Anno T, Kawasaki F, et al. A rare case of large pyosalpinx in an elderly patient with well-controlled type 2 diabetes mellitus: a case report. J Med Case Rep 2018;12(1):286.

96. Korn AP. Pelvic inflammatory disease in women infected with HIV. AIDS Patient Care STDS 1998;12(6):431–4.

97. Igra V. Pelvic inflammatory disease in adolescents. AIDS Patient Care STDS 1998;12(2):109–24.

98. Maraqa T, Mohamed M, Coffey D, et al. Bilateral recurrent pyosalpinx in a sexually inactive 12-year-old girl secondary to rare variant of Mullerian duct anomaly. BMJ Case Rep 2017;2017. https://doi.org/10.1136/bcr-2016-218924.

99. Champion JD, Piper JM, Holden AEC, et al. Relationship of abuse and pelvic inflammatory disease risk behavior in minority adolescents. J Am Acad Nurse Pract 2005;17(6):234–41.

100. Blanchard AC, Pastorek JG 2nd, Weeks T. Pelvic inflammatory disease during pregnancy. South Med J 1987;80(11):1363–5.

101. Kaiser IH. Fertilization and physiology and development of fetus and placenta. In: Danforth DN, Scott JR, DiSaia PJ, et al, editors. Obstetrics and gynecology, edition 5. Philadelphia, PA: Lipincott; 1986. Chapter 17.

102. Yip L, Sweeny PJ, Bock BF. Acute suppurative salpingitis with concomitant intra-uterine pregnancy. Am J Emerg Med 1993;11(5):476–9.
103. Grimes DA. Intrauterine device and upper-genital-tract infection. Lancet 2000; 356(9234):1013–9.
104. Jatlaoui TC, Simmons KB, Curtis KM. The safety of intrauterine contraception initiation among women with current asymptomatic cervical infections or at increased risk of sexually transmitted infections. Contraception 2016;94(6): 701–12.
105. Centers for Disease Control and Prevention (CDC). U S. medical eligibility criteria for contraceptive use, 2010. MMWR Recomm Rep 2010;59(RR-4):1–86.
106. Tepper NK, Steenland MW, Gaffield ME, et al. Retention of intrauterine devices in women who acquire pelvic inflammatory disease: a systematic review. Contraception 2013;87(5):655–60.
107. Levin G, Dior UP, Gilad R, et al. Pelvic inflammatory disease among users and non-users of an intrauterine device. J Obstet Gynaecol 2021;41(1):118–23.
108. Curtis KM, Jatlaoui TC, Tepper NK, et al. U.S. Selected Practice Recommenda-tions for Contraceptive Use, 2016. MMWR Recomm Rep 2016;65(4):1–66.
109. Caddy S, Yudin MH, Hakim J, et al, INFECTIOUS DISEASE COMMITTEE, SPE-CIAL CONTRIBUTOR. Best practices to minimize risk of infection with intrauter-ine device insertion. J Obstet Gynaecol Can 2014;36(3):266–74.
110. Levgur M, Duvivier R. Pelvic inflammatory disease after tubal sterilization: a re-view. Obstet Gynecol Surv 2000;55(1):41–50.
111. Goller JL, De Livera AM, Fairley CK, et al. Characteristics of pelvic inflammatory disease where no sexually transmitted infection is identified: a cross-sectional analysis of routinely collected sexual health clinic data. Sex Transm Infect 2017;93(1):68–70.
112. Lipscomb GH, Ling FW. Tubo-ovarian abscess in postmenopausal patients. South Med J 1992;85(7):696–9.
113. Gil Y, Capmas P, Tulandi T. Tubo-ovarian abscess in postmenopausal women: a systematic review. J Gynecol Obstet Hum Reprod 2020;49(9):101789.
114. Wang KG, Chen TC, Wang TY, et al. Accuracy of frozen section diagnosis in gy-necology. Gynecol Oncol 1998;70(1):105–10.
115. McElligott KA. Mortality from sexually transmitted diseases in reproductive-aged women: United States, 1999-2010. Am J Public Health 2014;104(8):e101–5.
116. Huang C-C, Huang C-C, Lin S-Y, et al. Association of pelvic inflammatory dis-ease (PID) with ectopic pregnancy and preterm labor in Taiwan: A nationwide population-based retrospective cohort study. PLoS One 2019;14(8):e0219351.
117. US Preventive Services Task Force, Davidson KW, Barry MJ, et al. Screening for chlamydia and gonorrhea: US preventive services task force recommendation statement. JAMA 2021;326(10):949–56.
118. Ness RB, Hillier SL, Kip KE, et al. Bacterial vaginosis and risk of pelvic inflam-matory disease. Obstet Gynecol 2004;104(4):761–9.
119. Intimate Partner Violence Screening. Agency for healthcare research and qual-ity. 2015. Available at: https://www.ahrq.gov/ncepcr/tools/healthier-pregnancy/fact-sheets/partner-violence.html. Accessed December 2021.

Sexual Assault/Domestic Violence

Ruth E.H. Yemane, MD[a],*, Nancy Sokkary, MD[b]

KEYWORDS

- Intimate partner violence • Sexual assault • Child sexual assault • Forensic

KEY POINTS

- Sexual assault and intimate partner violence (IPV) are prevalent in the United States.
- Pregnant women and women of color are particularly high-risk populations for sexual assault and IPV.
- Systematic forensic evaluation and treatment of sexual assault and IPV victims are important aspects of care for these patients.

INTRODUCTION

Sexual assault and intimate partner violence (IPV) affect millions of women each year in the United States.[1] Although sexual assault and IPV occur in people of all ages, races, and socioeconomic backgrounds, women of color are disproportionately impacted.[1] Furthermore, pregnant women are vulnerable to physical violence, with homicide as one of the leading causes of maternal mortality.[2] The health care costs of sexual assault and IPV are significant, and sequalae include financial, medical, and psychological harm. Assessment and treatment by an obstetrician and gynecologist may be essential in an acute care setting for victims of sexual assault and IPV. Appropriate, timely intervention may also prevent future negative outcomes associated with this violence.

Background

Definitions

The Centers for Disease Control and Prevention (CDC) defines intimate partner violence (IPV), commonly known as domestic violence, as "abuse or aggression that occurs in a romantic relationship."[3] IPV can be episodic or chronic in nature, and it includes physical violence, stalking, sexual violence, and psychological

---

[a] University of Wisconsin-Madison, West Clinic, 451 Junction Road, Madison, WI 53717, USA;
[b] Emory University School of Medicine, Children's Healthcare of Atlanta, 1400 Tully Drive, Atlanta GA 30329, USA
* Corresponding author.
E-mail address: ryemane@wisc.edu

Obstet Gynecol Clin N Am 49 (2022) 581–590
https://doi.org/10.1016/j.ogc.2022.02.020
0889-8545/22/© 2022 Elsevier Inc. All rights reserved.

obgyn.theclinics.com

aggression. Sexual violence is defined as a "sexual act that is committed or attempted by another person without freely given consent of the victim or against someone who is unable to consent or refuse."[4]

The National Intimate Partner and Sexual Violence Survey (NISVS) reports more than one-third of women in the United States have been victims of rape, physical violence, and/or stalking by an intimate partner in their lifetime, which translates into 42.4 million women.[1] NISVS further reports 1 in 3 women has experienced physical violence; 1 in 10 women has been raped by an intimate partner, and half of women have experienced sexual violence victimization at some time in their lives.[3] There are also racial disparities associated with IPV and sexual assault. Analysis of homicide data by the National Violent Death Reporting System of nearly 10,000 women aged 18 and older demonstrated non-Hispanic black and American Indian/Alaska Native women experience the highest rates of homicide (4.4 and 4.3, per 100,000 population, respectively).[5] Furthermore, 55.3% of all reported homicides were IPV-related, and 11.2% of these victims were subject to some form of violence in the month before their deaths. In addition, evaluation of IPV among pregnant women showed increased risk for homicide in pregnancy was greatest in younger women and non-Hispanic black women.[2]

IPV in pregnancy has both detrimental maternal and neonatal effects. Women experiencing IPV during pregnancy have increased risk of insufficient prenatal care, poor weight gain, higher rates of smoking and alcohol abuse, and substance abuse.[6] They also incur higher rates of intrapartum and postpartum depression.[6] Pregnant women who sustained physical assault had higher rates of prematurity, maternal death, fetal death, and uterine rupture compared with women who did not experience assault.[7] Recent findings further revealed that homicide is the leading cause of death during pregnancy and the postpartum period in the United States.[2] Most pregnancy-associated homicides occurred at home, implying IPV may have contributed to these horrific maternal outcomes.

Health Care Costs/Public Health Impact

The direct financial and tangible impacts of domestic violence and sexual assault in the United States are significant. The National Center for Injury Prevention and Control reports that intimate partner rape, stalking, and physical assault cost more than $5.8 billion annually and nearly $4.1 billion in direct medical and mental health services.[8] IPV also costs nearly $1 billion in lost productivity and nearly $1 billion in lost lifetime earnings for victims of nonfatal IPV.[8] Overall, health care is the largest portion of IPV-related costs.

Screening

Health care providers have a unique position to both assess and help treat patients at risk of IPV. For this reason, IPV screening should be done routinely. The US Preventative Services Task Force recommends clinicians screen for IPV in all women of reproductive age.[9] Although well-woman examinations, prenatal care visits, and postpartum visits are all opportunities for obstetrician-gynecologist providers to screen patients in routine settings, it should also be done in urgent and acute settings, such as the emergency department or obstetric triage units.

Furthermore, the nature of the obstetrician-gynecologist provider-patient relationship presents several opportunities when IPV or sexual assault concerns may be addressed. Chronic pelvic pain, sexual dysfunction, recurrent sexually transmitted infections (STIs) or testing for STIs, depression, substance abuse, multiple pregnancy tests in a patient not desiring pregnancy, and fear in discussing condoms with a partner, are all clinical scenarios that may reflect IPV. The American College of

Obstetricians and Gynecologists (ACOG) advises screening patients in a private, safe setting using clear communication tools. Introducing the topic with a framing statement can be very useful to smoothly transition into this subject and avoid alarming the patient. ACOG uses the following as an example, "We've started talking to all of our patients about safe and healthy relationships because it can have such a large impact on your health."[10] Take-home materials, including printed resources of local services and national hotlines, should be openly available in the clinical setting and privately available, such as in clinic and emergency room restrooms. It is imperative to avoid assumptions and biased language. How obstetrician-gynecologist providers communicate with patients helps to build a trusting relationship and create a physically and psychologically safe space that is vital in caring for patients with a history of trauma.

Evaluation

It is imperative to provide timely, compassionate, and comprehensive care for victims of IPV and sexual assault. A coordinated, multidisciplinary approach to treatment is important and very well may include obstetrician-gynecologist providers. A Sexual Assault Nurse Examiner (SANE), also known as a forensic nurse or Sexual Assault Forensic Examiner (SAFE), is a provider who has completed training in forensic medical care for victims of sexual assault. Ideally, a SANE collects a forensic history and performs a medical forensic examination after other health care providers have evaluated and stabilized an assault victim in an acute care setting. The historical and physical data collected by a SANE have proven to be more comprehensive and effective than a non-SANE provider.[11] If the acute care setting does not have immediate access to a SANE or SAFE, it is advisable to create an order set or protocol to assure key aspects of evaluation and treatment are addressed.

History

A victim-centered approach ensuring informed consent, clear communication, confidentiality, and immediate safety is imperative when it comes to history taking in this situation. It is also important to attain as much accurate information regarding the perpetration as possible. Important initial questions for victims of sexual assault include "who, what, when, with what, and how."[11]

Physical examination

A physical examination is ideally completed by a SANE provider, as this optimizes the chances of performing the examination in a standardized fashion that avoids interruptions, minimizes retraumatization of the victim, and collects findings for both medical and legal purposes. Details of the examination are beyond the scope of this article; however, in an emergent situation, a general physical examination should be performed to assess any injuries that require immediate intervention. This may include genital examination, speculum, or rectal examination, depending on location and severity of injuries. Providers interested in learning more details of the physical examination may reference "A National Protocol for Sexual Assault Medical Forensic Examinations" or "Evaluation and Management of Female Sexual Assault Victims."[11,12]

Pregnant patients who are victims of direct abdominal trauma as a result of IPV or sexual assault require additional testing and often multidisciplinary support depending on severity of injuries and hemodynamic stability of the patient. These patients are at risk for placental abruption, preterm birth, premature rupture of membranes, uterine rupture, amniotic fluid embolus, and pelvic fracture.[13] Once a pregnant patient has been stabilized, a secondary survey to assess for fetal well-being can be performed with fetal Doppler, bedside ultrasound, or continuous external fetal monitoring depending on the gestational age. If a patient is presenting with vaginal bleeding or leaking fluid, a sterile speculum examination should be performed. Studies have demonstrated that uterine contractions are the single most important predictor of placental abruption, so a tocometer should be placed to assess uterine activity if appropriate for gestational age.[13] Bedside ultrasound can quickly assess for fetal heart tones, gestational age, amniotic fluid index, placental location, and any evidence of placental separation.

Laboratory assessment

Several routine laboratory tests may be initiated by any provider or facility without access to a SANE provider. Following a sexual assault, testing should include screening for STIs (**Table 1**).

Additional serum laboratory tests to consider if the victim is pregnant include a complete blood count, type and screen, fibrinogen, fetal maternal hemorrhage screen with flow cytometry, serum creatinine, and coagulation profile.[12] Rh D immune globulin is indicated in Rh-negative pregnant patients who have direct abdominal trauma, with dosage dependent on results of the fetal-maternal hemorrhage screen.[12] Extended monitoring is warranted if uterine contractions, uterine tenderness, vaginal bleeding, rupture of membranes, nonreassuring fetal heart rate patterns, or more extensive maternal trauma is present."[13]

Treatment

STI exposure risk and risk of pregnancy may be significant concerns for sexual assault victims. Access to appropriate evaluation and treatment should be made available. The CDC reports the most common infections found on forensic examinations are chlamydia, gonorrhea, trichomonas, and bacterial vaginosis.[14] Although the source of these infections may remain unknown, a forensic examination is an opportunity to screen and treat patients who are victims of sexual assault.

CDC 2021 STI treatment guidelines advise the following[15]:

Empiric treatment for chlamydia and gonorrhea should be offered, with consideration for treatment of trichomonas and provision of emergency contraception. Postexposure hepatitis B and human papilloma virus (HPV) vaccination should be offered. If a victim is fully vaccinated, no additional treatment is necessary. If the perpetrator is known hepatitis B positive, unvaccinated victims should receive hepatitis B immunoglobulin and begin hepatitis B vaccination series. HPV vaccination should be offered to victims aged 9 to 26 years who have not been vaccinated or incompletely

Table 1
Post-sexual assault STI Evaluation

Recommended	Source Site
NAAT for *C.trachomatis* and *N.gonorrhoeae*	Site of assault or attempted assault
NAAT for *T.vaginalis*	Urine or vaginal sample
Wet prep for bacterial vaginosis and candidiasis	Vaginal
HIV	Serum
HBsAg	Serum
RPR	Serum

Per the CDC "2021 STI Treatment Guidelines-Sexual Assault, Abuse, and STIs"
Abbreviation: HBsAg, Hepatitis B surface Antigen; HIV, Human Immunodeficiency Virus; NAAT, Nucleic Acid Amplification Test; RPR, Rapid Plasma Reagin.

vaccinated. The first dose should be administered at the time of initial examination, then routine dose scheduling should be followed thereafter (**Table 2**).

Recommendations for HIV postexposure prophylaxis (PEP) should be individualized. Per 2021 CDC STI Treatment Guidelines, a 3- to 7-day starter pack or 28-day course of zidovudine can significantly reduce risk of acquiring HIV.[14] If the patient agrees to HIV testing, baseline testing should be performed within 72 hours of potential exposure. Factors to consider in determining if PEP is advisable include local epidemiology of HIV, time elapsed since potential exposure, probability that perpetrator has HIV, and nature of exposure event. Furthermore, risks and benefits of PEP should be addressed. Consider consulting with an HIV specialist if PEP is being seriously considered. If PEP therapy is initiated, order laboratory tests to assess baseline renal and hepatic function, including serum creatinine, aspartate aminotransferase, and alanine aminotransferase. For assistance with PEP-related decisions, the National Clinicians Post Exposure Prophylaxis Hotline may be contacted (888-448-4911).

The CDC advises follow-up examinations for STI testing, vaccination, and counseling 1 to 2 weeks after a sexual assault, and repeat HIV and syphilis testing is advised 6 weeks, 3 months, and 6 months after an assault, if initial screening was negative.[15]

Risk of pregnancy may be a grave concern for victims of sexual assault. Pregnancy testing (serum or urine pregnancy test) should be offered to all victims of reproductive age after informed consent, per SANE guidelines; if initial pregnancy testing is negative, emergency contraception should be discussed.[12] Emergency contraception options include copper intrauterine device, levonorgestrel tablets (plan B), or ulipristal acetate. Levonorgestrel tablets may be prescribed up to 72 hours following assault, and the copper IUD and ulipristal acetate are effective up to 120 hours after the assault.[16] It is also important to discuss efficacy, risks, benefits, and side effects of each option with the patient. States may have conscience statutes to protect health care providers with moral/religious objections to contraception. However, a provider with these objections must still refer the patient to a prescriber or facility that offers these services.[12]

Reporting

Per the 2013 National Protocol for Sexual Assault Medical Forensic Examinations, "reporting the crime provides the criminal justice system with the opportunity to offer immediate protection to victims, collect evidence from all crime scenes, investigate cases, prosecute if there is sufficient evidence, and hold offenders accountable for crimes committed."[12] However, victims must have autonomy to decide to report.

Table 2 Postsexual assault treatment	
Recommended	**Consider**
Doxycycline 100 mg po bid × 7 d	HBIG 5 mL IM[a]
Ceftriaxone 500 mg IM × 1	Hepatitis B vaccine (routine scheduled)[b]
Metronidazole 500 mg po bid × 7 d	Human papilloma virus vaccine (routine schedule)[b]
	Zidovudine po for 3–7 d
	Copper intrauterine device, levonorgestrel tablets, or ulipristal acetate

[a] If victim not vaccinated and perpetrator suspected to be positive.
[b] If victim unvaccinated.

Risks and benefits of reporting should be discussed with the patient, including the option to report at a later time, recognizing this may make prosecution more challenging.

Child Sexual Assault

Background
Definition. Sexual assault in a minor, or child sexual assault (CSA), is defined as attempted or completed contact or noncontact sexual interaction in an individual who legally cannot give consent, is unprepared for developmentally, cannot comprehend, and/or that violates the law of society.[17]

The perpetrator of sexual assault in most cases of CSA is a relative or acquaintance. In the emergency setting, a child may present as a result of trauma or injury attained during sexual assault, or it may be disclosed to a health care provider during a visit for another ailment.[17,18]

According to the US Department of Health and Human Services (DHHS), there are more than 60,000 reported cases of child sexual abuse annually.[19] However, this is likely an underestimate, as 15% to 30% of girls are estimated to experience some type of sexual abuse. Children with disabilities and developmental delay are at increased risk of sexual assault and other forms of abuse.[18,20,21]

Screening
Several screening tools exist to evaluate for CSA, specifically in the emergency department. Gynecologic evaluation should include confidential sexual abuse screening, regardless of the setting. Approaching the topic in an objective and routine manner that is incorporated into the greater social history assures that no biases play a role in the patients who are screened. Children presenting with nonspecific symptoms and signs should be questioned carefully and in a nonleading manner about any stressors, including abuse, in their life.[17] Introducing the subject as something that applies to all patients, similar to the approach as previously outlined for adults, is also recommended. It is imperative to screen both the parent and the child in private.

Evaluation
In an acute care setting, sexual abuse examination facilities and victim advocates should be alerted immediately upon presentation of a victim. Most institutions do have existing protocols for these teams. The goal of evaluation in the acute setting is to identify injuries, evaluate for suicidal ideation or human trafficking, screen for or diagnose STIs, and reduce risk of pregnancy.[22] Although it is recommended for CSA evaluations to be performed at a center with expertise and familiarity with this scope of practice, urgent or emergent evaluations are appropriate for the following situations: abuse that occurred within 72 to 96 hours, physical injuries that require treatment, collection of obvious forensic evidence, or if the child is in imminent danger either from the perpetrator or from self. If the victim's situation does not meet any of these criteria, then delay in evaluation until the patient can be seen at a specialized center should be strongly considered.[17,23]

It is beyond the scope of this article to review in depth recommendations for Sexual Assault Nurse Evaluations or forensic interviewing, but the following will outline key points and recommendations. Please see "A National Protocol for Sexual Abuse Medical Forensic Examinations Pediatric" for full details regarding evaluation of CSA victims.[12]

History
A forensic interview is part of a comprehensive investigation and is performed by a trained professional. It is imperative that the history be taken from the child in an

unbiased fashion, giving both the caregiver and the child an opportunity to disclose information in private and together, if appropriate.[24]

The history should address the chief complaint, injury, or report of sexual abuse and include a basic medical and surgical history. When asking about the event or events in question, it is important to illicit if the caregiver (or other responsible party) has any concerns. When interviewing the child, it is advisable to collect information in a simple, objective manner, while maintaining a safe and caring demeanor. It may be appropriate to ask the child if they know why they are there and what words they use to describe their private parts. This should be followed by asking specific questions, as addressed in the adult section, in reference to who, what, when, with what, and how.[11] In the emergent setting, it is important to evaluate for pain, bleeding, and ability to void. A formal forensic interview will illicit where the assault took place, how many times the victim has been assaulted, over what period of time, and details of the manner of the assault. In the acute setting, it is important to know the details and timing of the most recent event.[17,24]

Review of systems should include change in bowel or bladder habits, such as new-onset enuresis or regression of potty training, change in sleep patterns or eating behavior. Social history is critical to identify factors surrounding safety of the child, including who they live with, caregivers, other support structures, school, and extra-curricular activities.[25]

Physical examination

A routine physical examination should be performed in an acute setting to address stability of the patients and assess for injuries requiring immediate attention. Repeat pelvic examinations should be avoided, if possible, and performed by a provider trained in SANE. An obstetrician-gynecologist may be called to perform an examination to assess for injury specific to the genital region. It is imperative to work with the emergency room providers as well as anesthesia personnel to provide the safest and most comfortable examination possible; sedation should be strongly considered. Examination should include inspection for vaginal discharge, bleeding, and odor. Although vulvar condyloma and herpetic lesions in the anogenital region should warrant investigation for sexual assault in a minor, they are not diagnostic for sexual abuse.[14]

Laboratory evaluation

Laboratory diagnosis of specific infections provides important evidence in the case of CSA and is also critical for the evaluation and appropriate treatment of the victim. It is imperative to have a uniform approach to test selection and collection technique that considers patient age, gender, and anatomic location.

Laboratory testing is challenging in prepubertal victims because of the low prevalence and lack of thorough test validation in this age group.[26] Routine laboratory testing should include the same as those recommended for adults (see **Table 1**). Nucleic acid amplification tests (NAAT) are the preferred tests given their superior sensitivity and specificity; however, CSA assessments may require more than 1 NAAT and a culture. Most institutions with sexual assault evaluation teams have protocols in place, but it does present an additional level of complexity to the evaluation.[26] Similar to adult victims, swabbing of various orifices (oral, genital, anal) should be carefully considered. In patients who are postpubertal, pregnancy testing should be performed, and possibly repeated in 2 to 4 weeks, depending on when the assault occurred. Clinical specimens reviewed by the laboratory may also reveal sperm, which would provide definitive forensic evidence of sexual assault.

Reporting

DHHS Children's Bureau considers certain persons "mandated reporters," and they are required to report suspected cases of child abuse and neglect to the appropriate agency in their area. Mandated reporters are typically provided immunity from liability with good-faith reporting. Circumstances in which a report should be placed, and in most cases is mandatory, varies widely but certainly applies to any situation in which child abuse or neglect is suspected. Information on reporting agencies in a specific region of the country can be found on the Child Welfare Information Gateway Web site.[27]

Treatment

Prophylactic treatment of postpubertal individuals is the same as that described for adults (see above). For prepubertal victims, the incidence of STIs is very low so prophylactic treatment is not recommended in this patient population unless there is elevated concern based on history or specific symptoms. HIV PEP is generally well tolerated in children but should only be performed after thorough evaluation of the child's risk and in consultation with a specialist in pediatric HIV cases. A repeat examination should be conducted 2 weeks after the most recent assault; diagnostic testing can also be repeated at that time if initial assessment was negative. HIV, hepatitis B, and syphilis serologic screening can be repeated again between 6 weeks and 3 months after the most recent assault.[14]

Outcomes

The morbidity of CSA invades far beyond physical injuries and trauma in childhood. A comprehensive review and meta-analysis found a substantial association between child sexual abuse, substance abuse, and posttraumatic stress disorder (PTSD).[28] Several additional health, psychiatric, and social ailments have been associated with victims of sexual assault.[28]

People who are victims of childhood sexual assault have higher risk of depression, self-injurious behavior, and attempted suicide well into adulthood.[18,28] There is also a statistically significant increase in the likelihood of experiencing anxiety, eating disorders, PTSD, and sleep disorders.[21,29] There are also data that suggest that penetrative trauma is linked to a higher risk of self-injurious behavior.[30]

CSA is also a risk factor for specific physical illnesses, including HIV and obesity. The cause of this may be due to psychosocial issues, such as increased "risky behavior," resulting in more or riskier sexual acts and higher risk of HIV acquisition, as well as disordered eating or depression leading to obesity.[28]

SUMMARY

IPV and sexual assault of a minor or adult are situations that every obstetrician and gynecologist will be exposed to in their career, both in outpatient clinics and in the emergency care setting. As a provider, the obstetrician-gynecologist can elicit a sensitive history, perform a thorough evaluation, and provide necessary therapy in a safe, objective, and appropriate manner. Several useful protocols and guidelines have been developed, in addition to specially trained personnel, to assist and consult when dealing with IPV and sexual assault.[11]

CLINICS CARE POINTS

- Sexual assault and intimate partner violence can have devastating medical, psychological, and financial effects on victims.

- Obstetrician-gynecologists should screen all patients, regardless of age, for sexual assault, including in emergency care settings.
- A multidisciplinary approach, including access to a Sexual Assault Nurse Examiner, can improve care for victims of assault.
- There are routine, standardized laboratory tests and prophylactic medical therapies for sexual assault victims, outlined by the Centers for Disease Control and Prevention.

National resources (number or Web sites for providers or victims)
www.rainn.org.
www.nsvrc.org.
National Sexual Assault Telephone Hotline, 1-800-656-4673.
National Clinicians Post Exposure Prophylaxis Hotline, 1-888-448-4911.

DISCLOSURE

The authors have no commercial or financial disclosures to report.

REFERENCES

1. Black MC, Basile KC, Smith SG, et al. National intimate partner and sexual violence survey: 2010 summary report. National Center for Injury Prevention and Control, Centers for Disease Control and Prevention; 2011. https://doi.org/10.1093/oxfordhb/9780199844654.013.0003. Published online.
2. Wallace M, Gillispie-Bell V, Cruz K, et al. Homicide during pregnancy and the postpartum period in the United States, 2018–2019. Obstet Gynecol 2021;5: 138. https://doi.org/10.1097/aog.0000000000004567.
3. Centers for Disease Control and Prevention. Preventing intimate partner violence. Available at: https://www.cdc.gov/violenceprevention/intimatepartnerviolence/fastfact.html. Accessed December 28, 2021.
4. Breiding M, Basile K, Smith S, et al. Intimate partner violence surveillance: uniform definitions and recommended data elements, version 2.0 2015. Available at: https://www.cdc.gov/violenceprevention/pdf/ipv/intimatepartnerviolence.pdf. Accessed December 20, 2021.
5. Petrosky E, Blair JM, Betz CJ, et al. Racial and ethnic differences in homicides of adult women and the role of intimate partner violence — United States, 2003–2014. MMWR Morb Mortal Wkly Rep 2017;66(28):741-6.
6. Alhusen JL, Ray E, Sharps P, et al. Intimate partner violence during pregnancy: maternal and neonatal outcomes. J Womens Health (Larchmt) 2015;24(1):100-6.
7. el Kady D, Gilbert WM, Xing G, et al. Maternal and neonatal outcomes of assaults during pregnancy. Obstet Gynecol 2005;105(2):357-63.
8. National Center for Injury Prevention and Control. Costs of intimate partner violence against women in the United States. Atlanta, Georgia: Centers for Disease Control and Prevention; 2003 (March).
9. Curry S. USPSTF intimate partner violence, elder abuse, and abuse of vulnerable adults: screening. Published October 23 2018. Available at: https://www.uspreventiveservicestaskforce.org/uspstf/recommendation/intimate-partner-violence-and-abuse-of-elderly-and-vulnerable-adults-screening#bootstrap-panel-11. Accessed December 28, 2021.
10. ACOG committee opinion 518: intimate partner violence. Obstet Gynecol 2012; 119(2 Pt 1):412-7. Available at: http://www.acog.org/About_ACOG/.

11. Vrees RA. Evaluation and management of female victims of sexual assault. Obstet Gynecol Surv 2017;72(1):39–53.

12. Little K. A national protocol for sexual assault medical forensic examinations - adults/adolescents. US Department of Justice; 2013. Available at: https://www.justice.gov/ovw/file/846856/download. Accessed October 12, 2021.

13. Greco PS, Day LJ, Pearlman MD. Guidance for evaluation and management of blunt abdominal trauma in pregnancy. Obstet Gynecol 2019;134(6):1343–57.

14. Centers for Disease Control and Prevention. Sexual assault and abuse and STIs-adolescents and adults 2021. Available at: https://www.cdc.gov/std/treatment-guidelines/sexual-assault-adults.htm. Accessed December 28, 2021.

15. Centers for Disease Control and Prevention. STI treatment guidelines. Available at: https://www.cdc.gov/std/treatment-guidelines/default.htm. Accessed December 18, 2021.

16. ACOG practice bulletin 152: emergency contraception. Obstet Gynecol 2015;126(3):e1–11.

17. Kellogg N. The evaluation of sexual abuse in children. Pediatrics 2005;116(2):506–12.

18. Gilbert R, Widom CS, Browne K, et al. Burden and consequences of child maltreatment in high-income countries. Lancet 2009;373(9657):68–81.

19. Kelly C. Child Maltreatment 2019. U.S. Department of Health & Human Services, Administration for Children and Families, Administration on Children, Youth and Families, Children's Bureau.

20. Christian CW, Crawford-Jakubiak JE, Flaherty EG, et al. The evaluation of suspected child physical abuse. Pediatrics 2015;135(5):e1337-54.

21. Kiefer R, Goncharenko S, Contractor AA, et al. Posttraumatic stress disorder symptoms moderate the relation between childhood sexual abuse and disordered eating in a community sample. Int J Eat Disord 2021;54(10):1819–28.

22. Adams JA, Kellogg ND, Farst KJ, et al. Updated guidelines for the medical assessment and care of children who may have been sexually abused. J Pediatr Adolesc Gynecol 2016;29(2):81–7.

23. Floyed RL, Hirsh DA, Greenbaum VJ, et al. Development of a screening tool for pediatric sexual assault may reduce emergency-department visits. Pediatrics 2011;128(2):221–6.

24. Strickland J, Adams JA. Medical evaluation of suspected child sexual abuse. J Pediatr Adolesc Gynecol 2004;17(3):191–7.

25. A national protocol for sexual abuse medical forensic examinations pediatric. 2016. Available at: https://www.justice.gov/ovw/file/846856/download. Accessed October 11, 2021.

26. Qin X, Melvin AJ. Laboratory diagnosis of sexually transmitted infections in cases of suspected child sexual abuse. J Clin Microbiol 2020;58(2):e01433-19.

27. Mandated reporting-child welfare information gateway. Available at: https://www.childwelfare.gov/topics/responding/reporting/mandated/. Accessed October 12, 2021.

28. Hailes HP, Yu R, Danese A, et al. Long-term outcomes of childhood sexual abuse: an umbrella review. Lancet Psychiatry 2019;6(10):830–9.

29. Chen LP, Murad MH, Paras ML, et al. Sexual abuse and lifetime diagnosis of psychiatric disorders: SYSTEMATIC review and meta-analysis. Mayo Clin Proc 2010;85(7):618–29.

30. Amado BG, Arce R, Herraiz A. Psychological injury in victims of child sexual abuse: a meta-analytic review. Psychosocial Intervention 2015;24(1). https://doi.org/10.1016/j.psi.2015.03.002.

Evaluation and Management of Heavy Vaginal Bleeding (Noncancerous)

Bridget Kelly, MD[a,b], Emily Buttigieg, MD[a,c],*

KEYWORDS

- Heavy vaginal bleeding • Bleeding disorders • Hysteroscopy
- Saline infusion sonohysterography • Hormonal management

KEY POINTS

- Heavy vaginal bleeding is a common, life-altering condition.
- Etiology is separated into structural (polyps, adenomyosis leiomyomas, malignancy) and nonstructural (coagulopathy, ovulatory, iatrogenic, endometrial, not yet classified) causes.
- Work-up involves sequential laboratory and imaging studies depending on patient history and examination findings.
- Treatment involves acute stabilization and long-term therapy with medical and surgical options.

Definitions of normal and abnormal menses are as follows:

- Normal menstrual flow[1]
  - 28 days ± 7 days; in adolescents, range is wider from 21 to 45 days
  - Lasts 5 days ± 3 days
  - 8 to 80 mL of blood loss total
- Abnormal menstrual flow
  - Approximately 30% of women experience abnormal uterine bleeding at some point during their lifetime resulting in decreased quality of life and productivity[1]
  - Abnormal menses is defined by volume, timing, and duration:
    - Volume
      - Greater than 80 mL
      - Difficult for patients to quantify
      - Changing pads every 1 to 2 hours, passing clots greater than one-inch in diameter, and/or having frequent flooding accidents[2–4]

a University of Wisconsin School of Medicine and Public Health, Madison, WI, USA; b University of Wisconsin Obstetrics and Gynecology Clinic, 2402 Winnebago Street, Madison, WI 53704, USA; c University of Wisconsin Obstetrics and Gynecology Clinic, 20 South Park, Madison, WI 53715, USA
* Corresponding author. University of Wisconsin Obstetrics and Gynecology Clinic, 20 South Park, Madison, WI 53715.
E-mail address: buttigieg@wisc.edu

Obstet Gynecol Clin N Am 49 (2022) 591–606
https://doi.org/10.1016/j.ogc.2022.02.021   obgyn.theclinics.com

- Validated self-assessment screening tools,[3] such as the menstrual blood loss questionnaire[5] and pictorial blood loss assessment chart,[4,6,7] available in paper and mobile application formats, are available to provide an objective screen of bleeding quantity
  - Timing
    - Intermenstrual bleeding: bleeding between menstrual cycles
    - Postcoital bleeding: bleeding after intercourse
  - Duration
    - Acute: less than 6 months duration
    - Chronic: greater than or equal to 6 months duration

EVALUATION OF HEAVY VAGINAL BLEEDING
International Federation of Gynecology and Obstetrics Classification

Abnormal uterine bleeding is bleeding that falls outside of these normal parameters, as outlined previously. It is further classified by duration (acute or chronic), amount (heavy vaginal bleeding), or timing (intermenstrual or postcoital bleeding).

Furthermore, in 2011, the International Federation of Gynecology and Obstetrics introduced a classification system for gynecologic bleeding abnormalities. In this system, bleeding is further classified as resulting from a structural cause (polyp, adenomyosis, leiomyoma, malignancy/hyperplasia) or a nonstructural cause (coagulopathy, ovulatory dysfunction, endometrial, iatrogenic, and not yet classified).[8,9] Examples of abnormal uterine bleeding caused by coagulopathy include von Willebrand disease and coagulopathy from medication, such as anticoagulants. Ovulatory dysfunction results from multiple causes. These are typically related to dysfunction in the hypothalamic-pituitary-ovarian axis, including immaturity, polycystic ovary syndrome, and the female athlete triad.[9]

Age Considerations

The most common cause of abnormal uterine bleeding is also stratified based on the patient's age[1]

- Adolescents (<18 year old): bleeding disorders, anovulation
- Adults (18–40 year old): structural (polyp, fibroid), ovulatory (polycystic ovary syndrome)
- Perimenopause (>40 year old): structural (polyp, fibroid, endometrial hyperplasia/malignancy), anovulation
- Postmenopausal: structural (polyp, endometrial hyperplasia/malignancy), atrophy

Patient Stability

Patient evaluation begins with assessing patient stability.[10] For acute episodes, it is critical to determine patient hemodynamic stability. On initial evaluation, patient condition should be assessed for alertness and orientation and skin pallor.[11] Vital signs should be assessed including heart rate, blood pressure, respiratory rate, oxygen saturation, and temperature. Volume status should be assessed through capillary refill time, with a normal time of less than 2 seconds,[12,13] and peripheral pulse assessment, feeling for presence and strength, along with urine output if available.[11] Together, these are used to assess for signs of hypovolemic shock (**Table 1**).

If the patient is found to be in hypovolemic shock, initial efforts should be focused on resuscitative efforts. This includes obtaining intravenous (IV) access with two large-

Table 1
Classes of hypovolemic shock

	Class 1	Class 2	Class 3	Class 4
Heart rate (beats/min)	<100	>100	>120	>140
Blood pressure	Normal	Normal	Decreased	Decreased
Respiratory rate (respirations/min)	14–20	20–30	30–40	>35
Mental status	Slightly anxious	Mildly anxious	Anxious, confused	Confused, lethargic
Urine output (mL/h)	>30	20–30	5–15	<5
Blood loss	<15%; 750 mL	15%–30%; 750–1500 mL	30%–40%; 1500–2000 mL	>40%; >2000 mL

Data from Brady PC, Carusi D. Vaginal Hemorrhage. In: Handbook of Consult and Inpatient Gynecology. Springer International Publishing; 2016:31-51; and Evans L, Rhodes A, Alhazzani W, et al. Surviving Sepsis Campaign: International Guidelines for Management of Sepsis and Septic Shock 2021. Critical Care Medicine. 2021;49(11):e1063-e1143.

bore IVs, fluid resuscitation, laboratory evaluation, medications, and possible blood transfusion.[10,11,13] See the evaluation and treatment sections for further description.

Medical History

For those patients who are hemodynamically stable, work-up begins with a comprehensive history. Specific questions include the following[10]:

- Age of menarche
- Menstrual patterns: length of cycle, duration of bleeding
- Amount of bleeding: number of heavy days, saturation rate on heavy days, passage of clots, and frequency of flooding accidents
- Pain: dysmenorrhea, dyspareunia, dyschezia, dysuria
- Intercourse: pain or bleeding
- Cervical cancer screening history
- Medical and surgical history
- Family history, including bleeding disorders and cancer history
- Current medications and supplements

Additionally, a bleeding history should be obtained assessing for every patient who presents with heavy menstrual bleeding (**Fig. 1**). This is especially important in adolescents given that bleeding disorders, such as von Willebrand disease and hemophilia, are identified in approximately 20% of adolescents who present with heavy menstrual bleeding, compared with 1% to 2% of the general population. This is further increased to 34% to 37% in adolescents who are hospitalized for heavy bleeding.[14,15] Of these, von Willebrand disease is the most common cause, with a prevalence of 1% in the general population and 38% in adolescents with heavy menstrual bleeding.[15]

If patients screen positive, work-up for a bleeding disorder should include complete blood count, ferritin level, prothrombin time, partial thromboplastin time, and fibrinogen.[2] Additionally, initial screening for von Willebrand disease should be performed with von Willebrand factor antigen, von Willebrand factor VIII activity, and von Willebrand factor assay (ristocetin cofactor assay).[2,15] Consultation with hematology is considered to guide this and further testing if a bleeding disorder is suspected based on the patient's history and laboratory evaluation.[1,2,15]

Menstrual and Bleeding Abnormalities Associated with Bleeding Disorders

Menstrual Abnormalities:
- Menstrual bleeding lasting >8 d
- Shortened cycles <24 d
- Flooding episodes
- Passage of clots > 2cm
- Saturation of hygiene product in < 2 h
- Iron deficiency anemia
- Need for blood transfusion
- Heavy periods since menarche

AND/OR

Bleeding Abnormalities:
- Postpartum hemorrhage
- Excessive/prolonged bleeding during surgery or dental procedures Prolonged cutaneous bleeding (lasting >10 min) and/or frequent bruising
- Spontaneous epistaxis 1–2 times per mo (lasting >10 min)
- Frequent oral/gingival bleeding (lasting >10 min)
- Family history of heavy bleeding
- Muscle/Joint bleeding
- Bleeding episode requiring blood transfusion

Fig. 1. Evaluation for bleeding disorders. Patients who report heavier menstrual bleeding should undergo further evaluation with a detailed menstrual and bleeding history. Those with multiple abnormalities should undergo a laboratory evaluation for bleeding disorders with consideration of referral to hematology for any abnormal findings. (*Data from* Refs.[2,14,15])

Physical Examination

After collecting a detailed history, evaluation should continue with a physical examination.[10] This should include a general skin examination (assessing for hirsutism, acne, acanthosis nigricans, petechiae, ecchymosis, pallor), thyroid examination, and a pelvic examination. More specifically, the pelvic examination should include an external examination, speculum examination to confirm the source of the bleeding (vagina, uterus, or cervix) with consideration for sexually transmitted infection testing, cervical cancer screening, and endometrial biopsy if indicated (**Fig. 2**). A bimanual examination should also be performed to assess the uterine size and shape and adnexa, which may reveal large uterine fibroids or adnexal masses. In adolescents, an external vulvar examination should be performed to assess for patency of the external orifice through gentle palpation with a cotton swab, to assess Tanner stage, and to look for signs of trauma.[2,15] However, a speculum examination is generally not required because sexually transmitted infection testing is obtained through urine and blood samples.[2,15]

After completion of the history and physical examination, the differential diagnosis is narrowed down further. Next steps typically include laboratory evaluation and/or imaging in a stable patient. In patients with hemodynamic instability with evidence of hypovolemic shock, as outlined in **Table 1**, initial efforts should focus on patient resuscitation and stabilization,[11,13] followed by medical and surgical treatment.

Laboratory Evaluation

Overview

Initial testing in all patients with reported heavy vaginal bleeding should include a pregnancy test, complete blood count, and thyroid-stimulating hormone level (see **Fig. 2**).[1]

Menstrual irregularity

Patients with menstrual cycle irregularity, such as oligomenorrhea, often present with heavy menstrual bleeding. This most commonly occurs because of ovulatory dysfunction, commonly caused by hypothalamic-pituitary-ovarian axis immaturity in adolescents and polycystic ovary syndrome in adolescents and adults.[9] Anovulatory cycles create an environment of unopposed estrogen stimulation and endometrial proliferation, without progestin-induced stabilization. The end result is disorderly shedding of the endometrial lining without prostaglandin-mediated vasoconstriction

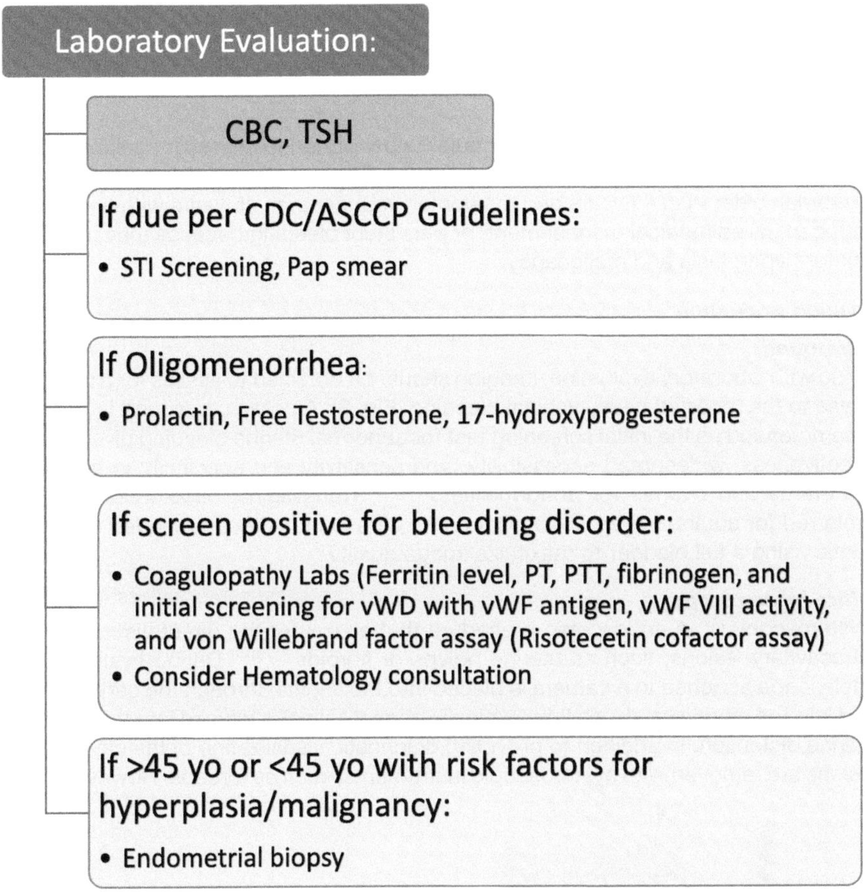

Laboratory Evaluation:

CBC, TSH

If due per CDC/ASCCP Guidelines:
- STI Screening, Pap smear

If Oligomenorrhea:
- Prolactin, Free Testosterone, 17-hydroxyprogesterone

If screen positive for bleeding disorder:
- Coagulopathy Labs (Ferritin level, PT, PTT, fibrinogen, and initial screening for vWD with vWF antigen, vWF VIII activity, and von Willebrand factor assay (Risotecetin cofactor assay)
- Consider Hematology consultation

If >45 yo or <45 yo with risk factors for hyperplasia/malignancy:
- Endometrial biopsy

Fig. 2. Algorithmic approach to the laboratory evaluation for heavy vaginal bleeding. CBC, complete blood count; CDC, Centers for Disease Control and Prevention; PT, prothrombin time; PTT, partial thromboplastin time; STI, sexually transmitted infection; TSH, thyroid-stimulating hormone; vWD, von Willebrand disease; vWF, von Willebrand factor; yo, years old. (*Data from* Refs.[1,2,10,15])

and platelet-plugging of arterioles.[16] This ultimately leads to episodes of heavy vaginal bleeding and sometimes urgent presentation to the office or emergency department. Work-up for this includes laboratory evaluation with a free testosterone level along with an examination assessing for signs of hyperandrogenism. In the adult patient, imaging can also be obtained to assess ovarian volume and antral follicle count, although imaging is not recommended for diagnosis of polycystic ovary syndrome in adolescents.[1,9] Prolactin and 17-hydroxyprogesterone should also be obtained to assess for more rare causes of oligomenorrhea including a prolactinoma or congenital adrenal hyperplasia, respectively.[1]

Bleeding disorders
If the patient is an adolescent or screens positive for a possible bleeding disorder (see **Fig. 1**), further work-up should be obtained including: ferritin level, prothrombin time, partial thromboplastin time, fibrinogen along with initial screening for von Willebrand

disease with von Willebrand factor antigen, von Willebrand factor VIII activity, and von Willebrand factor assay (ristocetin cofactor assay).[2,15] Hematology consultation should be considered for abnormal values or concern for bleeding disorders.[2,10,15]

Endometrial sampling

Additionally, an endometrial biopsy should be performed to assess for cellular abnormalities, such as endometrial hyperplasia and malignancy. This should be obtained for all women older than 45 years and for women younger than 45 years with unopposed estrogen, failed medical management, or persistent bleeding because they may be at risk for hyperplasia and malignancy.[1]

Imaging Evaluation

Ultrasound

Along with laboratory evaluation, imaging should be obtained to assess for a structural cause to the reported heavy vaginal bleeding (**Fig. 3**). A pelvic ultrasound is generally recommended as the initial screening test for abnormal uterine bleeding given its cost effectiveness, widespread accessibility, and sensitivity and specificity in evaluating the uterus and ovaries for abnormalities.[1,17,18] Transvaginal ultrasound (TVUS) is preferred for adults, but an abdominal pelvic ultrasound is recommended in adolescents, using a full bladder to maximize image quality.[2]

Office hysteroscopy

Hysteroscopy is an endoscopic procedure that allows for the direct visualization of intracavitary lesions, such as uterine polyps or fibroids.[1,19,20] During hysteroscopy, a telescope attached to a camera is placed into the vagina, through the cervical canal and into the uterine cavity, as fluid (typically normal saline) is infused into the cavity for uterine distention. In addition to providing diagnostic visualization of the cavity, small lesions are removed with hysteroscopic instruments, such as forceps. However, given

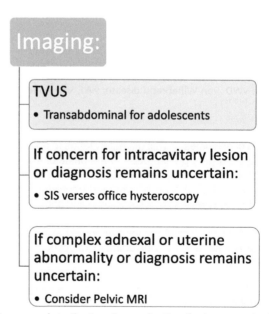

Imaging:

TVUS
- Transabdominal for adolescents

If concern for intracavitary lesion or diagnosis remains uncertain:
- SIS verses office hysteroscopy

If complex adnexal or uterine abnormality or diagnosis remains uncertain:
- Consider Pelvic MRI

Fig. 3. Algorithmic approach to the imaging evaluation for heavy vaginal bleeding. SIS, saline infusion sonohysterography; TVUS, transvaginal ultrasound. (*Data from* Refs.[1,17–20,22])

intracavitary location, hysteroscopy does not allow for evaluation of the myometrium, ovaries, or fallopian tubes.[19]

Saline infusion sonohysterography

Saline infusion sonohysterography (SIS) involves placing a balloon catheter into the vagina, through the cervix and into the uterine cavity, followed by infusion of fluid (typically normal saline) to distend the uterine cavity. TVUS is then performed simultaneously to evaluate the distended uterine cavity. This allows for the visualization of intracavitary lesions, typically endometrial polyps and fibroids, and extracavitary lesions with evaluation of the myometrium, ovaries, and fallopian tubes.[19] However, it does not allow for treatment of the identified lesions.

Choosing among transvaginal ultrasound, hysteroscopy, and saline infusion sonohysterography

A systematic review of the three imaging modalities, TVUS, hysteroscopy, and SIS, found hysteroscopy to be the most sensitive and specific for intracavitary lesions with a pooled sensitivity and specificity of 0.95 and 0.9, respectively.[20] This is significantly superior to SIS ($P = .007$) and TVUS ($P < .001$).[20] SIS remains highly diagnostic, although slightly less so when compared with hysteroscopy, with a pooled sensitivity and specificity of 0.93 and 0.9, respectively.[20] It is noteworthy that although TVUS is the preferred imaging modality for abnormal bleeding, it is the least accurate at identifying intracavitary lesions, with a pooled sensitivity of 0.6 and specificity of 0.85.[1,19,20] TVUS sensitivity for diagnosing polyps was particularly low (0.51).[19,20]

Based on this, if the patient has a thickened or irregular-appearing endometrial lining or any suspicion for intracavitary lesion, such as polyp or fibroid, on TVUS, further cavitary evaluation should be performed with either SIS or hysteroscopy. Choosing between the two methods depends on availability, cost, patient preference, and suspected pathology.[19] Although both modalities allow for evaluation of intracavitary lesions, only SIS evaluates the myometrium, ovaries, and fallopian tubes concurrently. Conversely, only hysteroscopy allows for the identification and treatment of small intracavitary lesions simultaneously. Indeed if an intracavity lesion is identified on SIS, hysteroscopy is subsequently required for removal.

Additionally, although all three imaging modalities are well-tolerated by patients, often without analgesia, patients report TVUS to be the least painful modality ($P < .0001$).[21] Patients also reported significantly less pain with SIS compared with hysteroscopy ($P < .0001$).[21] Although many procedures are able to be completed without analgesia, if desired, patients may be given oral or IV anxiolytic pain medication, such as nonsteroidal anti-inflammatory medications or narcotics, before the procedure, although this requires trained providers and support staff along with patient transportation to and from the clinic. Hysteroscopy may also be performed in an operating room, although this has significantly increased costs along with anesthetic risks.

MRI

Pelvic MRI is generally reserved for complex masses that cannot be fully characterized on ultrasound.[1,17] This can include complex ovarian masses, with an accuracy of 91% in evaluating for malignancy[22] and fallopian tube abnormalities. Additionally, MRI allows for the evaluation of adenomyosis, with a sensitivity of 78% and specificity of 93%,[22] in cases that are inconclusive following ultrasound evaluation. Fibroids can also be further characterized, including size, location, number, and blood supply, which is helpful in planning for embolization procedures, as detailed later. Pelvic MRI can also assess the endometrium for abnormalities including endometrial polyps or cancer, with a sensitivity of 79% and specificity of 89% for the detection of malignancy.[17,22] Pelvic MRI should be performed with and without IV gadolinium-based contrast, and diffusion-weighted sequences should be obtained.[22] Consultation with radiology before ordering the imaging is useful to ensure the correct imaging sequence is obtained.[17]

Age considerations

Age of the patient can also help to direct the work-up of heavy vaginal bleeding (**Fig. 4**). Heavy vaginal bleeding in adolescents is generally secondary to hypothalamic-pituitary-ovarian axis immaturity (ovulatory) or bleeding disorders (coagulopathy).[1] Therefore, evaluation should include screening for bleeding disorders, with appropriate laboratory testing if the screening test is positive (see **Fig. 1**). Pelvic imaging is rarely indicated given that the incidence of structural anomalies in this age group is rare.[2] Indications for a pelvic ultrasound in this population include persistent bleeding that does not respond to initial management or severe pelvic pain. When a pelvic ultrasound is ordered, a transabdominal approach is preferred.[2]

Similarly, postmenopausal bleeding has a different list of possible etiologies, including vaginal atrophy, endometrial polyps, endometrial hyperplasia, and endometrial malignancy. Work-up in this age group should include imaging with a pelvic ultrasound. If the endometrial thickness is greater than 4 mm or persistent episodes of bleeding occur, regardless of imaging findings,[1] endometrial sampling should be performed.

MANAGEMENT OF HEAVY VAGINAL BLEEDING
Overview

Management of heavy vaginal bleeding has a two-fold approach; first, to stop the acute episode of heavy bleeding; and second, to manage subsequent episodes to prevent further heavy bleeding. The two general options for the approach to management of heavy bleeding are medical and surgical. Most often, surgery is not needed.

Deciding on the best treatment option is specific to each patient. Questions to consider include[10]

- How heavy is the bleeding?
- Is the patient hemodynamically stable?

Workup of Heavy Vaginal Bleeding by Age

Adolescents (<18 yo)	Adults (18-40 yo)	Perimenopause (>40 yo)	Postmenopausal
History: medical, surgical, bleeding history	**History:** medical, surgical, bleeding history	**History:** medical, surgical, bleeding history	**History:** medical, surgical, bleeding history
Exam: Defer pelvic examination	**Exam:** Pelvic examination	**Exam:** Pelvic examination	**Exam:** Pelvic examination
Laboratory Evaluation: Pregnancy test, CBC, TSH, prolactin and free testosterone if irregular cycles, STI screening if sexually active, bleeding disorder evaluation	**Laboratory Evaluation:** Pregnancy test, CBC, TSH, prolactin and free testosterone if irregular cycles, STI and cervical cancer screening if due, bleeding disorder evaluation if positive history	**Laboratory Evaluation:** Pregnancy test, CBC, TSH, prolactin if irregular cycles, STI and cervical cancer screening if due, endometrial biopsy (>45 yo or risk factors for hyperplasia/malignancy), bleeding disorder evaluation if positive history	**Laboratory Evaluation:** CBC, cervical cancer screening if due, endometrial biopsy (endometrial thickness >4mm or recurrent bleeding), bleeding disorder evaluation if positive history
Imaging: Consider abdominal ultrasound if diagnosis is uncertain	**Imaging:** TVUS, consider SIS vs office hysteroscopy for endometrial abnormalities	**Imaging:** TVUS, consider SIS vs office hysteroscopy for endometrial abnormalities	**Imaging:** TVUS, consider SIS vs office hysteroscopy for endometrial abnormalities

Fig. 4. Work-up of heavy vaginal bleeding including history, examination, laboratory evaluation, and imaging stratified by age of the patient. STI, sexually transmitted infection.

- Does the patient need to be admitted to the hospital?
- What is the cause for the heavy vaginal bleeding?
- Does the patient have a bleeding disorder?
- What comorbidities does the patient have?
- Are there contraindications to estrogen use?
- What are the patient's future reproductive goals?

Medical Treatment Options

Most medical treatment options include hormonal medications, specifically estrogen or progesterone or a combination of both. The only treatment option approved by the Food and Drug Administration for acute bleeding is IV conjugate equine estrogen. However, there are several other options commonly used.[2,10] The treatment course is considered in three phases:

- Phase 1: acute endometrial stabilization
- Phase 2: hormone taper
- Phase 3: maintenance therapy (**Fig. 5**)

Options for phase 1 are listed in **Table 2**.

IV estrogen is generally recommended when the patient is not tolerating oral intake and/or is hemodynamically unstable. It is important to start a progesterone either in combined pill or alone within 24 to 48 hours of IV estrogen to avoid estrogen withdrawal bleeding from cessation of high-dose IV estrogen.[25] Additionally, monophasic combined pills are used.[2,10,26] In monophasic combined pills, the dosage of estrogen and progesterone is constant, whereas in multiphasic combined pills, the dosage of estrogen and progesterone varies.[27] Progesterone options are preferred for those patients with contraindications to estrogen. The Centers for Disease Control and Prevention's Medical Eligibility Criteria for Contraceptive Use is used to provide a complete list of medical contraindications to estrogen.[28] Generally, patients with high-risk for venous thromboembolism, such as a prior history of venous thromboembolism, hypertension, or migraines with auras, should not receive estrogen therapy. Additionally, high doses of hormones can cause significant nausea and vomiting for patients. Consider administering an antiemetic an hour before prescribing high-dose hormonal medications to help to alleviate this side effect.[2,10]

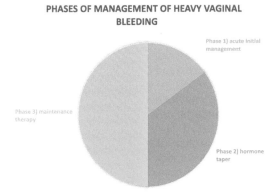

PHASES OF MANAGEMENT OF HEAVY VAGINAL
BLEEDING

Phase 1) acute initial
management

Phase 3) maintenance
therapy

Phase 2) hormone
taper

Fig. 5. The phases of management of heavy vaginal bleeding including acute initial management, hormone taper, and maintenance therapy.

Table 2
Phase 1 hormonal medications for acute initial management

Medication	Dose and Route	Initial Frequency
Estrogen only		
Conjugated equine estrogen[23]	25 mg IV	4–6 h for 24 h
Combination estrogen-progesterone[2,10,24]	30–50 μg of ethinyl estradiol + progesterone orally	6–8 h
Progesterone only		
Medroxyprogesterone acetate[2,10,24]	10–20 mg, maximum of 80 mg/d, orally	4–6 h
Norethindrone acetate[2,24]	5–10 mg orally	4–6 h

A nonhormonal medication option is tranexamic acid, which inhibits fibrinolysis to decrease menstrual bleeding. Patients are prescribed tranexamic acid 10 mg/kg IV (maximum, 600 mg/dose) or 1.3 g orally every 8 hours for up to 5 days.[2,10,24] It can decrease heavy menstrual bleeding by 30% to 55%.[10] Tranexamic acid should not be given to patients with thromboembolism, macroscopic hematuria, or color blindness.[10,24] Furthermore, concomitant use of tranexamic acid with combined oral contraceptive pills is contraindicated according to the Food and Drug Administration prescribing information because of the theoretic risk of thrombosis; however, this combination has still been suggested for those with heavy bleeding who have failed hormonal therapy alone, especially for those with a bleeding disorder, because the overall risk is observed to be low.[2] In reviews of existing literature, Thorne and colleagues[29] stated the beneficial effects of decreased heavy menstrual bleeding for women taking combination oral contraceptives with tranexamic acid for a short course outweigh the potential risks generally, but they caution that women with increased risk of venous thromboembolism, such as immobility, obesity, and coagulopathy, should not use these medications in combination.

Once the acute bleeding has decreased substantially or stopped, phase 2 begins and a hormonal taper is initiated. The goal with a hormonal taper is to slowly decrease the hormonal dose to minimize endometrial withdrawal bleeding, and establish a low-dose hormonal regimen long term to minimize medication side effects and maximize patient compliance. Multiple regimens exist and are effective.[2,10] Some options for phase 2 hormone tapers are listed in **Table 3**. It should be noted that none of these medications have been compared with placebo and limited comparative studies exist to guide recommendations.

Of note, when prescribing a hormonal taper of combination oral contraceptive pills, the placebo pills should be skipped and continuous hormonal medication maintained throughout the taper regimen to decrease the risk of further menstrual bleeding.

After bleeding has stopped and the hormonal taper has been finished, it is time to move into phase 3, maintenance therapy. There are fortunately many options for maintenance therapy as listed in **Box 1**. Given the multiple single-dose options available, specific medication selection is often tailored to minimize patient side effects, improve ease of use, and comply with insurance formularies.

A new medication class, an oral gonadotropin-releasing hormone antagonist, is an option for those with heavy bleeding secondary to leiomyomas.[33] There are two medications on the market, elagolix and relugolix, approved for use by the Food and Drug Administration for up to 24 months. Both medications are prescribed with add-back

Table 3
Phase 2 hormonal taper regimens

Medication	Dose	Taper
Combination estrogen-progesterone	35 μg ethinyl estradiol + progesterone orally[2,10,26]	Every 8 h for 7 d
	30–50 μg of ethinyl estradiol + progesterone orally[9]	Every 8 h for 2 d and up to 7 d Every 12 h for 2 d and up to 7 d Then daily
Progesterone only		
Medroxyprogesterone	10 mg orally[24]	Every 6 h for 4 d Every 8 h for 3 d Every 12 h for 2 d to 2 wk Then daily
	20 mg orally[2,10,26]	Every 8 h for 7 d
Norethindrone acetate	5–10 mg orally[24]	Every 6 h for 4 d Every 8 h for 3 d Every 12 h for 2 d to 2 wk Then daily

therapy, specifically 1 mg of estradiol and 0.5 mg of norethindrone acetate. Elagolix is 300 mg twice daily dosing, whereas relugolix is 40 mg once daily.[30,31] In clinical trials, the change in bone mineral density was not different for women who took placebo and those who took elagolix with add-back therapy.[34] Similarly, with relugolix, bone mineral density was preserved.[35] These medications offer longer-term options than gonadotropin-releasing hormone agonists, which use is limited to 6 months without add-back therapy and 12 months with add-back therapy.[33]

Nonhormonal medication
Nonsteroidal anti-inflammatory medications can also provide a nonhormonal option to reduce menstrual bleeding. A Cochrane review found this medication reduced bleeding more than placebo but was less effective than tranexamic acid or the levonorgestrel intrauterine system.[32]

Box 1
Phase 3 maintenance treatment options

Combination estrogen-progesterone options[2,10]
    Combination estrogen-progesterone pills
    Combination estrogen-progesterone patch
    Combination estrogen-progesterone vaginal ring

Progesterone-only options[2,10]
    Medroxyprogesterone acetate pills
    Medroxyprogesterone acetate depot injection
    Norethindrone acetate pills
    Levonorgestrel intrauterine system

Gonadotropin-releasing hormone antagonist[30,31]

Nonhormonal options[32]
    Nonsteroid anti-inflammatory pills
    Cyclic antifibrinolytics

Surgical Treatment Options

If nonsurgical options fail or if the patient is not a candidate for medical therapy, there are several different surgical options, including[2,10,24]

- Intrauterine balloon tamponade
- Dilation and curettage
- Hysteroscopy with dilation and curettage
- Hysteroscopy with myomectomy or polypectomy
- Uterine artery embolization
- Endometrial ablation
- Hysterectomy

When considering surgical options, a patient's future reproductive goals are of utmost importance. Hysterectomy removes the option for future childbearing. Additionally, pregnancy is contraindicated after endometrial ablation. The safety of pregnancy and fertility after uterine artery embolization is uncertain and therefore is not a first-line treatment of those desiring future childbearing.[10,24]

Intrauterine balloon tamponade
Uterine tamponade can provide control of acute menstrual bleeding. A Foley catheter with a 30-mL balloon is inserted into the vagina, through the cervix, and into the uterine cavity. Cervical dilation is typically not necessary, even in adolescents. The balloon is then inflated until resistance from the myometrium is felt, which can occur after the instillation of 10 mL of normal saline. TVUS is also helpful to guide placement. It is generally recommended for the balloon to be left in place for up to 24 hours, whereas hormonal and nonhormonal medications are continued.[2,10,33]

Dilation and curettage/hysteroscopy
Dilation and curettage (D&C) and hysteroscopy are minimally invasive surgical treatment options to help control menstrual bleeding. D&C alone can provide a means to obtain an endometrial tissue sample for evaluation and a potential temporary improvement in acute bleeding, but the subsequent episode of bleeding will be unchanged and likely heavy again. Because of likely recurrent bleeding in addition to the risks of anesthesia and endometrial scarring, D&C alone is not the first-line treatment of acute bleeding.

However, D&C is performed at the time of hysteroscopy, especially when intracavitary lesion, such as polyp and/or fibroid, is suspected as the cause of chronic bleeding. Hysteroscopy is diagnostic and therapeutic; it is a tool used to directly assess the intrauterine cavity and at the same time, treat and remove any structural lesion that is identified. A levonorgestrel intrauterine system is placed at the same time at these procedures, providing additional long-term hormonal management.[10,24]

Uterine artery embolization
Uterine artery embolization is a procedure performed by interventional radiology. An embolic medication is injected into the uterine artery under fluoroscopic guidance to decrease menstrual bleeding. Uterine artery embolization is most commonly used in patients with heavy vaginal bleeding secondary to uterine fibroids, or as a final, potentially reversible option before needing to proceed with hysterectomy in the setting of acute and severe menstrual bleeding. However, the effect on future reproductive potential is uncertain.[2,10,33]

Endometrial ablation

Endometrial ablation results in destruction of the endometrium to decrease menstrual bleeding. Appropriate patients are premenopausal with heavy bleeding, have a normal uterine cavity, have failed or do not tolerate medical therapy, do not desire pregnancy, and accept a normalization in bleeding but not necessarily amenorrhea. It is crucial to evaluate for malignancy before ablation with endometrial tissue sampling. Pregnancy is contraindicated after endometrial ablation; however, endometrial ablation is not a form of contraception and thus an appropriate method of contraception should be used.[36]

Risks of endometrial ablation include injury to the cervix and vagina, perforation of the uterus with damage to surrounding structures, infection, malignancy, pregnancy with increased risk for abnormal placentation, postablation tubal ligation syndrome, and fluid overload (for resectoscopic ablation only). Postablation tubal ligation syndrome occurs in patients who have had prior or concomitant tubal ligation and results in cyclical pain caused by residual endometrium in the cornua. The incidence of this is approximately 10%.[36]

Overall, there is similar reduction in bleeding and overall patient satisfaction with endometrial ablation as compared with the levonorgestrel-intrauterine system. Additionally, in the 4 years following the endometrial ablation procedure, about one-quarter (24%) of patients go on to have a hysterectomy.[36] Patients more likely to fail treatment with endometrial ablation are younger than age 45, have parity of five or more, had prior tubal ligation, or reported a history of dysmenorrhea.[37]

Hysterectomy

Hysterectomy may ultimately be indicated as definitive treatment of heavy bleeding when other temporary measures have failed or if the patient has completed childbearing.[38]

Route of hysterectomy includes transvaginal, laparoscopic, and abdominal. To determine the best route of hysterectomy, several factors need to be considered, such as the size of the vagina, size and shape of and accessibility to the uterus, adnexal pathology, and surgeon comfort. The American College of Obstetricians and Gynecologists recommends vaginal hysterectomy as the preferred route.[38] Laparoscopic hysterectomy is the second option because it remains minimally invasive. Abdominal hysterectomy may still be needed for certain patients and is a valid option when vaginal and laparoscopic hysterectomy are not feasible.[38]

IMPORTANT ADJUNCTS

Some patients with acute menstrual bleeding may require a blood transfusion, although this is not necessary for all patients. Criteria for blood transfusion include hemodynamic instability, symptomatic anemia, or hemoglobin less than 7 g/dL.[3,39]

Table 4 Iron supplementation options		
	Tablet (mg)	Elemental Iron (mg)
Ferrous sulfate	325	65
Ferrous gluconate	300	38
Ferrous fumarate	324	106

Data from Short MW, Domagalski JE. Iron deficiency anemia: evaluation and management. American family physician. 2013;87(2):98-104.

Many patients develop iron deficiency from heavy menstrual bleeding. A ferritin level reflects iron stores and should be used to assess for iron deficiency. Experts disagree on the specific cutoff for the diagnosis of iron deficiency, ranging from ferritin less than 15 to 30 ng/mL.[40] Prevention and treatment of iron deficiency anemia is an important component in the management of heavy vaginal bleeding. This is accomplished with iron supplementation.[2] The recommended supplementation is 60 to 120 mg per day of iron according to the Centers for Disease Control and Prevention.[41] Ferrous sulfate is most frequently used, but ferrous gluconate and ferrous fumarate are also other options (**Table 4**).[42] Recent research suggests alternate day, single dosing of iron supplementation may improve absorption of iron rather than daily, multiple-dose regimens.[43] After reduction in bleeding, the iron supplementation should be continued for at least 3 months. At that time, ferritin should be rechecked to assess if iron deficiency has resolved.[42]

CLINICS CARE POINTS

- Heavy vaginal bleeding is a common complaint in reproductive-age women.
- Initial evaluation should confirm patient stability.
- In a stable patient, a comprehensive history with a focus on menstrual and bleeding history should be obtained. A physical examination should be performed in all patients, with an internal speculum examination reserved for adults.
- Laboratory evaluation should include a urine pregnancy test, complete blood count, ferritin, and thyroid-stimulating hormone with additional testing as indicated based on the patient's clinical presentation.
- Imaging should include a pelvic ultrasound, except in adolescents, with additional imaging based on the patient's clinical presentation.
- Medical treatment involves acute stabilization with hormonal treatment, hormone taper once symptoms improve, and maintenance treatment to prevent recurrence.
- Surgical treatment is performed for refractory or unstable cases, with the modality depending on the cause of bleeding and the patient's future childbearing plans.

DISCLOSURE

No commercial or financial disclosures.

REFERENCES

1. ACOG Practice Bulletin No. 128: diagnosis of abnormal uterine bleeding in reproductive-aged women. Obstet Gynecol 2012;120(1):197–206.
2. ACOG Committee Opinion No. 785: screening and management of bleeding disorders in adolescents with heavy menstrual bleeding. Obstet Gynecol 2019;134(3):e71–83.
3. Magnay JL, O'Brien S, Gerlinger C, et al. Pictorial methods to assess heavy menstrual bleeding in research and clinical practice: a systematic literature review. BMC Womens health. 2020;20(1):24.
4. Wyatt KM, Dimmock PW, Walker TJ, et al. Determination of total menstrual blood loss. Fertil Steril 2001;76(1):125–31.
5. Toxqui L, Pérez-Granados AM, Blanco-Rojo R, et al. A simple and feasible questionnaire to estimate menstrual blood loss: relationship with hematological and gynecological parameters in young women. BMC Womens Health 2014;14(1):71.

6. Janssen CA, Scholten PC, Heintz AP. A simple visual assessment technique to discriminate between menorrhagia and normal menstrual blood loss. Obstet Gynecol 1995;85(6):977–82.
7. Reid PC, Coker A, Coltart R. Assessment of menstrual blood loss using a pictorial chart: a validation study. BJOG 2000;107(3):320–2.
8. Munro MG, Critchley HOD, Broder MS, et al. FIGO classification system (PALM-COEIN) for causes of abnormal uterine bleeding in nongravid women of reproductive age. Int J Gynecol Obstet 2011;113(1):3–13.
9. ACOG Practice Bulletin No. 136: management of abnormal uterine bleeding associated with ovulatory dysfunction. Obstet Gynecol 2013;122(1):176–85.
10. ACOG Committee Opinion No. 557: management of acute abnormal uterine bleeding in nonpregnant reproductive aged women. Obstet Gynecol 2013; 121(4):891–6.
11. Brady PC, Carusi D. Vaginal hemorrhage. In: Handbook of consult and inpatient gynecology. Springer International Publishing; 2016. p. 31–51.
12. Falotico JM, Shinozaki K, Saeki K, et al. Advances in the approaches using peripheral perfusion for monitoring hemodynamic status. Front Med 2020;7.
13. Evans L, Rhodes A, Alhazzani W, et al. Surviving Sepsis Campaign: international guidelines for management of sepsis and septic shock 2021. Crit Care Med 2021;49(11):e1063–143.
14. Kouides PA, Conard J, Peyvandi F, Lukes A, Kadir R. Hemostasis and menstruation: appropriate investigation for underlying disorders of hemostasis in women with excessive menstrual bleeding. Fertil Steril. 2005 Nov;84(5):1345-51. doi: 10. 1016/j.fertnstert.2005.05.035. PMID: 16275228.
15. Borzutzky C, Jaffray J. Diagnosis and management of heavy menstrual bleeding and bleeding disorders in adolescents. JAMA Pediatr 2020;174(2):186.
16. Cowan BD, Morrison JC. Management of abnormal genital bleeding in girls and women. New Engl J Med 1991;324(24):1710–5.
17. Bennett GL, Andreotti RF, Lee SI, et al. ACR Appropriateness Criteria on abnormal vaginal bleeding. J Am Coll Radiol 2011;8(7):460–8.
18. Williams PL, Laifer-Narin SL, Ragavendra N. US of abnormal uterine bleeding. Radiographics 2003;23(3):703–18.
19. Bingol B, Gunenc Z, Gedikbasi A, et al. Comparison of diagnostic accuracy of saline infusion sonohysterography, transvaginal sonography and hysteroscopy. J Obstet Gynaecol 2011;31(1):54–8.
20. Mahewux-Lacroix S, Li F, Laberge P, et al. Imaging for polyps and leiomyomas in women with abnormal uterine bleeding: a systematic review. Obstet Gynecol 2016;128:1425–36.
21. Van Den Bosch T, Verguts J, Daemen A, et al. Pain experienced during transvaginal ultrasound, saline contrast sonohysterography, hysteroscopy and office sampling: a comparative study. Ultrasound Obstet Gynecol 2008;31(3):346–51.
22. Hubert J, Bergin D. Imaging the female pelvis: when should MRI be considered? J Pract Med Imag Management 2011;37(1):9–22.
23. DeVore GR, Owens O, Kase N. Use of intravenous Premarin in the treatment of dysfunctional uterine bleeding: a double-blind randomized control study. Obstet Gynecol 1982;59(3):285–91.
24. James AH, Kouides PA, Abdul-Kadir R, et al. Evaluation and management of acute menorrhagia in women with and without underlying bleeding disorders: consensus from an international expert panel. Eur J Obstet Gynecol Reprod Biol 2011;158(2):124–34.

25. Emans SJ, Laufer M, DiVasta A. Abnormal vaginal bleeding in the adolescent. In: Emans, Laufer, editors. Goldstein's pediatric and adolescent Gynecology. 6th edition. Lippincot Williams and Wilkins; 2011. p. 159–67.

26. Munro MG, Mainor N, Basu R, et al. Oral medroxyprogesterone acetate and combination oral contraceptives for acute uterine bleeding. Obstet Gynecol 2006; 108(4):924–9.

27. Speroff L, Darney P. Oral contraception. In: Clinical guide for contraception. 5th edition. Lippincott Williams & Wilkins; 2010. p. 19–152.

28. Curtis KM, Tepper NK, Jatlaoui TC, et al. U.S. medical eligibility criteria for contraceptive use, 2016. MMWR Recomm Rep 2016;65(3):1–103.

29. Thorne J, James P, Reid R. Heavy menstrual bleeding: is tranexamic acid a safe adjunct to combined hormonal contraception? Contraception 2018;98(1):1–3.

30. AbbVie Inc. Oriahnn (elagolix, estradiol, and norethindrone capsules) [package insert]. U.S Food and Drug Administration website. 2020. Available at: https://www.accessdata.fda.gov/drugsatfda_docs/label/2020/213388s000lbl.pdf. Accessed January 11, 2022.

31. Pantheon Inc. Myfembree (relugolix, estradiol, and norethindrone acetate). U.S. Federal Drug Administration website. 2021. Available at: https://www.accessdata.fda.gov/drugsatfda_docs/label/2021/214846s000lbl.pdf. Accessed January 11, 2022.

32. Bofill Rodriguez M, Lethaby A, Farquhar C. Non-steroidal anti-inflammatory drugs for heavy menstrual bleeding. Cochrane database Syst Rev 2019;9:CD000400.

33. ACOG Practice Bulletin No. 228: management of symptomatic uterine leiomyomas. Obstet Gynecol 2021;137(6):e100–15.

34. Schlaff WD, Ackerman RT, Al-Hendy A, et al. Elagolix for heavy menstrual bleeding in women with uterine fibroids. New Engl J Med 2020;382(4):328–40.

35. Al-Hendy A, Lukes AS, Poindexter AN, et al. Treatment of uterine fibroid symptoms with relugolix combination therapy. N Engl J Med 2021;384(7):630–42.

36. ACOG Practice Bulletin No. 81: endometrial ablation. Obstet Gynecol 2007; 109(5):1233–48.

37. El-Nashar SA, Hopkins MR, Creedon DJ, et al. Prediction of treatment outcomes after global endometrial ablation. Obstet Gynecol 2009;113(1):97–106.

38. ACOG Committee Opinion No. 701: choosing the route of hysterectomy for benign disease. Obstet Gynecol 2017;129(6):155–9.

39. Napolitano LM, Kurek S, Luchette FA, et al. Clinical practice guideline: red blood cell transfusion in adult trauma and critical care. Crit Care Med 2009;37(12): 3124–57.

40. Short MW, Domagalski JE. Iron deficiency anemia: evaluation and management. Am Fam Physician 2013;87(2):98–104.

41. Recommendations to prevent and control iron deficiency in the United States. Centers for Disease Control and Prevention. MMWR Recomm Rep 1998; 47(RR-3):1–29.

42. Powers JM, Buchanan GR. Diagnosis and management of iron deficiency anemia. Hematol Oncol Clin North Am 2014;28(4):729–45.

43. Stoffel NU, Cercamondi CI, Brittenham G, et al. Iron absorption from oral iron supplements given on consecutive versus alternate days and as single morning doses versus twice-daily split dosing in iron-depleted women: two open-label, randomised controlled trials. Lancet Haematol 2017;4(11):524–33.

Bleeding from Gynecologic Malignancies

Megan L. Hutchcraft, MD*, Rachel W. Miller, MD

KEYWORDS

- Vaginal hemorrhage • Gynecologic malignancy • Vaginal bleeding
- Gynecologic oncology emergencies

KEY POINTS

- Bleeding in gynecologic malignancy is common, and the best treatment modality depends on site of disease and current disease status.
- Early discussion of patient goals of care is imperative to providing optimal and individualized patient-centered care.
- Following hemodynamic stabilization, patients should be managed as inpatients at a facility with available radiation, intensive care, and gynecologic oncology services.
- Vaginal bleeding in gynecologic malignancy may be treated surgically, medically, with radiation, or with interventional radiology services.

INTRODUCTION

Vaginal bleeding is a common presenting symptom of several gynecologic malignancies. Postmenopausal vaginal bleeding occurs in 90% of women diagnosed with endometrial cancer.[1] The incidence of vaginal bleeding in cervical cancer ranges from 0.7% to 100%, and it is responsible for death in 6% of women with the disease.[2] Similarly, 80% to 90% of patients with gestational trophoblastic disease present with vaginal bleeding in the setting of current or recent pregnancy.[3] Although abnormal vaginal bleeding may occur with other gynecologic cancers, bleeding is less common. Acute vaginal hemorrhage may be seen in advanced disease secondary to tumoral angiogenesis, local tumor invasion, or systemic effects related to the disease or cancer treatments.[4] Additionally, bleeding in gynecologic malignancies can be exacerbated by medications that cancer patients frequently are prescribed, including anticoagulants and nonsteroidal anti-inflammatory drugs.

PATIENT EVALUATION

Standard work-up of vaginal hemorrhage in the setting of gynecologic malignancy begins with a thorough history and physical examination (**Table 1**). A detailed history

Division of Gynecologic Oncology, Department of Obstetrics and Gynecology, University of Kentucky Markey Cancer Center, 800 Rose Street, Lexington, KY 40536, USA
* Corresponding author.
E-mail address: megan.hutchcraft@uky.edu

Obstet Gynecol Clin N Am 49 (2022) 607–622
https://doi.org/10.1016/j.ogc.2022.02.022
0889-8545/22/© 2022 Elsevier Inc. All rights reserved.

obgyn.theclinics.com

Table 1	
Approach to the work-up of bleeding in gynecologic malignancy	
History	Thorough medication history, including the use of herbs and supplements
	Disease history
	Current/prior cancer treatment
	Comorbid conditions
Physical examination	Overall assessment
	Vital signs
	Skin examination
	Lymph node evaluation
	Cardiovascular examination
	Pulmonary examination
	Abdominal examination
	External and internal pelvic examination
	Lower extremity examination
Laboratory evaluation	Type and screen
	Complete blood cell count with differential
	Complete metabolic profile
	Prothrombin time, international normalized ratio
	Partial thromboplastin time
	Fibrinogen
	Lactate dehydrogenase [a]
	Cardiac troponins [a]
	hCG quantitative level [a]
Radiographic evaluation	Computerized tomography of chest, abdomen, and pelvis with contrast
	Transvaginal ultrasound [a]
	Echocardiogram [a]
Other	ECG [a]

Components of each aspect of the work-up should be performed for all patients, unless specified.
[a] Useful in select situations.

reveals the primary disease site and treatment history in patients previously diagnosed with malignancy; however, in patients without prior diagnosis, risk factors may suggest the primary disease site. Bleeding may be a symptom of recurrent or metastatic disease, in which case the patient's goals of care should be considered to ensure treatment aligns accordingly. The history may identify contributory factors, such as medications contributing to coagulopathy (eg, anticoagulants, nonsteroidal anti-inflammatory drugs, and herbs/supplements), cancer treatment agents (eg, anti-angiogenic anticancer agents), adverse effects of antineoplastic agents (eg, thrombocytopenia from systemic or radiation therapy), or comorbid conditions (eg, hepatic dysfunction). Consideration should be given to how the treatment may have an impact on a patient's quality of life, because some treatments may be highly invasive and undesirable for a patient who desires comfort measures only.

Physical examination should begin with an overall assessment to determine hemodynamic stability. Vital signs may indicate the presence of compensated or decompensated hypovolemic shock, including severe hypotension and tachycardia. Other systemic findings may be present in the setting of acute anemia: a skin evaluation may identify pallor, or a cardiovascular examination may reveal signs of underlying heart failure, including tachycardia or a systolic murmur.[5,6]

In the setting of a hemodynamically stable patient, attention should be given to a thorough examination of disease status. This includes a lymph node evaluation—in particular, supraclavicular and inguinal lymph nodes, because those are common sites of metastases for cervical, vaginal, and vulvar cancers. A pulmonary examination may identify pleural effusions or the presence of metastases. An abdominal examination may be unremarkable or may identify a pelvic mass or ascites in the setting of more advanced malignancies. A pelvic examination, including speculum, bimanual, and rectovaginal examinations, may reveal the origin of bleeding, which may help with treatment decision making. Finally, evaluation of the lower extremities is critical because patients with advanced pelvic malignancies often are diagnosed concurrently with venous thromboembolic disease.

Although etiology of hemorrhage may be gleaned from physical examination, laboratory evaluation may be beneficial to determine the presence of coagulopathy, need for volume or blood product resuscitation, and identification of systemic sequelae of acute hypovolemic shock. A biopsy for tissue diagnosis should be obtained if primary disease site has not yet been established, because this drives treatment decision making. Human chorionic gonadotropin (hCG) quantitative level also should be obtained in patients bleeding from gestational trophoblastic disease. Comprehensive radiographic imaging may demonstrate origin of bleeding and allows assessment of a patient's disease status. Although pelvic ultrasonography can identify abnormalities in the gynecologic organs contributing to vaginal bleeding, computerized tomography of the chest, abdomen, and pelvis, with contrast, if renal function permits, is preferable.

In patients with hemodynamic compromise, initial stabilization is imperative (**Fig. 1**). Obtaining vascular access and early communication of anticipated needs from the blood bank are critical early interventions. Concurrently, obtaining samples for a blood typing and cross matching, complete blood cell count, and coagulation profile may identify need for additional blood products. Initial stabilization includes discontinuing contributing factors, correction of coagulopathy, and hemodynamic support, including blood pressure support. Once medically stable, patients with acute vaginal bleeding from gynecologic malignancy should be transferred to a center with intensive care, gynecologic oncology, and radiation oncology services.

Following hemodynamic stabilization, serial laboratory evaluation can identify the need for additional fluid and blood product resuscitation as well as sequelae of acute

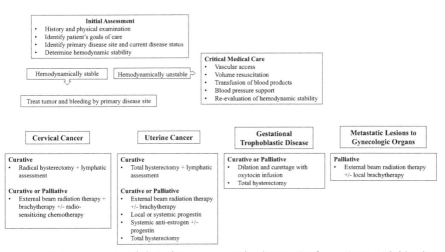

Fig. 1. Initial assessment and clinical management by disease site for patients with bleeding from gynecologic malignancies.

hypovolemia, including ischemic kidney or liver injuries. Acute kidney injuries can be identified from elevated blood urea nitrogen (BUN) and creatinine values. A BUN:creatinine ratio and functional excretion of sodium may identify prerenal azotemia or intrinsic renal disease related to acute tubular necrosis. Ischemic hepatitis, also known as shock liver or hypoxic hepatitis, can occur in the setting of hypovolemic shock. Laboratory findings include elevated alanine aminotransferase (ALT), aspartate transaminase (AST), and lactate dehydrogenase (LDH). Finally, some patients may develop cardiac demand ischemia, resulting in elevated serum troponins and electrocardiogram (ECG) changes. Demand ischemia may occur in the setting of acute hypovolemia and anemia when the myocardial oxygen demand exceeds its available supply in the absence of coronary thrombosis.[7] A type 2 myocardial infarction occurs when there is a mismatch in supply and demand, resulting in myocardial ischemia, elevated serum troponins, ischemic ECG changes, and cardiac imaging abnormalities suggestive of ischemia.[7]

CLINICAL MANAGEMENT

For most patients with vaginal hemorrhage related to gynecologic cancer, the primary goal is to ensure hemodynamic stability. Stabilization may include obtaining vascular access, supporting the patient with fluids or blood products, and discontinuing offending agents. Additional management strategies are aimed at treating the underlying cause and are dependent on the primary site of disease. Treatment strategies may include surgery, medical management with systemic or local therapies, and/or the use of radiation therapy. Although one therapy may provide adequate treatment of bleeding, many patients require multimodal therapy.

Medical Treatment Options

Systemic medical management targeting the hematologic system may improve bleeding in gynecologic malignancy, especially in the setting of coagulopathy or anticoagulation (**Table 2**). Although originally developed for use in trauma patients,[8] mass transfusion protocols may be used in patients with significant blood loss, including malignancy-related hemorrhage,[9] when aggressive measures are required. Mass transfusion protocols vary by institution but historically include transfusion of greater than 10 U of packed red blood cells,[10] often in a 1:1:1 ratio with platelets and fresh frozen plasma.[11]

Guidelines are available that summarize appropriate use of nonmassive transfusion of individual blood products, which may be used to correct coagulopathy or obtain hemodynamic stability.[10,12,13] In general, patients with hemoglobin under 7 g/dL without underlying cardiovascular disease require transfusion of packed red blood cells.[13] Patients with cardiovascular disease[13] or patients actively receiving external beam radiation therapy[14] also should be transfused if hemoglobin values remain under 8 g/dL. Similarly, patients with symptomatic anemia (eg, tachycardia, fatigue, near syncope, or syncope) also are candidates for red blood cell transfusion.[13] Transfusion of red blood cells also may be used in advanced cancer patients for control of anemia-related symptoms in the palliative setting.[15] Platelet transfusion should be considered in patients with thrombocytopenia when values are less than 10,000 cells/μL, due to the risk of spontaneous bleeding, or less than 50,000 cells/μL in patients undergoing surgical procedures.[12] Transfusion of fresh frozen plasma is indicated in the setting of mass transfusion and may be considered in patients requiring rapid reversal of warfarin with acute life-threatening bleeding.[10]

Gynecologic cancer patients often are prescribed anticoagulants for prevention or treatment of thromboembolic disease.[16] For patients taking these drugs,

Table 2 General pharmacologic management of bleeding in gynecologic malignancy	
Anticoagulant reversal	Vitamin K (reverses warfarin) Idarucizumab (reverses dabigatran) Andexanet alfa (reverses factor Xa inhibitors) Protamine sulfate (reverses unfractionated and low-molecular-weight heparins)
Systemic hemostatic agents	Tranexamic acid
Topical hemostatic agents	Porcine gelatin ± thrombin Bovine collagen, thrombin Oxidized regenerated cellulose Polysaccharide spheres Pooled/individual human plasma Fibrin sealant
Local hemostatic agents	Monsel ferric subsulfate solution Mohs zinc chloride paste Silver nitrate Formalin Kaolin-impregnated gauze
Progestins	Levonorgestrel intrauterine device Megestrol acetate Medroxyprogesterone acetate
Antiestrogens	Aromatase inhibitor Fulvestrant Tamoxifen + progestin

discontinuation of the offending agent and supportive measures usually are required in the setting of major bleeding.[17] Although specific reversal agents exist for direct thrombin and factor Xa inhibitors, their use should be reserved for life-threatening bleeding and when there is a high index of suspicion that the anticoagulant in question is contributing to the bleeding.[17] In the setting of dabigatran-associated major bleeding, idarucizumab, a humanized monoclonal anti-dabigatran antibody fragment, may be administered intravenously. In the setting of factor Xa inhibitor–associated major bleeding, andexanet alfa (modified recombinant factor Xa) may be used intravenously on-label, for rivaroxaban- or apixaban-associated bleeding, or off-label, for patients taking edoxaban or betrixaban.[17] When specific reversal agents are not available, activated or inactive prothrombin complex concentrate, which contains factors II, IX, and X and occasionally factor VII, may be used either in a weight-based or fixed dosing for patients bleeding from direct oral anticoagulants.[17]

Similarly, administration of vitamin K may be used in patients anticoagulated with vitamin K antagonist therapy; however, fresh frozen plasma may be indicated for patients requiring more rapid reversal than can be obtained using vitamin K.[10] Patients anticoagulated with heparin or low-molecular-weight heparin also may require reversal; however, the half-life of these drugs is shorter than that of their oral counterparts, and discontinuation of the drug often is adequate.[18] Protamine sulfate completely neutralizes unfractionated heparin; however, it neutralizes low-molecular-weight heparin only partially. This drug is administered via slow intravenous infusion; rapid infusion is associated with hypotension and anaphylactoid reactions.[19] Dosing is determined based on time of last dose and the most recent heparin dose.[19] Care should be taken in patients with fish allergies, because the protamine protein is derived from fish sperm.[19]

Tranexamic acid, an antifibrinolytic drug, decreases acute vaginal bleeding in benign conditions[20,21] and the risk of death in trauma-related bleeding[22]; currently, it is under investigation for treatment of acute bleeding from gastrointestinal malignancies.[23] Although its use has been studied inadequately in gynecologic malignancies,[2] its use may be considered when no other effective treatment options are available. In the setting of hemorrhage, tranexamic acid is administered intravenously. This medication forms a reversible complex that displaces plasminogen and fibrin, inhibiting fibrinolysis. It also reduces plasmin's proteolytic activity.[24] This medication may not be efficacious for patients who are pharmacologically anticoagulated, because the mechanism of action of heparins, factor Xa inhibitors, direct thrombin inhibitors, and vitamin K antagonists all function proximal to the production of fibrin clots. In this scenario, it may be more efficacious to consider anticoagulation reversal.

Although most episodes of acute kidney injury, shock liver, and cardiac demand ischemia related to acute anemia and hypovolemia improve with treatment of the underlying disorder, additional management considerations may be necessary. The goal of resuscitation includes restoring adequate perfusion to these organs, which requires adequate cardiac output. Although transfusion of blood products and intravenous fluid administration may be adequate, occasionally vasopressor support and critical care treatment are needed. Supportive care, avoidance of additional exacerbation, and treatment of the underlying hypovolemia usually are sufficient treatment of these sequelae, which often are self-limited. In severe cases, significant injury may occur, and involvement of specialized teams, including nephrology, hepatology, and cardiology, may be necessary.

Avoidance of prolonged hypotension is necessary to avoid progression of a prerenal insult to acute tubular necrosis. In these cases, it is critical that nephrotoxins are avoided and medications are dosed renally. Similarly, serum ALT, AST, and LDH rise dramatically within the first 3 days after ischemic insult to the liver; however, once adequate perfusion is obtained, gradual return to normal values occurs within 10 days.[25] Avoidance of additional hepatic insults is necessary. Although synthesis of hepatic proteins is compromised infrequently, patients with shock liver may require continued monitoring of coagulation profiles because the prothrombin time and international normalized ratio also may be impaired.[25,26] In the setting of demand cardiac ischemia, treatment of underlying hypovolemia and anemia is critical; however, additional measures to avoid cardiac injury are necessary and include careful control of heart rate and blood pressure. Type 2 myocardial infarction may occur in patients with underlying coronary artery disease, and, in some situations, coronary artery assessment (eg, coronary angiography and cardiac catheterization) may be indicated. In patients with coronary artery disease, standard risk reduction strategies (eg, aspirin, statin) are indicated; however, there is uncertain benefit in patients without coronary artery disease.[7]

Uterine Cancer: Surgical/Interventional Treatment Options

Surgical management is the mainstay of treatment of most uterine cancers. In patients with acutely bleeding uterine cancer, surgical management of disease by a gynecologic oncologist is preferred because data indicate patients with uterine cancer experience improved survival outcomes when treated by high-volume gynecologic oncologists at cancer centers.[27,28] In cases suitable for primary surgery, management includes total hysterectomy, bilateral salpingo-oophorectomy, and lymph node assessment, which includes sentinel lymphadenectomy or selective pelvic lymphadenectomy with or without para-aortic lymphadenectomy.[29] Although surgical management of clinically early-stage uterine cancer may be performed safely via laparotomy or via minimally invasive techniques with no impact on survival,[30,31] acute vaginal hemorrhage may dictate the fastest approach, which may vary by surgeon.

In cases that are not suitable for primary surgical therapy, management may include external beam radiation therapy with or without radiation-sensitizing chemotherapy and/or vaginal brachytherapy.[29] Radiation therapy decreases vaginal bleeding and may be delivered in the inpatient setting for hemostasis. This therapy often provides hemostasis within 24 hours to 48 hours and may be delivered at various dosages and fractionation schedules, ranging from 5 Gy to 45 Gy over the course of 1 to 18 fractions.[32–35] Scheduling and dosing for hemostatic purposes differ from standard treatment doses, which generally range from 45 Gy to 50 Gy over 25 to 28 fractions for neoadjuvant and adjuvant radiotherapy.[29]

Uterine Cancer: Medical Treatment Options

Progesterone opposes estrogen-driven endometrial hyperplasia and adenocarcinoma[36] and may be used as medical management of endometrial cancer for patients who are not surgical candidates or who desire attempts at fertility-sparing treatment. A fertility-sparing approach to treatment of endometrial cancer requires patients to have grade one disease or demonstrate positive estrogen receptor status on immunohistochemical testing, have disease with minimal or no myometrial invasion, and have no evidence of metastatic disease.[29] Progestational agents that could be used in this setting include megestrol acetate, levonorgestrel intrauterine device, or high-dose medroxyprogesterone acetate.[29] Alternative antiestrogen therapies may include aromatase inhibitors and fulvestrant or tamoxifen alternating with a progestin.[29] Although not standard of care, these medications may be used for the acute treatment of vaginal bleeding from endometrial cancer because a temporizing measure until definitive treatment is possible.

Patient selection is an important component in fertility-sparing hormonal treatment of uterine cancer. Patients must understand that hormonal therapy may not provide definitive treatment but that it may be appropriate in selective circumstances for a period of time. This approach requires serial endometrial sampling every 3 months to 6 months, and consideration of definitive surgical management if disease clearance does not occur within 6 months to 12 months.[29] Patients who respond to hormonal treatment usually respond within 6 months; however, approximately half of patients have persistent disease despite this approach.[37]

Cervical Cancer: Surgical/Interventional Treatment Options

Patients presenting with acute bleeding from cervical cancer or other gynecologic tumors involving the cervix often are not candidates for primary surgical therapy because most cervical cancers presenting in this fashion are a more advanced stage[2] and are treated with definitive chemoradiation therapy.[38] Similar to uterine cancer, hemostatic radiation treatments may be administered to patients with bleeding cervical cancer[2,34,35] prior to definitive treatment, which includes external beam radiation therapy with concurrent radio-sensitizing chemotherapy, followed by vaginal brachytherapy.[38]

Although most patients who present with vaginal hemorrhage from cervical cancer are not candidates for primary surgical therapy, patients with early-stage (eg, IA1, with lymphovascular space invasion–IIA) cervical cancer may be treated with radical hysterectomy, which involves removal of the uterus, cervix, parametrial tissue, and upper portion of the vagina[39,40] and pelvic lymphadenectomy with or without para-aortic lymphadenectomy,[38] which is performed via laparotomy.[41]

Cervical Cancer: Medical Treatment Options

Because few community medical centers have readily available radiation services, interim management of acute bleeding from cancers involving the uterine cervix may require tamponade and the use of topical hemostatic agents for initial patient stabilization, with subsequent transfer to a capable facility. Tamponade of the cervix may be performed using vaginal gauze packing or a balloon tamponade device.[42] Vaginal packing could be soaked in formalin[43] and used with Mohs zinc chloride paste,[44] Monsel ferric subsulfate solution,[45] or topical hemostatic agents used in the surgical setting (eg, oxidized regenerated cellulose, topical thrombin, and fibrin sealants).[46] Vaginal packing with kaolin-impregnated gauze also is an option.[47] In the event of an isolated bleeding mucosal lesion, chemical cautery with silver nitrate also may provide hemostasis.[48]

Gestational Trophoblastic Disease: Combination Therapies

Patients with hydatidiform mole often present with vaginal bleeding and should be managed primarily with dilation and suction curettage. When possible, this procedure should be performed with a 12-mm to 14-mm suction curette and under ultrasound guidance to ensure complete evacuation of the uterus.[49] Importantly, these patients are at increased risk of continued hemorrhage after evacuation, and, although administration of intravenous oxytocin during and after this procedure aids the uterus in contraction and minimizes blood loss,[49–51] empiric use prior to complete evacuation remains controversial due to the theoretic risk of tumor embolization.[52] Initiation of oxytocin infusion at the time of anesthesia induction or upon start of cervical dilation is recommended because many anesthetics induce uterine relaxation. Although no standard rate for oxytocin infusion has been determined, 10 U to 20 U of oxytocin should be admixed with 1 L of crystalloid fluid and infused to achieve uterine contraction.[53,54] A starting dose of 25 mU/min has been suggested.[54] Uterine fundal massage should be performed at time of uterine evacuation to aid in myometrial contraction.[54] Although this option usually is sufficient for treatment of molar pregnancies or bleeding gestational trophoblastic disease, occasionally, urgent hysterectomy, uterine artery embolization, or ligation is necessary.[55]

For patients who do not desire fertility-sparing management or whose hemodynamic status dictates more aggressive management, hysterectomy may be indicated.[55] Hysterectomy may be performed safely via laparotomy or laparoscopy; however, uterine size and other technical issues may dictate the optimal approach.[56,57] Consultation with a gynecologic oncologist in this situation is recommended. Although this procedure often is effective in controlling acute vaginal hemorrhage, it does not eliminate the possibility of metastatic disease and should be performed only for women at high risk of persistent disease or in those in whom bleeding cannot be controlled with less invasive techniques.[50,58]

Patients who present with vaginal bleeding in the setting of persistent gestational trophoblastic disease or postmolar gestational trophoblastic neoplasia may be managed with repeat suction dilation and curettage. Although this procedure often is effective in controlling bleeding,[59] it is curative for only approximately 40% of patients with nonmetastatic, low-risk disease (World Health Organization score 0–4).[59]

In addition to standard patient preparation and work-up, additional considerations are important for this unique disease. Identification and treatment of disease-related complications include preeclampsia and thyroid storm. Because RhD antigen is expressed in trophoblasts, determination of patient Rh status and concurrent administration of Rh immunoglobulin to those with Rh-negative blood type prevents isoimmunization. Preoperative measurement of hCG aids in disease risk stratification.[50,58]

TREATMENT RESISTANCE AND COMPLICATIONS

In cases that are refractory to radiation or medical management and not amenable to surgical management, interventional radiology procedures may be used to embolize a bleeding vessel. Uterine artery embolization often is used to decrease bleeding from symptomatic uterine fibroids or preoperatively to decrease complications of hysterectomy for uterine fibroids. Although it does not treat the underlying cancer, arterial embolization of the uterine or internal iliac artery also may be a palliative option to control vaginal hemorrhage related to malignancy.[60,61] This procedure places an embolic agent (eg, gelatin sponge, polyvinyl alcohol beads, or coils) through an arterial catheter into the femoral artery and guides it into the bleeding vessel using real-time computerized tomography.[62] This procedure may be used prior to or concurrent to cancer radiotherapy or at the end of life in the palliative setting.

Although interventional radiology provides an effective and minimally invasive approach to control of acute bleeding in cancer patients, postembolization syndrome is common and includes pain, fever, nausea, and vomiting for up to 3 days following the procedure.[63] For premenopausal patients undergoing hormonal-sparing cancer treatment, uterine or internal iliac arterial embolization also may compromise ovarian function [ARTHUR 2014 [1]]; however, this is of minimal functional consequence in postmenopausal patients or those who have oophorectomy as a component of their cancer care. Although there are reports of patients who have undergone successful embolization of pelvic vessels who currently were receiving or later received radiation therapy for gynecologic cancers, oncologic outcomes for these patients remain unknown.[60,61,64] The use of vascular embolization theoretically could alter the efficacy of radiation because local hypoxia results in resistance to radiation treatment, so this approach should remain a last resort in patients undergoing active radiation treatment or who are scheduled to start radiation treatment in the future.

When interventional radiology services are unavailable, surgical ligation of the uterine or internal iliac artery may be indicated. The decision for surgical intervention should consider a patient's overall disease status and life expectancy because surgical intervention may be inappropriate for patients with limited life expectancies.[2,4,65]

NEW DEVELOPMENTS

A wide variety of topical hemostatic agents are available and increasingly used in surgery; current estimates suggest that more than one-third of patients undergoing major surgery receive a hemostatic agent.[66] These agents may provide mechanical tamponade, clotting factors to produce a fibrin clot, or both. Although these agents are approved for use in surgery, their use is not limited to the operating room and could be used to address friable vaginal, vulvar, or cervical lesions and may be used in combination with vaginal packing.

Although the increase in use of topical hemostatic agents has coincided with an overall decrease in need for perioperative transfusion,[66] they are not without risk. The most commonly reported risk of their use is the demonstration of postoperative abscess[67] — or mimicry of abscess on imaging.[68] In fact, their use is contraindicated in the setting of a known infection. Consideration of the origin of the topical hemostatic is important and should be considered for individualized treatment. Prior to their use, a discussion of allergies and ethical beliefs is required because some of these procoagulant agents are derived from bovine, porcine, or human tissue.[69] Additional consideration should be given to agents containing bovine thrombin, because these may stimulate a strong immunologic response, which can lead to coagulopathy and death. Patients also should be informed about receipt of agents containing human thrombin because these are not without infectious risk (eg, human immunodeficiency virus and hepatitis viruses).

SPECIAL CONSIDERATIONS
Nongynecologic Metastatic Cancers

Although most cancers presenting with vaginal or uterine bleeding are gynecologic in origin, several other disease sites may metastasize to the gynecologic organs and present with vaginal bleeding. Tumors that commonly metastasize to the gynecologic tract may present with similar symptoms to gynecologic malignancies, including acute vaginal bleeding. Abnormal uterine bleeding has been associated with Krukenberg tumors arising from intestinal malignancies,[70] vaginal metastases of renal cell carcinoma,[71] and cervical metastases from breast cancers.[72] Vaginal hemorrhage also has been described in vaginal lymphoma.[73] In general, patient evaluation and initial supportive measures are the same as for suspected primary gynecologic malignancy; however, these examples stress the importance of obtaining a tissue diagnosis to provide the appropriate definitive treatment.

Prior Radiation Treatment

Patients who previously have been treated with external beam radiation therapy often are not candidates for retreatment due to risk of toxicity to adjacent organs at risk (eg, rectum and bladder). The decision for retreatment in a previously irradiated field must consider a patient's life expectancy. For example, patients at the end of life may benefit from retreatment for palliative bleeding control because they may not survive to experience radiation toxicities; however, those with longer life expectancies may experience excess toxicity, and alternative treatment options should be considered.[65]

Records should be obtained from prior radiation treatments because these describe the previously irradiated field and the approximate dose each organ received, which helps radiation oncologists determine the feasibility and safety of retreatment. Although some patients may be offered secondary external beam radiation therapy, dosing and fractionation options are more limited. Retreatment usually is limited to a single site of persistent disease, which may be delivered using stereotactic body radiation therapy, which delivers a high dose of external beam radiation in 5 or fewer fractions.[74] A bleeding vaginal lesion could be treated similarly with lesion-directed brachytherapy; however, the invasiveness of this approach may outweigh its utility in a purely palliative setting. In patients with longer life expectancy, lesion-directed brachytherapy may be beneficial; however, patients with prior radiation experience lower rates of disease control than patients who are radiation naïve.[75]

Refusal of Blood Products

Some patients may decline transfusion of blood products for personal, religious, or ethical reasons. In acute hemorrhage settings, this presents an additional layer of complexity. The best way to approach patients who decline blood transfusion is to treat bleeding aggressively, be respectful of the patient's wishes, and discuss acceptable treatments with patients as early as possible.[76] Several options to treat bleeding aggressively include the use of hemostatic agents, including tranexamic acid, recombinant coagulation factors, and topical hemostatic agents.[76] Some patients may be amenable to the use of autologous blood cell salvage; however, this treatment is not universally acceptable to all patients who decline blood products.[76] Although hemostatic agents may be used to prevent the need for transfusion of blood products, it is important to discuss which specific hemostatic agents to which patients are agreeable because some hemostatic agents are derived from human blood products.[69]

If there is time to prepare for a procedure that may coincide with a risk for bleeding, preoperative medications may be used to boost the hemoglobin and hematocrit levels. Most patients who decline blood products often are amenable to the use of intravenous iron, which can be administered for patients with iron deficiency anemia. Patients who receive intravenous iron often experience a rise in hemoglobin value by 2 g/dL 3 weeks following treatment.[77] Some perioperative bloodless surgery protocols include the use of erythropoietin,[78] which requires adequate stores of iron, vitamin B_{12}, and folate.[79] This medication should be used with extreme caution in the setting of cancer because erythropoiesis-stimulating agents have been demonstrated to shorten overall survival and may increase the risk of tumor progression in some cancer patients.[79]

End of Life

In patients with bleeding from malignancy at the end of life, treatment goals are aimed at addressing the symptoms that are most bothersome to the patient and her family. A direct conversation with the patient and her family helps identify the symptoms that are most distressing. Early consultation with palliative care and hospice teams may help guide these discussions. Vaginal bleeding at the end of life can be disturbing, and supportive measures may be simple and include discontinuation of exacerbating medications and vaginal packing or may include procedures, such as interventional radiology embolization or radiation treatments. Patients also may experience symptoms related to anemia resulting from heavy bleeding, which can be supported with oxygen supplementation or position changes.

SUMMARY

Bleeding is a common complaint in women with gynecologic malignancies and may occur at any stage in a patient's cancer journey. Similar approaches to bleeding from trauma or after surgery should be employed, including assurance of hemodynamic stability and avoidance of exacerbating agents. Important considerations from bleeding related to cancer is a careful determination of disease status to determine optimal approach to bleeding and a discussion of goals of care to ensure a patient-focused treatment plan.

CLINICS CARE POINTS

- Vaginal bleeding is common in gynecologic malignancy.
- A detailed history and physical examination guide patient-centered treatments that align with patient goals of care and site and extent of disease.
- Patients with heavy bleeding require discontinuation of anticoagulants and may require transfusion of blood products, critical care services, and supportive care for treatment of sequelae of hemorrhagic shock.
- Bleeding from uterine cancer is treated primarily with total hysterectomy; however, some patients may be treated with radiation or antiestrogen therapy.
- Bleeding from cervical cancer frequently is treated with chemoradiation; however, early-stage disease may be treated surgically via radical abdominal hysterectomy.
- Bleeding from gestational trophoblastic disease generally is treated surgically with dilation and curettage; however, some patients may require total hysterectomy.

- Alternative treatment modalities include interventional radiology vascular embolization; however, this approach treats bleeding without treating the underlying cancer.
- Topical hemostatic agents may be used for mucosal bleeding or in conjunction with vaginal packing.
- Consultation with radiation oncology may be helpful when considering re-irradiation to patients who previously have received radiation treatments.
- Early shared decision making is important to determine safe care plans for patients who decline blood transfusions.
- Vaginal bleeding may be a disturbing symptom at the end of life and must be addressed.

DISCLOSURE

The authors have nothing to disclose.

REFERENCES

1. Clarke MA, Long BJ, Del Mar Morillo A, et al. Association of endometrial cancer risk with postmenopausal bleeding in women: a systematic review and meta-analysis. JAMA Intern Med 2018;178:1210–22.
2. Eleje GU, Eke AC, Igberase GO, et al. Palliative interventions for controlling vaginal bleeding in advanced cervical cancer. Cochrane Database Syst Rev 2019;3(3):Cd011000.
3. Lurain JR. Gestational trophoblastic disease I: epidemiology, pathology, clinical presentation and diagnosis of gestational trophoblastic disease, and management of hydatidiform mole. Am J Obstet Gynecol 2010;203:531–9.
4. Pereira J, Phan T. Management of bleeding in patients with advanced cancer. Oncologist 2004;9(5):561–70.
5. Luisada AA. The functional murmur: the laying to rest of a ghost. Dis Chest 1955; 27:579–81.
6. Mozos I. Mechanisms linking red blood cell disorders and cardiovascular diseases. Biomed Res Int 2015;2015:682054.
7. Thygesen K, Alpert JS, Jaffe AS, et al. Fourth universal definition of myocardial infarction (2018). J Am Coll Cardiol 2018;72:2231–64.
8. Holcomb JB, Tilley BC, Baraniuk S, et al. Transfusion of plasma, platelets, and red blood cells in a 1:1:1 vs a 1:1:2 ratio and mortality in patients with severe trauma: the PROPPR randomized clinical trial. JAMA 2015;313:471–82.
9. Knopfelmacher AM, Martinez F. Massive transfusion protocols (MTPs) in cancer patients. In: Nates JL, Price KJ, editors. Oncologic critical care. Cham (Switzerland): Springer International Publishing; 2020. p. 1205–11.
10. Roback JD, Caldwell S, Carson J, et al. Evidence-based practice guidelines for plasma transfusion. Transfusion 2010;50:1227–39.
11. Holcomb JB, Wade CE, Michalek JE, et al. Increased plasma and platelet to red blood cell ratios improves outcome in 466 massively transfused civilian trauma patients. Ann Surg 2008;248:447–58.
12. Kaufman RM, Djulbegovic B, Gernsheimer T, et al. Platelet transfusion: a clinical practice guideline from the AABB. Ann Intern Med 2015;162:205–13.
13. Carson JL, Guyatt G, Heddle NM, et al. Clinical practice guidelines from the AABB: red blood cell transfusion thresholds and storage. JAMA 2016;316: 2025–35.

14. Zayed S, Nguyen TK, Lin C, et al. Red blood cell transfusion practices for patients with cervical cancer undergoing radiotherapy. JAMA Netw Open 2021;4: e213531.

15. Monti M, Castellani L, Berlusconi A, et al. Use of red blood cell transfusions in terminally ill cancer patients admitted to a palliative care unit. J Pain Symptom Manage 1996;12:18–22.

16. Key NS, Khorana AA, Kuderer NM, et al. Venous thromboembolism prophylaxis and treatment in patients with cancer: ASCO clinical practice guideline update. J Clin Oncol 2020;38:496–520.

17. Cuker A, Burnett A, Triller D, et al. Reversal of direct oral anticoagulants: guidance from the Anticoagulation Forum. Am J Hematol 2019;94:697–709.

18. Thomas S, Makris M. The reversal of anticoagulation in clinical practice. Clin Med (Lond) 2018;18:314–9.

19. Kabi Fresenius. Protamine Sulfate Injection, USP [prescribing information]. 2016. Available at: http://editor.fresenius-kabi.us/PIs/US-PH-Protamine_Sulfate_FK-45848G_12_2016-PI.pdf. Accessed December 12, 2021.

20. ACOG committee opinion no. 557: management of acute abnormal uterine bleeding in nonpregnant reproductive-aged women. Obstet Gynecol 2013;121: 891–6.

21. James AH, Kouides PA, Abdul-Kadir R, et al. Evaluation and management of acute menorrhagia in women with and without underlying bleeding disorders: consensus from an international expert panel. Eur J Obstet Gynecol Reprod Biol 2011;158:124–34.

22. Shakur H, Roberts I, Bautista R, et al. Effects of tranexamic acid on death, vascular occlusive events, and blood transfusion in trauma patients with significant haemorrhage (CRASH-2): a randomised, placebo-controlled trial. Lancet 2010;376:23–32.

23. Brenner A, Afolabi A, Ahmad SM, et al. Tranexamic acid for acute gastrointestinal bleeding (the HALT-IT trial): statistical analysis plan for an international, randomised, double-blind, placebo-controlled trial. Trials 2019;20:467.

24. Pharmacia & Upjohn Company LLC. Cyklokapron (tranexamic acid) [prescribing information]. 2021. Available at: https://labeling.pfizer.com/showlabeling.aspx?id=556. Accessed December 12, 2021.

25. Gitlin N, Serio KM. Ischemic hepatitis: widening horizons. Am J Gastroenterol 1992;87:831–6.

26. Strassburg CP. Gastrointestinal disorders of the critically ill. Shock liver. Best Pract Res Clin Gastroenterol 2003;17:369–81.

27. Practice Bulletin No. 149. Endometrial cancer. Obstet Gynecol 2015;125: 1006–26.

28. Díaz-Montes TP, Zahurak ML, Giuntoli RL 2nd, et al. Uterine cancer in Maryland: impact of surgeon case volume and other prognostic factors on short-term mortality. Gynecol Oncol 2006;103:1043–7.

29. Abu-Rustum NR, Yashar CM, Bradley K, et al. National Comprehensive Cancer Network clinical practice guidelines in oncology: uterine cancer. Version 1.2022. Available at: https://www.nccn.org/professionals/physician_gls/pdf/uterine.pdf. Accessed December 12, 2021.

30. Walker JL, Piedmonte MR, Spirtos NM, et al. Laparoscopy compared with laparotomy for comprehensive surgical staging of uterine cancer: Gynecologic Oncology Group Study LAP2. J Clin Oncol 2009;27:5331–6.

31. Janda M, Gebski V, Davies LC, et al. Effect of total laparoscopic hysterectomy vs total abdominal hysterectomy on disease-free survival among women with stage I endometrial cancer: a randomized clinical trial. JAMA 2017;317:1224–33.

32. Cihoric N, Crowe S, Eychmüller S, et al. Clinically significant bleeding in incurable cancer patients: effectiveness of hemostatic radiotherapy. Radiat Oncol 2012; 7:132.

33. Onsrud M, Hagen B, Strickert T. 10-Gy single-fraction pelvic irradiation for palliation and life prolongation in patients with cancer of the cervix and corpus uteri. Gynecol Oncol 2001;82:167–71.

34. Shuja M, Nazli S, Mansha MA, et al. Bleeding in locally invasive pelvic malignancies: is hypofractionated radiation therapy a safe and effective non-invasive option for securing hemostasis? A single institution perspective. Cureus 2018; 10:e2137.

35. Butala AA, Lee DY, Patel RR, et al. A retrospective study of rapid symptom response in bleeding gynecologic malignancies with short course palliative radiation therapy: less is more. J Pain Symptom Manage 2021;61:377–83.e372.

36. Kim JJ, Chapman-Davis E. Role of progesterone in endometrial cancer. Semin Reprod Med 2010;28:81–90.

37. Gunderson CC, Fader AN, Carson KA, et al. Oncologic and reproductive outcomes with progestin therapy in women with endometrial hyperplasia and grade 1 adenocarcinoma: a systematic review. Gynecol Oncol 2012;125:477–82.

38. Abu-Rustum NR, Yashar CM, Bradley K, et al. National Comprehensive Cancer Network clinical practice guidelines in oncology: cervical cancer. Version 1.2022. Available at: https://www.nccn.org/professionals/physician_gls/pdf/cervical.pdf. Accessed December 12, 2021.

39. Piver MS, Rutledge F, Smith JP. Five classes of extended hysterectomy for women with cervical cancer. Obstet Gynecol 1974;44:265–72.

40. Querleu D, Morrow CP. Classification of radical hysterectomy. Lancet Oncol 2008; 9:297–303.

41. Ramirez PT, Frumovitz M, Pareja R, et al. Minimally invasive versus abdominal radical hysterectomy for cervical cancer. N Engl J Med 2018;379:1895–904.

42. Sonoo T, Inokuchi R, Yamamoto M, et al. Severe hemorrhage from cervical cancer managed with foley catheter balloon tamponade. West J Emerg Med 2015;16: 793–4.

43. Fletcher H, Wharfe G, Mitchell S, et al. Treatment of intractable vaginal bleeding with formaldehyde soaked packs. J Obstet Gynaecol 2002;22:570–1.

44. Yanazume S, Douzono H, Yanazume Y, et al. New hemostatic method using Mohs' paste for fatal genital bleeding in advanced cervical cancer. Gynecol Oncol Case Rep 2013;4:47–9.

45. Attarbashi S, Faulkner RL, Slade RJ. The use of Monsel's solution and vaginal pack for haemostasis in cold knife cone biopsy. J Obstet Gynaecol 2007;27:189.

46. Duenas-Garcia OF, Goldberg JM. Topical hemostatic agents in gynecologic surgery. Obstet Gynecol Surv 2008;63:389–94 [quiz: 405].

47. Vilardo N, Feinberg J, Black J, et al. The use of QuikClot combat gauze in cervical and vaginal hemorrhage. Gynecol Oncol Rep 2017;21:114–6.

48. Arzol Chemical Co. Arzol silver nitrate applicators (75% silver nitrate/25% potassium nitrate) [prescribing information]. 2002. Available at: https://www.drugs.com/pro/silver-nitrate-applicators.html. Accessed December 26, 2021.

49. Ngan HYS, Seckl MJ, Berkowitz RS, et al. Update on the diagnosis and management of gestational trophoblastic disease. Int J Gynaecol Obstet 2018;143(Suppl 2):79–85.

50. Berkowitz RS, Goldstein DP. Clinical practice. Molar pregnancy. N Engl J Med 2009;360:1639–45.
51. Soper JT. Gestational trophoblastic disease: current evaluation and management. Obstet Gynecol 2021;137:355–70.
52. Management of gestational trophoblastic disease: green-top guideline No. 38 - June 2020. BJOG 2021;128:e1–27.
53. Gestational trophoblastic disease. In: Hoffman BL, Schorge JO, Schaffer JI, et al, editors. Williams gynecology. 2nd edition. Chicago (IL): McGraw Hill Medical; 2012. p. 898–915.
54. Berkowitz RS, Horowitz NS, Elias KM. Hydatidiform mole: treatment and follow-up. 2021. Available at: https://www.uptodate.com/contents/hydatidiform-mole-treatment-and-follow-up?search=molar%20pregnancy%20&sectionRank=2&usage_type%20=default&anchor=H432805321&source=machineLearning&selectedTitle=1%7E48&display_rank=1. Accessed December 19, 2021.
55. Tse KY, Chan KK, Tam KF, et al. 20-year experience of managing profuse bleeding in gestational trophoblastic disease. J Reprod Med 2007;52:397–401.
56. Sugrue R, Foley O, Elias KM, et al. Outcomes of minimally invasive versus open abdominal hysterectomy in patients with gestational trophoblastic disease. Gynecol Oncol 2021;160:445–9.
57. Patel M, Stuparich M, Nahas S. Total laparoscopic hysterectomy in combination with dilation and evacuation of an 18-week-sized uterus with gestational trophoblastic neoplasia: a novel treatment approach. Am J Obstet Gynecol 2021;224:314–5.
58. Schink JC, Lurain JR. Gestational trophoblastic disease: molar pregnancy and gestational trophoblastic neoplasia. In: Chi DS, Berchuck A, Dizon DS, et al, editors. Principles and practice of gynecologic oncology. 7th edition. Philadelphia (PA): Wolters Kluwer; 2017. p. 744–65.
59. Osborne RJ, Filiaci VL, Schink JC, et al. Second curettage for low-risk nonmetastatic gestational trophoblastic neoplasia. Obstet Gynecol 2016;128:535–42.
60. Nogueira-García J, Moreno-Selva R, Ruiz-Sánchez ME, et al. [Uterine artery embolization as palliative treatment in cervical cancer]. Ginecol Obstet Mex 2015;83:289–93.
61. Field K, Ryan MJ, Saadeh FA, et al. Selective arterial embolisation for intractable vaginal haemorrhage in genital tract malignancies. Eur J Gynaecol Oncol 2016;37:736–40.
62. Hague J, Tippett R. Endovascular techniques in palliative care. Clin Oncol (R Coll Radiol) 2010;22:771–80.
63. Revel-Mouroz P, Mokrane FZ, Collot S, et al. Hemostastic embolization in oncology. Diagn Interv Imaging 2015;96:807–21.
64. Alméciga A, Rodriguez J, Beltrán J, et al. Emergency embolization of pelvic vessels in patients with locally advanced cervical cancer and massive vaginal bleeding: a case series in a Latin American oncological center. JCO Glob Oncol 2020;6:1376–83.
65. Johnstone C, Rich SE. Bleeding in cancer patients and its treatment: a review. Ann Palliat Med 2018;7:265–73.
66. Wright JD, Ananth CV, Lewin SN, et al. Patterns of use of hemostatic agents in patients undergoing major surgery. J Surg Res 2014;186:458–66.
67. Anderson CK, Medlin E, Ferriss AF, et al. Association between gelatin-thrombin matrix use and abscesses in women undergoing pelvic surgery. Obstet Gynecol 2014;124:589–95.

68. Frati A, Thomassin-Naggara I, Bazot M, et al. Accuracy of diagnosis on CT scan of Surgicel® Fibrillar: results of a prospective blind reading study. Eur J Obstet Gynecol Reprod Biol 2013;169:397–401.
69. Stachowicz AM, Whiteside JL. Topical hemostatic agents in gynecologic surgery for benign indications. Obstet Gynecol 2020;135:463–8.
70. Zhang JJ, Cao DY, Yang JX, et al. Ovarian metastasis from nongynecologic primary sites: a retrospective analysis of 177 cases and 13-year experience. J Ovarian Res 2020;13:128.
71. Moradi A, Shakiba B, Maghsoudi R, et al. Vaginal bleeding as primary presentation of renal cell carcinoma. CEN Case Rep 2020;9:138–40.
72. Abdalla AS, Lazarevska A, Omer MM, et al. Metastatic breast cancer to the cervix presenting with abnormal vaginal bleeding during chemotherapy: a case report and literature review. Chirurgia (Bucur) 2018;113:564–70.
73. Nohuz E, Kullab S, Ledoux-Pilon A, et al. Vaginal lymphoma: a possible cause of genital hemorrhage. Turk J Haematol 2016;33:259–60.
74. Kunos CA, Brindle J, Waggoner S, et al. Phase II clinical trial of robotic stereotactic body radiosurgery for metastatic gynecologic malignancies. Front Oncol 2012;2:181.
75. Beriwal S, Heron DE, Mogus R, et al. High-dose rate brachytherapy (HDRB) for primary or recurrent cancer in the vagina. Radiat Oncol 2008;3:7.
76. Rogers DM, Crookston KP. The approach to the patient who refuses blood transfusion. Transfusion 2006;46:1471–7.
77. Vadhan-Raj S, Strauss W, Ford D, et al. Efficacy and safety of IV ferumoxytol for adults with iron deficiency anemia previously unresponsive to or unable to tolerate oral iron. Am J Hematol 2014;89:7–12.
78. Jo KI, Shin JW, Choi TY, et al. Eight-year experience of bloodless surgery at a tertiary care hospital in Korea. Transfusion 2013;53:948–54.
79. Ortho Biotech Products L.P. Procrit (Epoetin alfa) for injection [product labeling]. 2000. Available at: https://www.accessdata.fda.gov/drugsatfda_docs/label/2008/103234s5196 pi.pdf. Accessed December 19, 2021.

First Trimester Miscarriage

Maria Shaker, MD[a,b,*], Ayanna Smith, MD, MPH[a]

KEYWORDS

- Miscarriage • Spontaneous abortion • Early pregnancy loss management
- Miscarriage complications

KEY POINTS

- Early pregnancy loss is the most common complication of pregnancy.
- Multiple modalities of management exist, which include expectant, medical, and surgical options. Patient preferences, clinical presentation, and comorbidities should be considered when counseling patients on these options.
- The most effective medical management regimen is a combination of mifepristone and misoprostol, but is limited by the availability of mifepristone. Misoprostol alone is an efficacious alternative.
- Rarely, complications of early pregnancy loss occur, with the most common complications including hemorrhage and infection. Quick recognition and implementation of interventions are critical to achieve fertility-preserving and life-saving outcomes.

INTRODUCTION

Early pregnancy loss (EPL) is an important clinical scenario encountered by a variety of health care providers, in various settings. Patients experiencing symptoms associated with first trimester miscarriage, such as vaginal bleeding and cramping, frequently seek care in emergency departments. An estimated 900,000 visits to the emergency department occur yearly in the United States related to EPL-associated care.[1] Pregnancy loss is also frequently encountered in the office setting. Acquiring the knowledge and skills to confirm the diagnosis and the finesse with which to counsel patients on management options are important clinical tools for obstetrician/gynecologists. Not only are there physical implications of EPL but also psychological sequelae that are important to consider. For these reasons, competence in addressing miscarriage compassionately and proficiently is important.

First trimester miscarriage is the most common complication of pregnancy.[2] Approximately 15% of clinical pregnancies will result in miscarriage during the first trimester, and 1 in 4 people capable of pregnancy will experience a miscarriage in their

[a] University Hospitals Cleveland Medical Center - MacDonald Women's Hospital, 11100 Euclid Avenue, Cleveland, OH 44106, USA; [b] Department of Reproductive Biology, Case Western Reserve University School of Medicine
* Corresponding author.
E-mail address: maria.shaker@uhhospitals.org

Obstet Gynecol Clin N Am 49 (2022) 623–635
https://doi.org/10.1016/j.ogc.2022.04.004
0889-8545/22/© 2022 Published by Elsevier Inc.

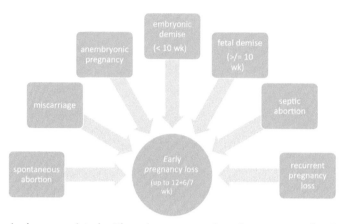

Fig. 1. Terminology associated with early pregnancy loss. Spontaneous abortion: General term, used interchangeably with miscarriage and EPL for pregnancy loss before 20 weeks gestational age. Miscarriage: General term, also used interchangeably with spontaneous abortion to up to 20 weeks gestational age. Anembryonic pregnancy: Intrauterine pregnancy with gestational sac but without evidence of an embryo. Embryonic demise: Intrauterine pregnancy at less than 10 weeks, with an embryo without cardiac activity; crown-rump length of the embryo measures at least 7 mm.[13] Fetal demise: Miscarriage diagnosed at or beyond 10 weeks gestational age. Septic abortion: Pregnancy before 20 weeks complicated by intrauterine infection or overt sepsis. Recurrent pregnancy loss: At least 2 consecutive pregnancy losses before 20 weeks gestational age.

lifetime. EPL and its treatments do not commonly lead to obstetric emergencies. However, it is necessary to be able to recognize these complications to curtail potentially life-altering, and even life-threatening, sequelae like hemorrhage, infection, and even death. Although these complications infrequently occur in developed countries, their potential implications in any socioeconomic setting necessitates competency in evaluation and management.

Terminology associated with first trimester miscarriage can lead to clinical confusion. EPL is used interchangeably with miscarriage and spontaneous abortion. Various terms address specific gestational age ranges, findings on ultrasonography, or other clinical factors in making the diagnosis of EPL (**Fig. 1**). **Table 1** lists additional terminology with more of a historical context, but these are still frequently used to identify various clinical scenarios based on examination findings. Language and terminology associated with EPL, although sometimes ambiguous and confusing, should always be compassionate. Patients prefer EPL and miscarriage to spontaneous abortion and early pregnancy failure.[3]

CAUSE AND RISK FACTORS

Chromosomal abnormalities account for up to 60% of all cases of EPL.[4] One of the most common risk factors for spontaneous miscarriage in the first trimester is advanced maternal age; prior pregnancy loss is also common.[5,6] The inflection point at which miscarriage risk increases is age 35 years.[4] Women older than 40 years experience pregnancy loss at a rate of approximately 50% of clinically recognized pregnancies.[4]

Other maternal risk factors for EPL include medical conditions such as infection,[7] endocrinopathies (eg, uncontrolled thyroid disorders and diabetes mellitus),

Table 1
Terminology of early pregnancy loss based on symptoms and clinical examination findings

Term	Cervical Os Examination	Definition
Complete abortion	Closed	Process completed, no evidence of gestational sac
Threatened abortion	Closed	Bleeding in the setting of inconclusive viability of pregnancy
Missed abortion	Closed	Gestational sac with embryo, without fetal cardiac activity
Incomplete abortion	Open	Miscarriage in process with retained products of conception
Inevitable	Open	Dilated cervix in early pregnancy, without passage of tissue

cardiovascular disease, and dose-related substance abuse. Obesity is another risk factor for first trimester miscarriage; however, the exact reason is unknown and not explained by oocyte abnormality or polycystic ovary syndrome.[8]

Black, indigenous, and other people of color have an increased risk of pregnancy loss when compared with white people,[9] with differences most likely reflective of systemic racism, social determinants of health, and environmental and/or occupational exposure.

Anatomic abnormalities such as uterine leiomyomas, polyps, intrauterine adhesions, or septa can be associated with pregnancy loss and should be medically or surgically addressed before attempting subsequent pregnancies. In addition, intrauterine devices (IUDs), although extremely effective methods of contraception, are risk factors for pregnancy loss if conception and intrauterine implantation occur with an IUD in place.[10]

Education on the interplay of these risk factors and health care providers' roles in helping patients reduce risks is important. The optimal timing for these conversations should be before conception so that patients can maximize pregnancy outcomes and ultimately, their general health.

PATIENT EVALUATION OVERVIEW

Symptoms of EPL exist on a spectrum, ranging from a complete absence of symptoms with the diagnosis made incidentally on routine ultrasonography to life-threatening hemorrhage and severe pain. Vaginal spotting or heavier bleeding with or without cramping alerts the patient that something may be abnormal. It is important to cast a wide differential diagnosis in a patient who presents with symptoms like vaginal bleeding and/or cramping in the first trimester to include those that can lead to adverse events (eg, ectopic pregnancy, molar pregnancy). It is also prudent to remember that symptoms of EPL can sometimes occur in normally progressing pregnancies.[5]

Confirmation of EPL before intervention is an imperative to avoid interrupting a normal pregnancy.[5,11] Therefore, evaluation of EPL should include a thorough medical history, physical examination, pelvic ultrasonography, and laboratory studies.[5] Serum human chorionic gonadotropin (β-hCG) can be helpful if an intrauterine pregnancy has not already been diagnosed. A complete blood cell count (CBC), with blood type and determination of Rh status, should also be obtained. A CBC is especially helpful in the setting of ongoing bleeding to determine the need for blood transfusion, and a white blood cell (WBC) count with differential can aid in the diagnosis when infection is suspected.

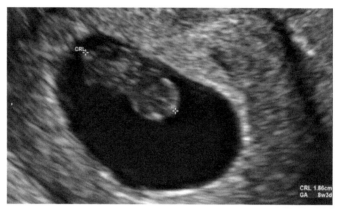

Fig. 2. Sonographic image demonstrating a missed abortion: a crown-rump length (CRL) of 7 mm without a heartbeat. (*Courtesy of* M. Shaker, MD, Cleveland, OH.)

On physical examination, a skilled practitioner should assess the patient's general appearance, their cardiac and respiratory status, and perform an abdominal examination. A thorough pelvic examination is also critical to the workup of EPL, which includes visualization of the vagina and cervix with a speculum to help quantify ongoing bleeding and a bimanual examination to assess cervical dilation and elicit uterine tenderness, if present.

Both hemorrhage and infection, if severe enough, can lead to hemodynamic instability. Severe hemorrhage necessitating hospitalization accounts for only 1% of EPL.[11] Evidence of hypotension, tachycardia, and orthostatic vitals are important clues to volume status and can be interpreted along with the CBC to assess for acute blood loss anemia. The speculum examination enables visualization and detection of products of conception (POC) possibly retained in the cervix. If present, removal of the tissue can result in quick resolution of ongoing bleeding.[2]

Infection is another potential complication. Derangements in WBC count and/or body temperature, together with physical examination findings like uterine or abdominal tenderness and purulent vaginal discharge are important clues in quickly making this diagnosis.

Pelvic ultrasonography is the preferred modality to verify intrauterine location and viability,[5] with preference for transvaginal approach when complications of early pregnancy are suspected. Compared with ultrasonograhic examination, digital and speculum examination are unreliable in the diagnosis of miscarriage.[2,12]

Various parameters have been studied to definitively diagnose EPL with sonographic evaluation. Previously, a crown-rump length (CRL) of 5 mm without cardiac activity and a mean gestational sac diameter (MSD) of 16 mm without an embryo were widely accepted as diagnostic criteria for EPL.[5] The Society of Radiologists in Ultrasound Multispecialty Panel on Early First Trimester Diagnosis of Miscarriage and Exclusion of a Viable Intrauterine Pregnancy has published more conservative guidelines to achieve nearly 100% specificity to make the diagnosis. These diagnostic criteria include[13]:

- CRL of at least 7 mm without cardiac activity (**Fig. 2**);
- MSD of 25 mm without an embryo (average of the gestational sac dimensions in craniocaudal, anteroposterior, and transverse views);
- Absence of embryo with fetal cardiac activity 2 weeks or more after ultrasonography, which demonstrates gestational sac without a yolk sac; or

- Absence of embryo with heartbeat 11 days or more after ultrasonography, which demonstrates gestational sac (**Fig. 3**).

When counseling patients about pregnancy viability and options for management, providers should consider these guidelines and other clinical factors, while exploring the patient's preferences and feelings about the pregnancy. Factors to consider include patient's desire to achieve 100% certainty of diagnosis, potential for unpredictable onset of EPL symptoms, and preferences for management. Shared decision-making between patient and provider should drive the creation of an individualized care plan.[5]

MANAGEMENT

The management of EPL consists of 4 different options: (1) expectant management, (2) medical management with misoprostol with or without mifepristone, (3) uterine aspiration in the office, or (4) uterine aspiration in the operating room. Counseling patients on options for EPL management should be patient centered, eliciting their preferences and priorities. Patients report higher satisfaction with care when these preferences are explored and considered during the counseling process.[14]

Aside from patient preference, there are other important factors to consider when counseling a patient on management options: gestational age, unpredictable onset of miscarriage-associated symptoms, duration of bleeding and cramping, as well as efficacy of method. Surgical management is the most efficacious, followed by medical management, with expectant management being the least efficacious method.[15,16] Importantly, a patient's medical comorbidities influence the safety profile of one method over another. Availability of certain resources, such as access to 24-h care also plays a role in the decision for management. All these factors, in addition to the risks, benefits, and expectations of each option, should be discussed with the patient to provide full informed consent.

EXPECTANT MANAGEMENT

The least invasive option, expectant management, allows for spontaneous expulsion of the POC, or the "watch and wait" approach. This option should depend on the availability of emergency care and surgical intervention, in the event of heavy bleeding or retained products.[17]

Expectant management has lower effectiveness in achieving complete evacuation of POC compared with other treatment modalities.[15] It is important to counsel patients regarding the possibility of prolonged follow-up, repeated hospital visits, and the need for surgical intervention for unsuccessful expectant management.

Blood loss associated with nonsurgical interventions can induce a drop in hemoglobin by at least 3 g/dL.[18] Therefore, contraindications to expectant management include certain medical comorbidities including anemia, cardiovascular disease, bleeding disorders, or anticoagulated status. Importantly, acute bleeding leading to hemodynamic instability or evidence of infection are also contraindications.

Patient education to set expectations surrounding pain and bleeding is important. Bleeding can be significant, and it can be difficult to know when to seek medical care. General recommendations for excessive bleeding requiring further evaluation include soaking 2 maxi pads per hour for 2 or more consecutive hours.[17] Educational materials with information regarding when and who to call can help support the expectantly managed patient. It is also important to provide nonsteroidal anti-inflammatory medications (NSAIDs) to address associated abdominal cramping.

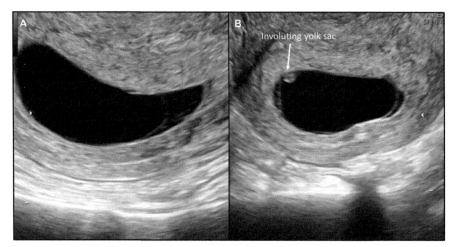

Fig. 3. Sonographic illustration of an anembryonic pregnancy, obtained 11 days after ultrasonography, demonstrated a gestational sac with yolk sac. (*A*) Sagittal view of uterus. (*B*). Transverse view. (*Courtesy of* M. Shaker, MD, Cleveland, OH.)

Follow-up should include assessment of the patient's symptoms and physical and emotional well-being. Absence of the gestational sac on ultrasonography and an endometrial thickness of less than 30 mm are commonly used criteria to confirm complete passage of pregnancy tissue, although no formal consensus exists.[18] Patient-reported symptoms and serial β-hCG values can also be used to determine a completed miscarriage.

PHARMACOLOGIC TREATMENT

Medical management, although mimicking a more natural route of treatment, expedites the process for those diagnosed with EPL and provides a method that potentially avoids surgical intervention. Contraindications to pharmacologic intervention mirror those of expectant management (eg, anemia, cardiovascular disease, bleeding disorders).

Historically, medical management relied solely on local or systemic administration of misoprostol. Misoprostol, a synthetic prostaglandin E_1 analogue, causes uterine contractions that work to expel the pregnancy tissue. Misoprostol is available via multiple routes: orally, sublingually, or vaginally, and is self-administered, an attractive characteristic to patients who seek patient-controlled environments for management. When prescribed at 800 μg via the vaginal or sublingual routes, the regimen has a complete expulsion rate of just more than 70%. If a second dose is indicated, the success rate increases to 84%.[5,18] The vaginal and sublingual routes are more effective and associated with lower gastrointestinal side effects when compared with sublingual administration.[19]

More recently, results from a 2018 randomized controlled trial demonstrated superiority of a combined regimen of mifepristone plus misoprostol when compared with misoprostol alone.[20] Mifepristone, a competitive progesterone-receptor antagonist, primes the uterine myometrium and cervix, readying these for the contractile activity induced by misoprostol. Patients with a confirmed anembryonic or missed abortion between 5 and 12 completed weeks' gestation were included in the trial. Patients were randomized to either pretreatment with mifepristone 200 mg orally plus vaginal misoprostol 800 µg administered 24 hours later, or misoprostol alone (800 µg vaginally). Outcomes between the 2 groups were compared. Rates of complete expulsion were higher and risks of surgical intervention were lower with the combined regimen.[20] Although this combination regimen is superior and recommended as the preferred regimen when available, the US Food and Drug Administration Risk Evaluation and Mitigation Strategy restrictions currently limit mifepristone administration in some areas.[21]

Counseling about expectations for medical management should parallel those given for expectant management, addressing bleeding and pain precautions. As with expectant management, NSAIDs are effective for pain management. Antibiotics are not recommended for routine medical management. Gastrointestinal side effects are common with misoprostol, so prescriptions for antinausea medications are prudent.

Follow-up is advised whether in person or via telehealth, with or without confirmatory imaging or laboratory testing. Imaging can be used to confirm absence of a gestational sac. Serial β-hCG levels can also be used if ultrasonography is not readily available.[5] Again, addressing the patient's emotional well-being provides a comprehensive approach to care.

SURGICAL TREATMENT OPTIONS

Historically, surgical management with uterine evacuation of the POC was offered as first-line treatment. This approach has since evolved as evidence has emerged regarding the safety and efficacy of the other treatment options. Surgical management with uterine aspiration is first line for patients who present with hemorrhage, hemodynamic instability, or signs of infection. Uterine aspiration is also preferred for patients with significant comorbidities including severe anemia, bleeding disorders, or cardiovascular disease, all of which necessitate the need for controlled clinical environments and potentially for additional resources. Patients may opt for surgical management if they desire immediate resolution of the miscarriage or want to avoid additional follow-up visits, 2 advantages over expectant and medical management options.

Surgical evacuation of the uterus can be performed either by electric or manual vacuum aspiration, the latter of which can be performed in any clinical setting. The American College of Obstetricians and Gynecologists, the Society for Family Planning, and the World Health Organization advise against the use of sharp curettage for surgical management of EPL. Sharp curettage increases the risks of uterine perforation, blood loss, pain, intrauterine adhesion formation, and need for greater cervical dilation compared with suction cannula. Depending on the gestational age of the pregnancy and the skill of the provider, manual uterine aspiration can be offered in the emergency department or office setting. This benefit has significant cost savings compared with procedures performed in an operating room.[1] In addition, manual uterine aspiration provides increased convenience in scheduling the procedure, allowing for the ability to provide care on the same day as the miscarriage diagnosis. Local anesthesia via an intracervical or paracervical block, in addition to oral pain medication, provides adequate pain control; an oral sedative may be added should the patient desire. Procedures performed in the operating room provide the added benefit of intravenous sedation, although at the expense of time and health care costs.

Briefly, with a speculum in place to visualize the entire cervix, a tenaculum is used to grasp the cervix for stabilization and traction purposes. Local anesthesia is administered. The cervix is then adequately dilated to ensure easy passage of a suction curette. The size of curette depends on the gestational age at which the miscarriage is measured. Vacuum is deployed to aspirate the pregnancy tissue. This procedure can be done under the guidance of ultrasound visualization. POC should be sent for pathologic evaluation. If the patient desires, genetic assessment of the trophoblastic tissue can sometimes elucidate the cause of the pregnancy loss.

The risk of infection associated with surgical management has been extrapolated from induced abortion data. Based on this evidence, prophylactic antibiotics are recommended before surgical management. A commonly accepted practice is the utilization of doxycycline 200 mg administrated orally 1 hour before the procedure. Evidence for prophylactic antibiotics in the setting of expectant or medical management does not exist and therefore, is not recommended.[22]

TREATMENT COMPLICATIONS

Known complications associated with EPL and treatment options include retained POC, infection, and hemorrhage.[5] Rarely, intrauterine adhesions can also form, leading to amenorrhea and secondary infertility.[5] Another more nuanced complication is hematometra, which is a collection of blood and/or retained POC within the uterus. Although serious complications are rare, they should not be discounted. It is important to remember that clinically significant bleeding can occur with expectant and medical management options, with greater than or equal to 3 g/dL drop in hemoglobin.[18] Tissue trauma like cervical laceration and uterine perforation are other potential complications in the setting of surgical management. Death is an extremely rare complication associated with EPL, especially with early diagnosis and management. Except for cervical laceration, uterine perforation, and intrauterine adhesion formation, complications of EPL are not specific to one treatment modality, and all should be discussed with patients as part of the informed consent process.

Clinical presentation depends on the type of complication that develops, but symptoms can frequently overlap. Common complaints that may suggest a complication include abdominal or pelvic pain, persistent or heavy bleeding, or fever. Hemorrhage is only a symptom or sign of an underlying cause that must be corrected to stop the bleeding.

Obtaining a thorough history and physical examination are the mainstays in working up potential complications. Laboratory tests include CBC; metabolic panel to assess for electrolyte abnormalities and renal or hepatic impairment; coagulation studies, including fibrinogen; blood type and cross-match, in case of the need for transfusion; blood cultures; and a lactate level if septic abortion is considered. Imaging may be helpful, especially if retained products are suspected, and therefore, pelvic ultrasonography should be obtained. Additionally, an abdominal radiograph can demonstrate free air in the abdomen and/or myometrium, whereas a computed tomography scan can be used to assess for bowel injury, fluid collections in the pelvis, or other structural abnormalities.

Crucial to quickly initiating life-saving interventions in the context of hemorrhage and/or septic abortion is the assessment of the patient's hemodynamic status. Fluid resuscitation is imperative, and the type of fluid is dictated by the underlying cause (ie, blood products for acute blood loss anemia vs intravenous fluids and possible vasopressors for septic shock).

The risk of infection with EPL is relatively low at approximately 2% to 3%, and there is no evidence to suggest a difference between miscarriage management options.[23] Increasing gestational age correlates with the risk of infection, due to a larger volume of tissue that can be infected. Although infection rates are low, septic abortion accounts for the vast majority of maternal death after spontaneous abortion (59%).[24,25] Most cases of maternal death due to sepsis occur in women without other medical comorbidities, when compared with other causes of maternal death.[24] Fetal death inevitably occurs with septic abortion. Therefore, treatment with uterine evacuation should not await the loss of fetal cardiac activity,[24] as the risk for rapid deterioration is high.

There are no standard criteria to diagnose maternal sepsis, but vital sign changes are usually the earliest indicators.[26] As in any case of sepsis, early initiation of antibiotics and fluid resuscitation (30 mL/kg) are critical, particularly if blood lactate level is greater than 4 mmol/L or mean arterial pressure is less than 65 mm Hg.[26] In addition, source control is warranted with uterine evacuation if retained POC are diagnosed. Providers should have a low threshold for hysterectomy if the patient does not improve within 6 hours of curettage, antibiotic therapy, and fluid resuscitation.[24,27]

Septic abortion is known to be polymicrobial in cause, commonly caused by vaginal flora and anaerobic bacteria, which are usually sensitive to antibiotics. Although commonly considered polymicrobial, septic abortions can also be caused by toxin-producing bacteria, most notably group A streptococci. Unrecognized infection by group A *Streptococcus* can be lethal, especially if the infection extends into the uterine tissue where antibiotics are futile in controlling the resultant tissue necrosis.[24]

Broad-spectrum antibiotics are indicated for septic abortion, remembering that anaerobic coverage is necessary. Drug availability and patient allergies drive antibiotic selection. Some commonly recommended antibiotic regimens include[24]:

- Gentamicin (5 mg/kg/d) and clindamycin (900 mg every 8 hours) with or without ampicillin
- Ampicillin (2 g every 4 hours) and gentamicin with metronidazole (500 mg every 8 hours)
- Piperacillin-tazobactam (4.5 g every 8 hours)

To align with antibiotic stewardship, drug selection is tailored once cultures result with bacterial identification and sensitivities. Toxin-producing bacteria are extremely sensitive to penicillin-containing regimens. Of note, clindamycin should be considered as an adjunct due to its in vitro efficacy against toxin-producing strains.[24]

Miscarriage-associated hemorrhage can be managed with some of the same pharmacologic interventions and surgical techniques used for postpartum hemorrhage. Of course, adequate treatment relies on identification and correction of the underlying cause. Uterotonic medications are used to reverse atony (methylergonovine, carboprost, and misoprostol), retained products are evacuated to expedite uterine involution, cervical lacerations are repaired primarily, and coagulopathies are corrected by repleting clotting factors with blood products. Tranexamic acid, which inhibits fibrinolysis, can also be considered for treatment. An intrauterine balloon (eg, a Foley catheter or Bakri balloon) can provide intrauterine tamponade, should the patient require transfer to a higher level of care or the operating room. Interventional radiology can be consulted for the possibility of uterine artery embolization if the patient is an appropriate candidate. Laparoscopy and/or laparotomy aid in investigation of the source and enable repair of tissue trauma, like a bleeding perforation. Refractory bleeding rarely occurs, but definitive management with hysterectomy may be required in certain cases.

NEW DEVELOPMENTS

Although the manual vacuum aspirator has been available for decades, which has increased access to a safe, effective method for surgical management of EPL, widespread adoption of in-office and emergency department procedures is still needed.[28] As mentioned previously, performing in-office procedures increases convenience and reduces general anesthesia risks. In addition, in-office manual uterine aspiration procedures may reduce costs by more than half when compared with the same procedure occurring in the operating room.[29]

Despite the evidence published in 2018 in support of the combined regimen of mifepristone plus misoprostol, the US Food and Drug Administration's Risk Evaluation and Mitigation Strategy restrictions[21] limit implementation of this regimen. Many organizations, including The American College of Obstetricians and Gynecologists, support lifting these restrictions to improve access to mifepristone to benefit reproductive health care for all.[5]

Last, in response to the severe acute respiratory syndrome coronavirus 2 pandemic, telehealth has become an important pathway for health care delivery. Specific to reproductive health, telehealth allows for appointments in which a physical examination or other testing is not necessarily indicated, such as with contraceptive counseling. Even abortion care can be provided remotely.[30] Therefore, telemedicine can be adopted for use in miscarriage management (for expectant and medical management counseling), as well as for follow-up.

LONG-TERM RECOMMENDATIONS

Frequently, patients are concerned about future pregnancy outcomes after experiencing a miscarriage. Patients were previously recommended to avoid pregnancy for several menstrual cycles after miscarriage occurred. This recommendation has no scientific basis, and since has become an abandoned practice pattern. Patients should be counseled that conception can happen quickly after miscarriage, yet the timing of the next ovulatory cycle may be difficult to predict. If pregnancy is desired, patients should be counseled to continue taking their folic acid supplementation and/or a prenatal vitamin.

For patients who wish to prevent pregnancy after miscarriage management, most methods of contraception are appropriate and can be initiated immediately after treatment. Any short-acting contraceptive method may be initiated after miscarriage.[31] An IUD can be inserted at the time of surgical management, unless septic abortion is diagnosed. Expulsion rates of an IUD after suction curettage do not reach clinical significance when compared with rates later in the postoperative period.[32] The patient's preferences and medical comorbidities should instead guide the appropriateness of contraceptive method, and the Centers for Disease Control's US Medical Eligibility Criteria is a useful tool in contraceptive counseling.[31]

RhD immune globulin should be considered in cases of EPL, even though risk of alloimmunization is low. Priority should be given to those undergoing surgical management.[5]

Variations exist in the definition of recurrent pregnancy loss (RPL). Workup for RPL is typically not recommended until after the second consecutive EPL.[4] Details of the workup are beyond the scope of this publication, but clinicians can access guidelines from the American College of Obstetricians and Gynecologists[5] and the American Society for Reproductive Medicine[4] in these clinical scenarios.

SUMMARY

First trimester miscarriage or EPL is a frequently encountered clinical condition by many women's health care and emergency medicine providers. Rarely, complications from EPL occur, but prompt recognition and management curb adverse outcomes that can be fertility ending or even life threatening, like hemorrhage or sepsis. Treatment modalities should be decided upon based on a patient's preference, along with pertinent medical comorbidities, and ability for emergent follow-up. Opportunities to expand surgical management to the emergency room and the outpatient setting improve health care delivery. Telemedicine is another option to increase patient satisfaction and efficiency. Screening for psychological well-being and reproductive life-planning are important components in EPL management.

CLINICS CARE PEARLS

- Surgical management is the most efficacious management option in complete uterine evacuation, followed by medical and then expectant management.
- Patient preference, together with medical comorbidities should be considered when counseling on options for management of EPL.
- Use of mifepristone, when available, combined with misoprostol increases efficacy of medical management.
- Complications associated with EPL are rare, but can be clinically significant. The same principles pertinent to peripartum hemorrhage management apply to bleeding in EPL.
- Early recognition of septic abortion and prompt initiation of management strategies (ie, administration of broad-spectrum antibiotics and fluid resuscitation) can be life saving.
- Essentially any method of contraception can be safely initiated after surgical management of EPL, and the CDC's MEC can help guide patient counseling.

DISCLOSURE

The authors have nothing to disclose.

REFERENCES

1. Benson LS, Magnusson SL, Gray KE, et al. Early pregnancy loss in the emergency department, 2006–2016. J Am Coll Emerg Physicians Open 2021;2(6): e12549.
2. Jurkovic D, Overton C, Bender-Atik R. Diagnosis and management of first trimester miscarriage. BMJ 2013;346:f3676.
3. Clement EG, Horvath S, McAllister A, et al. The language of first-trimester nonviable pregnancy: patient-reported preferences and clarity. Obstet Gynecol 2019; 133(1):149.
4. Evaluation and treatment of recurrent pregnancy loss: a committee opinion. Practice committee of the american society for reproductive medicine. Fertil Steril 2012;98:1103–11.
5. ACOG Practice Bulletin No. 200: Early Pregnancy Loss. Obstet Gynecol 2018; 132(5):e197–207.
6. Magnus MC, Wilcox AJ, Morken NH, et al. Role of maternal age and pregnancy history in risk of miscarriage: prospective register based study. BMJ 2019;364: l869.
7. Giakoumelou S, Wheelhouse N, Cuschieri K, et al. The role of infection in miscarriage. Hum Reprod Update 2016;22(1):116–33.

8. Lashen H, Fear K, Sturdee DW. Obesity is associated with increased risk of first trimester and recurrent miscarriage: matched case-control study. Hum Reprod 2004;19(7):1644–6.

9. Mukherjee S, Velez Edwards DR, Baird DD, et al. Risk of miscarriage among black women and white women in a U.S. Prospective Cohort Study. Am J Epidemiol 2013;177(11):1271.

10. Ozgu-Erdinca AS, Tasdemir UG, Uygura D, et al. Outcome of intrauterine pregnancies with intrauterine device in place and effects of device location on prognosis. Contraception 2014;89(5):426–30.

11. Barnhart KT. Early pregnancy failure: beware of the pitfalls of modern management. Fertil Steril 2012;98:1061–5.

12. Wieringa-de Waard M, Bonsel GJ, Ankum WM, et al. Threatened miscarriage in general practice: diagnostic value of history taking and physical examination. Br J Gen Pract 2002;52:825–9.

13. Doubilet PM, Benson CB, Bourne T, et al. Diagnostic criteria for nonviable pregnancy early in the first trimester. Society of Radiologists in Ultrasound Multispecialty Panel on Early First Trimester Diagnosis of Miscarriage and Exclusion of a Viable Intrauterine Pregnancy. N Engl J Med 2013;369:1443–51.

14. Wallace RR, Goodman S, Freedman LR, et al. Counseling women with early pregnancy failure: utilizing evidence, preserving preference. Patient Educ Couns 2010;81:454–61.

15. Ghosh J, Papadopoulou A, Devall AJ, et al. Methods for managing miscarriage: a network meta-analysis. Cochrane Database Syst Rev 2021;6(6):CD012602.

16. Luise C, Jermy K, May C, et al. Outcome of expectant management of spontaneous first trimester miscarriage: observational study. BMJ 2002;324(7342): 873–5.

17. Paul M, Lichtenberg ES, Borgatta L, et al. Management of unintended and abnormal pregnancy: comprehensive abortion care. Hoboken (NJ): Wiley-Blackwell; 2009.

18. Zhang J, Giles JM, Barhart K, et al. A comparison of medical management with misoprostol and surgical management for early pregnancy failure. N Engl J Med 2005;353(8):761.

19. Kim C, Barnard S, Neilson JP, et al. Medical treatments for incomplete miscarriage. Cochrane Database Syst Rev 2017;31(1):CD007223.

20. Schreiber CA, Creinin MD, Atrio J, et al. Mifepristone Pretreatment for the Medical Management of Early Pregnancy Loss. N Engl J Med 2018;378(23):2161–70.

21. U.S. Food and Drug Administration. Mifeprex (mifepristone information). Postmarket drug safety information for patients and providers. Silver Spring (MD): FDA; 2018.

22. Achilles SL, Reeves MF. Prevention of infection after induced abortion. Contraception 2011;83(4):295–309.

23. Trinder J, Brocklehurst P, Porter R, et al. Management of miscarriage: expectant, medical, or surgical? Results of randomised controlled trial (miscarriage treatment (MIST) trial). BMJ 2006;332(7552):1235–40.

24. Eschenbach DA. Treating spontaneous and induced septic abortions. Obstet Gynecol 2015;125(5):1042–8.

25. Saraiya M, Green C, Berg C, et al. Spontaneous abortion-related deaths among women in the United States—1981–1991. Obstet Gynecol 1999;94:172–6.

26. Shields A, de Assis V, Halscott T. Top 10 Pearls for the recognition, evaluation and management of maternal sepsis. Obstet Gynecol 2021;138(2):289–304.

27. Reid DE. Assessment and management of the seriously ill patient following abortion. JAMA 1967;199:141–8.
28. Rausch MD, Lorch S, Chung K, et al. A cost-effectiveness analysis of surgical versus medical management of early pregnancy loss. Fertil Steril 2012;97(2): 355–60.
29. Quinley KE, Chong D, Prager S, et al. Manual uterine aspiration: adding to the emergency physician stabilization toolkit. Ann Emerg Med 2018;72(1):86–92.
30. Upadhyay U, Koenigh LR, Meckstroth KR. Safety and efficacy of telehealth medication abortions in the US during the COVID-19 pandemic. JAMA Netw Open 2021;4(8):e2122320.
31. Curtis KM, Tepper NK, Jatlaoui TC, et al. U.S. Medical eligibility criteria for contraceptive use, 2016. MMWR Recomm Rep 2016;65(RR-3):1–104.
32. Roe AH, Bartz D. Society of family planning clinical recommendations: contraception after surgical abortion. Contraception 2019;99:2–9. https://doi.org/10. 1016/j.contraception.2018.08.

Simulation in Obstetric Emergencies

Jean-Ju Sheen, MD[a], Dena Goffman, MD[a], Shad Deering, MD, CHSE, COL(ret) USA[b],*

KEYWORDS

- Simulation • Obstetric emergencies • Hemorrhage • Cardiac arrest • Training
- Patient safety

KEY POINTS

- Simulation is critical for individual skill acquisition in obstetric emergency management.
- Teamwork and communication are best taught through multidisciplinary simulation exercises.
- Practicing for obstetric emergencies with simulation is recommended by national organizations and required by the Joint Commission.

INTRODUCTION, HISTORY, AND BACKGROUND

Simulation has been defined as a situation in which an artificial representation of a real-world condition is created to achieve educational goals via experiential learning.[1] Although simulation was incorporated into surgical training as early as 2500 years ago,[2] the use of simulation in obstetric training dates back centuries as wooden, leather, or cloth midwifery training models thought to be from the sixteenth century are displayed in South American and European museums.[3] In fact, the mid-eighteenth century surgeon Giovanni Antonio Galli designed a pelvis with a glass uterus and flexible fetus birthing simulator to provide childbirth training to midwives and surgeons.[4] Indeed, multiple medical institutions worldwide have historically incorporated obstetric simulation in their curricula. J. Whitridge Williams, Associate Professor of Obstetrics at Johns Hopkins, presented to the 1898 Association of American Medical Colleges annual meeting that "exercises upon the manikin should form an integral part of the obstetric course . . . that the students be taught the rudiments . . . upon the manikin, so that they will know exactly what they are to do when they

[a] New York-Presbyterian Sloan Hospital for Women, Columbia University Irving Medical Center, 622 West 168th Street PH 16-66, New York, NY 10032, USA; [b] Baylor College of Medicine, Children's Hospital of San Antonio, 315 North San Saba, Suite 1135, San Antonio, TX 78207, USA
* Corresponding author. 315 North San Saba, Suite 1135, San Antonio, TX 78207.
E-mail address: Shad.Deering@christushealth.org

Obstet Gynecol Clin N Am 49 (2022) 637–646
https://doi.org/10.1016/j.ogc.2022.04.005
0889-8545/22/© 2022 Elsevier Inc. All rights reserved.

examine the patients in the wards, whereby clinical material is economized, and the patients saved considerable annoyance."[5]

Around the same time that Williams made his recommendation to the Association of American Medical Colleges, William Stewart Halsted, the first Chief of Surgery at Johns Hopkins, was transforming surgical education via the creation of the residency training program, with formalized teaching based on the concept of "see one, do one, teach one."[6] The system he developed essentially remained unchanged for the subsequent century. As births moved from the home to hospitals in the 1900s, there was an apparent decreased need for obstetric simulation as trainees now had access to a large diverse group of patients instead.[7] Thus, despite the advances in simulation in Europe and in the United States between the seventeenth and the early twentieth century, much of the twentieth century became a "dark age" for simulation, during which students and trainees obtained their initial training on patients instead of simulators, with some inevitable results.[2]

TWENTIETH CENTURY REVITALIZATION OF OBSTETRIC SIMULATION

Toward the end of the twentieth century, interest in medical simulation was revitalized. The advent of modern obstetric simulation was driven by contemporaneous changes in medical education and patient safety concerns, in addition to the decreasing frequency of exposure to certain obstetric clinical procedures and scenarios. In 1999, the Institute of Medicine published a landmark report, To Err Is Human, which estimated that 44,000 to 98,000 Americans die each year owing to preventable harm from human error.[8] Shortly thereafter, in 2003, the Accreditation Council for Graduate Medical Education set restricted duty-hour standards for all accredited medical training institutions in the United States.[9] These work-hour reductions posed additional challenges to ensuring adequate clinical experience, especially for trainees in obstetrics and gynecology, who require broad exposure to increasingly complex clinical situations.[10]

The initial revival of obstetric simulation began with training residents to perform task-specific procedures that have had an increasingly low frequency of occurrence with shifts in obstetric practice, such as repairing fourth-degree perineal lacerations, performing singleton breech deliveries, and performing forceps-assisted vaginal deliveries. Residency programs recognized that time constraints and the unpredictable nature of obstetric lacerations warranted improved education regarding perineal repair; thus, surgical models such as a sponge perineum or beef tongue model with structured assessments could provide trainees the initial experience, constructive feedback and improved confidence.[11,12] In 2000, the Term Breech Trial concluded that planned cesarean deliveries yielded less neonatal morbidity and mortality than vaginal birth,[13] resulting in a stark decrease in singleton vaginal breech births and the potential for increased suboptimal outcomes as trainees became less familiar with the maneuvers to achieve a successful breech vaginal birth. Subsequent studies have shown that simulation training is helpful in improving resident performance and comfort in the management of a simulated vaginal breech birth with retention of skills within a limited timeframe.[14,15] Similarly, in a recent commentary, Dildy and colleagues[16] noted that, in the United States, both resident training in obstetric forceps and forceps deliveries have experienced drastic declines, such that "attempts by experienced teaching faculty to provide residents with experience in a few forceps deliveries are of little value and may do more harm than good." They recommended prioritizing the development of high-fidelity simulation models to allow residents to obtain sufficient experience in understanding the appropriate circumstances to proceed with a forceps birth.[16] The needs of obstetrics and gynecology residency training drove the acceptance of simulation such that nearly every skill required to be learned during residency has been addressed through simulation.[7] Indeed, simulation makes the abstract concrete and cements concepts into reflexive learning.

EMERGENCY TEAM TRAINING IN OBSTETRICS

The early success and ease of adaptability of simulation in obstetrics curricula resulted in an expansion of its use to include more complicated and emergent scenarios, such as shoulder dystocia and postpartum hemorrhage (PPH). Subsequent increased emphasis on team training and safety initiatives has driven the necessary inclusion of higher level learners, such as fellows and attending physicians,[7] and the expansion of scenario complexity to include critical care and multidisciplinary participants. In 2012, a joint publication titled "Quality Patient Care in Labor and Delivery: A Call to Action," endorsed by 7 different societies including the American College of Obstetricians and Gynecologists and the Society for Maternal Fetal Medicine, recommended simulation training as part of a comprehensive strategy to improve outcomes in obstetrics.[17] Interdisciplinary team training was specifically recognized as one strategy for improving perinatal care, because highly reliable teams decrease the number of clinical errors and improve patient outcomes.[17]

As teamwork training became more mainstream in medical education and patient safety initiatives, it was integrated into simulation curricula for obstetric emergencies. Simulated emergencies have included common situations such a PPH to the less common shoulder dystocia and eclampsia to rare occurrences such as anaphylactoid syndrome of pregnancy and maternal cardiac arrest. Most recently, the coronavirus disease 2019 (COVID-19) pandemic has prompted an increased need for preparedness and simulated scenarios incorporating enhanced safety protocols for both clinicians and patients. In this review, we focus on obstetric emergency simulation literature concerning shoulder dystocia, PPH, maternal cardiac arrest from anaphylactoid syndrome of pregnancy, pre-eclampsia, eclampsia, and COVID-19.

SHOULDER DYSTOCIA

Shoulder dystocia is a result of the fetal anterior shoulder being obstructed by the pubic symphysis or the fetal posterior shoulder being impacted on the maternal sacral promontory, requiring additional obstetric maneuvers to achieve birth.[18,19] Its reported incidence among cephalic-presenting fetuses undergoing vaginal births ranges from 0.2% to 3.0%.[20,21] Simulation training has been shown to improve outcomes and documentation for this unpredictable and unpreventable obstetric emergency.[18] In fact, data from shoulder dystocia training has yielded the most evidence of any single obstetrics emergency simulation for simulation training improving outcomes.[22]

Multiple studies have shown that shoulder dystocia training decreases the incidence of neonatal injury. Draycott and colleagues[23] published a large retrospective observational study from the UK that reviewed neonatal outcomes from all births complicated by shoulder dystocia 4 years before and after mandatory yearly shoulder dystocia training. Although the incidence of shoulder dystocia stayed constant, the risk of neonatal injury was decreased by almost 4-fold.[23] In a subsequent review by the same group 12 years after the introduction of training, fetal morbidity from shoulder dystocia remained low.[24] Inglis and colleagues[25] and Grobman and colleagues[26] also published findings from separate institutions demonstrating significant decreases in brachial plexus injuries after training program implementation.

In addition to improvements in neonatal morbidity, shoulder dystocia simulation training has demonstrated improvements in clinical management above traditional didactic education and in documentation. Deering and colleagues[27] in 2004 showed that resident performance during simulated shoulder dystocia cases after simulation training was significantly better in all evaluation categories than performance after didactic education, including intervention timing, maneuver performance, and birth time. Shoulder dystocia simulation sessions were also able to determine common and recurrent errors, such as inadequate documentation of the event, delayed or no episiotomy, ineffective suprapubic pressure, and incorrect McRoberts technique.[28] Additionally, shoulder dystocia training has demonstrated the added benefit of improved documentation, which is important both for patient care and medical–legal risk mitigation.[29]

POSTPARTUM HEMORRHAGE

The American College of Obstetricians and Gynecologists defines PPH as cumulative blood loss of greater than or equal to 1000 mL or blood loss with signs or symptoms of hypovolemia within 24 hours after birth (including intrapartum blood loss).[30] In the United States, hemorrhage requiring blood transfusion is the leading cause of severe maternal morbidity, followed closely by disseminated intravascular coagulation, which is often a sequela of PPH.[31] Because postpartum patients are often able to compensate for blood loss until the loss is substantial, earlier recognition of PPH before vital sign deterioration should be the aim.[32] Because recent data indicate that the rates of PPH are increasing in developed countries and there are significant racial/ethnic disparities in pregnancy-related mortality, the Joint Commission introduced 2 new standards effective July 1, 2020, addressing both maternal hemorrhage and severe hypertension and pre-eclampsia (to be discussed elsewhere in this article), including the use of safety bundles and multidisciplinary annual drills.[33]

Like simulation in shoulder dystocia, simulation in PPH has shown significant potential in multiple areas. In 2007, Maslovitz and colleagues[28] were able to demonstrate common and recurrent errors detected by PPH simulation, such as underestimation of blood loss, lack of familiarity with prostaglandin use, and later transition to the operating room. In 2009, Deering and colleagues[34] were able to identify significant deficiencies in resident PPH management via simulation, including medication errors and delayed response time. Furthermore, Birch and colleagues[35] demonstrated that simulated PPH management participants improved their teamwork skills in communication, confidence, and interdisciplinary relationships when compared with those who had lecture-based training alone. Last, PPH simulation has been able to demonstrate improvements in the accuracy of blood loss estimation, which is critical to the appropriate resuscitation of the hemorrhaging patient. Maslovitz and colleagues[36] reported improved accuracy of blood loss estimation through simulation, recognizing that large volume blood loss was more frequently underestimated than lower volumes. Dildy and colleagues[37] followed with having learners undergo pre- and postdidactic simulations for estimating blood loss, finding significantly fewer error after the intervention.

Although PPH simulation has demonstrated improvements in many areas, such as teamwork, communication, blood loss estimation, and error reduction in simulated scenarios, there are limited data demonstrating improvement in clinical outcomes. A 2021 study by Dillon and colleagues[38] set out to determine if simulation improves clinical performance in PPH. This study demonstrated that the use of a multidisciplinary PPH simulation program was associated with faster times for uterotonic administration and blood transfusion.[38] Because a major cause of preventable maternal death in the setting of PPH is delayed treatment, these results provided clinical evidence that simulation training may improve patient outcomes in such emergencies.[38]

MATERNAL CARDIAC ARREST

Approximately 1 in 12,000 birth hospitalizations is complicated by cardiac arrest, with survival being highly dependent on the etiology of the arrest.[39] An analysis of cardiac arrest in pregnancy in the United States between 1998 and 2011 revealed that, although hemorrhage was the leading potential etiology (contributing to 38.1% of all cases), fewer than 1 in 1000 patients who experienced hemorrhage also had a cardiac arrest.[39] Amniotic fluid embolism (more recently termed anaphylactoid syndrome of pregnancy) was the diagnosis that was most frequently complicated by cardiac arrest (252.7 per 1000), despite an incidence of only approximately 1 in 40,000 births.[39,40] Cardiac arrest in pregnancy poses unique medical challenges, not only owing to its rarity, but also owing to the physiologic changes of pregnancy and considerations for both the patient and the fetus, leading to prompt resuscitative cesarean birth if initial resuscitative attempts are unsuccessful. The American Heart Association only started including pregnancy in its advanced cardiac life support algorithms in 2020.[41] Thus, even members of the medical team who regularly renewed their advanced cardiac life support certifications would not necessarily be familiar with considerations unique to pregnancy. In fact, Lipman and colleagues[42] demonstrated that, despite labor and delivery staff having current advanced cardiac life support certification, there were multiple deficiencies in cardiopulmonary resuscitation during simulated cardiac arrests in pregnant patients.

Simulation training for cardiac arrest in pregnancy has been noted to improve medical management by obstetric providers. Dijkman and colleagues[43] from the Netherlands demonstrated an increase in the rate of resuscitative cesarean birth after the 2004 introduction of emergency skills training, but outcomes remained poor, thought to be because of procedural delay with no cesareans being done within the recommended 5 minutes of the cardiac arrest being diagnosed. A subsequent study by Fisher and colleagues[44] performed pre– and post–maternal cardiac arrest simulation evaluations of maternal–fetal medicine staff, demonstrating improvements in the timing of the initiation of cardiopulmonary resuscitation, in addition to improvements in promptness of cesarean birth when indicated, with the more experienced providers and those who had participated in the management of a previous cardiac arrest performing better postintervention. Although a relatively uncommon emergency, there is an obvious need for more formal training programs specific to the management of cardiac arrest in obstetric patients.

PRE-ECLAMPSIA AND ECLAMPSIA

Pre-eclampsia is a pregnancy disorder associated with new-onset hypertension, most often occurring after 20 weeks gestation and frequently near term, complicating 2% to 8% of pregnancies worldwide.[45,46] Eclampsia, a severe manifestation of pre-eclampsia, is defined as new-onset seizures in the absence of other causes such as epilepsy, cerebral arterial ischemia and infarction, intracranial hemorrhage, or substance use.[45] Although eclampsia occurs in only 2% to 3% of patients with pre-eclampsia with severe features not receiving antiseizure prophylaxis, its significant maternal and perinatal morbidity and mortality prompted the Joint Commission to require institutions to conduct multidisciplinary drills, including a team debrief at least annually to determine system issues, as a part of ongoing quality improvement efforts for severe hypertension and pre-eclampsia.[47,48]

Studies have shown that simulations for pre-eclampsia and eclampsia are more effective than lecture alone, and, as in the other simulation topics mentioned elsewhere in this article, also have identified recurrent mistakes and improved performances of repeat learners. Maslovitz and colleagues[28] in 2007 demonstrated common and recurrent errors seen in eclamptic seizure simulations, including inappropriate ventilation technique, incorrect treatment or underdetection of magnesium sulfate intoxication, and not performing ventilation on an apneic patient. Fisher and colleagues[49] demonstrated that residents participating in a simulation of eclampsia and associated complications performed better than residents in a lecture-only group. When assessing potentially harmful actions in the same study, the simulation group demonstrated decreases in magnesium sulfate overdose, decision to perform unwarranted cesareans, and medication errors.[49] Similarly, Ellis and colleagues[50] in the UK performed a randomized, controlled trial evaluating simulation training in eclampsia management across 6 large hospitals. Results showed that simulation training improved rates of completion for basic tasks, decreased time to magnesium sulfate administration and improved teamwork.[50]

CORONAVIRUS DISEASE 2019 PANDEMIC PREPAREDNESS

COVID-19 is caused by severe acute respiratory syndrome coronavirus 2. On March 11, 2020, the World Health Organization declared the COVID-19 pandemic, which has presented unprecedented challenges to the health care system, requiring urgent effective implementation of new and rapidly evolving protocols for clinical care and infection prevention and control while balancing the need for social distancing and thoughtful utilization of scarce personal protective equipment.[51,52] The pandemic has been particularly challenging for obstetric providers to navigate; data suggest that pregnant patients infected with COVID-19 are at an increased risk for severe illness compared with nonpregnant patients, with an increased need for intensive care unit admissions, invasive ventilation, and extracorporeal membrane oxygenation.[53] In addition, there is an increased risk of poor perinatal outcomes and maternal death.[53]

Previous disasters and pandemics have demonstrated simulation to be one of the most effective ways to practice new protocols and identify knowledge and preparedness gaps while improving teamwork, communication and process efficiency.[54] The most recent large-scale contagious outbreak before COVID-19 was that of the highly infectious Ebola virus in 2014 to 2016, which prompted recognition of the need for disaster preparedness and planning for protecting providers in addition to improving patient care, although the infection was limited in the United States.[54] However, at the time of this writing, the COVID-19 virus continues to evolve rapidly, with different virus variants and variably timed surges affecting clinical management and hospital protocols. Unlike our previous examples of simulated obstetric emergencies, simulations of COVID-19 management in the obstetric patient may not only concentrate on a specific emergent clinical event, but rather may involve wider management considerations during an entire hospital stay. Few publications to date discuss the effectiveness of COVID-19 simulation training in obstetrics, but several important considerations should be taken into account, including precautions to prevent occupational spread, given that transmission of the severe acute respiratory syndrome coronavirus 2 virus is thought to be both by droplet and airborne means. Appropriate signage placement and isolation procedures for patients with suspected or confirmed COVID-19 infection should be included in the simulation. Staff should practice donning and doffing appropriate personal protective equipment, if supply allows, and should practice maintaining appropriate social distancing whenever possible. Scenarios should take into account initial patient screening/evaluation environment, inpatient management (including recognition of patient compromise and preparation for providing obstetric management on nonobstetric units), and handling obstetric emergencies.[52,54] If using spatial separation to maintain social distancing during training is not possible, temporal separation (via sequential training of smaller numbers of participants), video recording, videoconferencing technologies, and virtual training may be considered.[52] In response to these identified needs, the American College of Obstetricians and Gynecologists Simulation Working Group created a COVID-19 simulation program that allows any size institution to run drills to prepare for pregnant COVID patients and it is available for free online (https://www.acog.org/education-and-events/simulations/covid-19-obstetric-preparedness-manual).

DISCUSSION

From these examples, it is clear that obstetric simulation training is versatile and adaptable to a wide range of scenarios. Training can be modified and tailored to the areas of greatest need. Obstetric simulations for emergencies allow for a safe space for learners to reflect on their management and practice skills where they may lack comfort. These simulations have shown not only direct benefits to patients but also to the learners and their institutions.

Because the resultant highly reliable teams after obstetric simulation sessions help to decrease the number of clinical errors, improve outcomes, and enhance satisfaction, there are now national obstetric emergencies simulation courses offered by various national organizations to address the need for obstetric simulation training and to assist in implementation.[17] The American College of Obstetrics and Gynecology sponsors the Emergencies in Clinical Obstetrics course, covering topics such as breech vaginal birth, shoulder dystocia, PPH, umbilical cord prolapse, and teamwork and communication.[55] The Council on Patient Safety in Women's Health Care also sponsors the Practicing for Patients Clinical Simulation Scenario Packages as a complement to its Obstetric In-Situ Drill Program Manual; at the time of this writing, the comprehensive scenario bundles include hypertension and PPH (which includes example simulation videos such as https://www.youtube.com/watch?v=-yvymXBYigY&t=2s and https://www.youtube.com/watch?v=H4zSQjPl95s).[56] The American Academy of Family Physicians helps facilitate Advanced Life Support in Obstetrics courses, which they describe as evidence-based, interprofessional, and multidisciplinary training programs that equip the entire maternity care team with skills to effectively manage obstetric emergencies.[57] Additionally, the Society for Maternal-Fetal Medicine runs both an online and an annual in-person course (in conjunction with Banner University Medical Center Phoenix) in critical care obstetrics. These and other organizations may help to provide resources to institutions who are interested in advancing their obstetric emergency simulation programs, particularly in light of inclusion of simulation as an institutional requirement by accreditation organizations such as the Joint Commission.

SUMMARY

- Obstetric simulation training is versatile and adaptable to a wide range of scenarios.
- Obstetric simulations for emergencies allow for a safe space for learners to reflect on their management and practice skills where they may lack comfort.

- Obstetric simulation training decreases the risk of adverse outcomes and decreases the number of errors that could contribute to these outcomes.
- Learners demonstrate improved performance in emergencies (especially if they are repeat learners), increased confidence, better teamwork and improved documentation after simulation training.

DISCLOSURE

The authors have no financial conflicts of interest to disclose.

REFERENCES

1. Flanagan B, Nestel D, Joseph M. Making patient safety the focus: crisis resource management in the undergraduate curriculum. Med Educ 2004;38:56–66.
2. Owen H. Early use of simulation in medical education. Simul Healthc 2012;7(2): 102–16.
3. Moran ME. Enlightenment via simulation: "crone-ology's" first woman. J Endourol 2010;24(1):5–8.
4. Markoviç D, Markoviç-Živkoviç B. Development of anatomical models—chronology. Acta Med Median 2010;49:56–62.
5. Williams JW. Teaching obstetrics. Proceedings of the Association of American Medical Colleges meeting at Denver. 1898. Available at: https://www.aamc.org/download/172580/data/aamc_proceedings_of_the_meeting_at_denver_1898.pdf.
6. Kotsis SV, Chung KC. Application of the "see one, do one, teach one" concept in surgical training. Plast Reconstr Surg 2013;131(5):1194–201.
7. Satin AJ. Simulation in obstetrics. Obstet Gynecol 2018;132(1):199–209.
8. Institute of Medicine (US) Committee on Quality of Health Care in America. In: Kohn LT, Corrigan JM, Donaldson MS, editors. To err is human: building a safer health system. Washington (DC): National Academies Press (US); 2000.
9. Philibert I, Friedmann P, Williams WT. ACGME Work Group on Resident Duty Hours. Accreditation Council for Graduate Medical Education. New requirements for resident duty hours. JAMA 2002;288(9):1112–4.
10. Sheen JJ, Goffman D. Emerging role of drills and simulations in patient safety. Obstet Gynecol Clin North Am 2019;46(2):305–15.
11. Siddiqui NY, Stepp KJ, Lasch SJ, et al. Objective structured assessment of technical skills for repair of fourth-degree perineal lacerations. Am J Obstet Gynecol 2008;199(6):676.e1–6.
12. Sparks RA, Beesley AD, Jones AD. The sponge perineum:" an innovative method of teaching fourth-degree obstetric perineal laceration repair to family medicine residents. Fam Med 2006;38(8):542–4.
13. Hannah ME, Hannah WJ, Hewson SA, et al. Planned caesarean section versus planned vaginal birth for breech presentation at term: a randomised multicentre trial. Term Breech Trial Collaborative Group. Lancet 2000;356(9239):1375–83.
14. Deering S, Brown J, Hodor J, et al. Simulation training and resident performance of singleton vaginal breech delivery. Obstet Gynecol 2006;107(1):86–9.
15. Stone H, Crane J, Johnston K, et al. Retention of vaginal breech delivery skills taught in simulation. J Obstet Gynaecol Can 2018;40(2):205–10.
16. Dildy GA, Belfort MA, Clark SL. Obstetric forceps: a species on the brink of extinction. Obstet Gynecol 2016;128(3):436–9.
17. Lawrence HC 3rd, Copel JA, O'Keeffe DF, et al. Quality patient care in labor and delivery: a call to action. Am J Obstet Gynecol 2012;207(3):147–8.

18. ACOG Practice Bulletin No 178: shoulder dystocia. Obstet Gynecol 2017;129(5): e123–33.
19. Resnik R. Management of shoulder girdle dystocia. Clin Obstet Gynecol 1980;23: 559–64.
20. Gherman RB, Chauhan S, Ouzounian JG, et al. Shoulder dystocia: the unpreventable obstetric emergency with empiric management guidelines. Am J Obstet Gynecol 2006;195:657–72.
21. Executive summary: neonatal brachial plexus palsy. Report of the American College of Obstetricians and Gynecologists' Task Force on Neonatal Brachial Plexus Palsy. Obstet Gynecol 2014;123(4):902–4.
22. Deering S, Rowland J. Obstetric emergency simulation. Semin Perinatol 2013; 37(3):179–88.
23. Draycott TJ, Crofts JF, Ash JP, et al. Improving neonatal outcome through practical shoulder dystocia training. Obstet Gynecol 2008;112(1):14–20.
24. Crofts JF, Lenguerrand E, Bentham GL, et al. Prevention of brachial plexus injury—12 years of shoulder dystocia training: an interrupted time-series study. BJOG 2016;123:111–8.
25. Inglis SR, Feier N, Chetiyaar JB, et al. Effects of shoulder dystocia training on the incidence of brachial plexus injury. Am J Obstet Gynecol 2011;204(4):322.e1–6.
26. Grobman WA, Miller D, Burke C, et al. Outcomes associated with introduction of a shoulder dystocia protocol. Am J Obstet Gynecol 2011;205(6):513–7.
27. Deering S, Poggi S, Macedonia C, et al. Improving resident competency in the management of shoulder dystocia with simulation training. Obstet Gynecol 2004;103(6):1224–8.
28. Maslovitz S, Barkai G, Lessing JB, et al. Recurrent obstetric management mistakes identified by simulation. Obstet Gynecol 2007;109(6):1295–300.
29. Goffman D, Heo H, Chazotte C, et al. Using simulation training to improve shoulder dystocia documentation. Obstet Gynecol 2008;112(6):1284–7.
30. Menard MK, Main EK, Currigan SM. Executive summary of the reVITALize initiative: standardizing obstetric data definitions. Obstet Gynecol 2014;124:150–3.
31. Creanga AA, Berg CJ, Ko JY, et al. Maternal mortality and morbidity in the United States: where are we now? J Womens Health (Larchmt) 2014;23(1):3–9.
32. ACOG Practice Bulletin No 76: postpartum hemorrhage. Obstet Gynecol 2006; 108(4):1039–47.
33. Proactive prevention of maternal death from maternal hemorrhage. Quick Safety. Issue 51. 2019. Available at: https://www.jointcommission.org/-/media/tjc/newsletters/qs-51-maternal-hemorrhage-10-25-19-final2.pdf. Accessed December 12, 2021.
34. Deering SH, Chinn M, Hodor J, et al. Use of a postpartum hemorrhage simulator for instruction and evaluation of residents. J Grad Med Educ 2009;1(2):260–3.
35. Birch L, Jones N, Doyle PM, et al. Obstetric skills drills: evaluation of teaching methods. Nurse Educ Today 2007;27(8):915–22.
36. Maslovitz S, Barkai G, Lessing JB, et al. Improved accuracy of postpartum blood loss estimation as assessed by simulation. Acta Obstet Gynecol Scand 2008; 87(9):929–34.
37. Dildy GA 3rd, Paine AR, George NC, et al. Estimating blood loss: can teaching significantly improve visual estimation? Obstet Gynecol 2004;104(3):601–6.
38. Dillon SJ, Kleinmann W, Fomina Y, et al. Does simulation improve clinical performance in management of postpartum hemorrhage? Am J Obstet Gynecol 2021; 225(4):435.e1–8.

39. Mhyre JM, Tsen LC, Einav S, et al. Cardiac arrest during hospitalization for delivery in the United States, 1998-2011. Anesthesiology 2014;120(4):810–8.
40. Shamshirsaz AA, Clark SL. Amniotic fluid embolism. Obstet Gynecol Clin North Am 2016;43(4):779–90.
41. Available at. https://cpr.heart.org/-/media/cpr-files/cpr-guidelines-files/highlights/hghlghts_2020_ecc_guidelines_english.pdf. Accessed December 19, 2021.
42. Lipman SS, Daniels KI, Carvalho B, et al. Deficits in the provision of cardiopulmonary resuscitation during simulated obstetric crises. Am J Obstet Gynecol 2010; 203(2):179.e1–5.
43. Dijkman A, Huisman CM, Smit M, et al. Cardiac arrest in pregnancy: increasing use of perimortem caesarean section due to emergency skills training? BJOG 2010;117(3):282–7.
44. Fisher N, Eisen LA, Bayya JV, et al. Improved performance of maternal-fetal medicine staff after maternal cardiac arrest simulation-based training. Am J Obstet Gynecol 2011;205(3):239.e1–5.
45. ACOG Practice Bulletin No 222. Gestational hypertension and preeclampsia. Obstet Gynecol 2020;135(6):e237–60.
46. Steegers EA, von Dadelszen P, Duvekot JJ, et al. Pre-eclampsia. Lancet 2010; 376:631–44.
47. Sibai BM. Magnesium sulfate prophylaxis in preeclampsia: lessons learned from recent trials. Am J Obstet Gynecol 2004;190(6):1520–6.
48. Available at: https://www.jointcommission.org/-/media/tjc/documents/standards/r3-reports/r3-issue-24-maternal-12-7-2021.pdf. Accessed January 3, 2022.
49. Fisher N, Bernstein PS, Satin A, et al. Resident training for eclampsia and magnesium toxicity management: simulation or traditional lecture? Am J Obstet Gynecol 2010;203(4):379.e1–5.
50. Ellis D, Crofts JF, Hunt LP, et al. Hospital, simulation center, and teamwork training for eclampsia management: a randomized controlled trial. Obstet Gynecol 2008; 111(3):723–31.
51. Fauci AS, Lane HC, Redfield RR. COVID-19 — navigating the uncharted. N Engl J Med 2020;382:1268–9.
52. Kiely DJ, Posner GD, Sansregret A. Health care team training and simulation-based education in obstetrics during the COVID-19 pandemic. J Obstet Gynaecol Can 2020;42(8):1017–20.
53. Society for Maternal-Fetal Medicine (SMFM). COVID-19 and pregnancy. What maternal-fetal medicine subspecialists need to know. Washington (DC): SMFM; 2020. Available at: https://www.smfm.org/covidclinical. Accessed January 3, 2022.
54. Eubanks A, Thomson B, Marko E, et al. Obstetric simulation for a pandemic. Semin Perinatol 2020;44(6):151294.
55. Available at: https://www.acog.org/education-and-events/simulations/eco. Accessed January 17 2022.
56. Available at: https://safehealthcareforeverywoman.org/clinical-scenario-packages/. Accessed April 14 2022.
57. Available at: https://www.aafp.org/cme/programs/also.html. Accessed January 17 2022.

Moving?

Make sure your subscription moves with you!

To notify us of your new address, find your **Clinics Account Number** (located on your mailing label above your name), and contact customer service at:

Email: journalscustomerservice-usa@elsevier.com

800-654-2452 (subscribers in the U.S. & Canada)
314-447-8871 (subscribers outside of the U.S. & Canada)

Fax number: 314-447-8029

Elsevier Health Sciences Division
Subscription Customer Service
3251 Riverport Lane
Maryland Heights, MO 63043

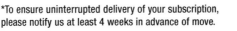

Printed and bound by CPI Group (UK) Ltd, Croydon, CR0 4YY

08/05/2025

01864723-0006